COMPLEMENTARY AND ALTERNATIVE MEDICINE FOR PTSD

Advance Praise for Complementary and Alternative Medicine for PTSD

"Wynn and Benedek's book on *Complementary and Alternative Medicine for PTSD* represents a landmark in trauma publishing. Never has there been such a thorough presentation of the use of CAM treatment of PTSD. Clinicians who oversell the effectiveness of the CAM techniques will be embarrassed by the clear lack of evidence for many CAM approaches, while those who seek to provide the best care possible to their patients will be encouraged to continue the necessary research required to change clinical practice. Wynn and Benedek's book on CAM for PTSD provides a much needed ballast towards ensuring clinicians provide the best care currently available for survivors of trauma, including sexual assault and combat-related PTSD. They are to be commended."

—Carl A. Castro, PhD, Director and Assistant Professor,
Colonel, U.S. Army (Retired),
Center for Innovation and Research on Veterans and Military Families (CIR),
USC School of Social Work, University of Southern California, Los Angeles, CA

"Recognizing the increasing need for more consolidated information on Complementary Alternative Medicine for the treatment of PTSD, Doctors Benedek and Wynn have contributed a ground-breaking and invaluable textbook for scholars and practitioners alike. The depth and comprehensiveness of this must-have desk reference is noteworthy, and the openness to additional research where robust evidence is currently lacking is a breath of fresh air. This book should go a long way toward contributing to better understanding of alternative modalities for addressing PTSD, and to helping mitigate PTSD related crisis among our military service men and women and their families."

—Keith G. Tidball, PhD, Senior Extension Associate,
Department of Natural Resources, Cornell University, Ithaca, NY

"Kudos to Gary Wynn and David Benedek for their groundbreaking book on the use of integrative, complementary, and alternative approaches for PTSD. Inspired by the needs, strengths, and suffering of patients following traumatic experiences, the authors and contributors of this work make a clear and compelling case for healing professionals to embrace a more comprehensive approach to the management of PTSD. Thus one must also credit America's sons and daughters in uniform and their families for their collective service and sacrifice, which no doubt catalyzed the conception of this timely work and enriched its content. This book and the decades of courageous service and selfless sacrifice it represents is a most welcome development for patients, family members, clinicians, CAM practitioners, advocates, and compassionate human beings - in short, all of us."

—Loree Sutton, MD, Brigadier General, U.S. Army (Ret.); Commissioner,
NYC Department of Veterans' Services, New York, NY

COMPLEMENTARY AND ALTERNATIVE MEDICINE FOR PTSD

Edited by

David M. Benedek, MD, DFAPA

Uniformed Services University of the Health Sciences Bethesda, MD

and

Gary H. Wynn, MD, FAPA

Uniformed Services University of the Health Sciences Bethesda, MD

OXFORD
UNIVERSITY PRESS

OXFORD
UNIVERSITY PRESS

Oxford University Press is a department of the University of Oxford. It furthers
the University's objective of excellence in research, scholarship, and education
by publishing worldwide. Oxford is a registered trade mark of Oxford University
Press in the UK and certain other countries.

Published in the United States of America by Oxford University Press
198 Madison Avenue, New York, NY 10016, United States of America.

Library of Congress Cataloging-in-Publication Data
Names: Benedek, David M., editor. | Wynn, Gary H., 1958– , editor.
Title: Complementary and alternative medicine for PTSD / edited by
David M. Benedek and Gary H. Wynn.
Description: Oxford ; New York : Oxford University Press, [2016] | Includes
bibliographical references and index.
Identifiers: LCCN 2016008309 | ISBN 9780190205959 (alk. paper)
Subjects: | MESH: Stress Disorders, Post-Traumatic—therapy | Complementary Therapies—methods
Classification: LCC RC552.P67 | NLM WM 172.5 | DDC 616.85/21—dc23 LC record available
at http://lccn.loc.gov/2016008309

This material is not intended to be, and should not be considered, a substitute for medical or other
professional advice. Treatment for the conditions described in this material is highly dependent on the
individual circumstances. And although this material is designed to offer accurate information with respect to
the subject matter covered, and to be current at the time it was written, research and knowledge about medical
and health issues is evolves constantly, and dose schedules for medications are being revised continuously,
with new side effects recognized and accounted for regularly. Readers must therefore always check the
product information and clinical procedures with the most up-to-date published product information and
data sheets provided by the manufacturers, and the most recent codes of conduct and safety regulation. The
publisher and the authors make no representations or warranties to readers, express or implied, regarding
the accuracy or completeness of this material. Without limiting the foregoing, the publisher and the authors
make no representations or warranties regarding the accuracy or efficacy of the drug dosages mentioned in
the material. The authors and the publisher do not accept, and expressly disclaim, any responsibility for any
liability, loss, or risk that may be claimed or incurred as a consequence of the use and/or application of any of
the contents of this material.

All opinions, interpretations, conclusions, and recommendations contained herein are those of the authors
and should not be construed as representing the positions or policies of an author's institution including,
but not limited to, the Uniformed Services University of the Health Sciences, the Veterans Affairs
Administration, and the United States Department of Defense.

1 3 5 7 9 8 6 4 2

Printed by Sheridan Books, Inc., United States of America

Contents

PART 5: CONCLUSION

Acknowledgments

Thank you to the men and women of the US Military whose personal sacrifices in the service of their nation inspire us to seek continuous improvement in the care we provide for them. Thanks, also, to my wife for consistently reminding me that healthy skepticism must not preclude an openness to alternative perspectives.

DMB

For Ripley and Ruby. May your curiosity and imagination always be vibrant, no matter your age.

GHW

Contributors

Amy B. Adler, PhD
Center for Military Psychiatry
   and Neuroscience
Walter Reed Army Institute of Research
Silver Spring, MD

Daniel J. Balog, MD
Center for the Study of Traumatic Stress
Department of Psychiatry
Uniformed Services University
   of the Health Sciences
Bethesda, MD

Bradley E. Belsher, PhD
Department of Defense Deployment
   Health Clinical Center
Bethesda, MD

David M. Benedek, MD, DFAPA
Center for the Study of Traumatic Stress
Department of Psychiatry
Uniformed Services University of
   the Health Sciences
Bethesda, MD

Nathaniel A. Brown, MD
Naval Medical Center San Diego
San Diego, CA

Perry R. Chumley, DVM, MPH
Department of Defense Veterinary
   Service Activity
Office of the Surgeon General
Falls Church, VA

Caroline Clark, MD
Department of Behavioral Health
Walter Reed National Military
   Medical Center
Bethesda, MD

Jeffrey Cole, PhD
National Intrepid Center of Excellence
Walter Reed National Military
   Medical Center
Bethesda, MD

Stephen J. Cozza, MD
Center for the Study of Traumatic Stress
Department of Psychiatry
Uniformed Services University of
   the Health Sciences
Bethesda, MD

JoAnn Difede, PhD
Department of Psychiatry
Weill Cornell Medical College
New York, NY

Charles C. Engel, MD, MPH
RAND Corporation
Santa Monica, CA

Daniel P. Evatt, PhD
Department of Defense Deployment
   Health Clinical Center
Bethesda, MD

Lucy Finkelstein-Fox, MD
Department of Psychological Sciences
University of Connecticut
Storrs, CT

Michael C. Freed, PhD
Department of Defense Deployment
   Health Clinical Center
Bethesda, MD

Geoffrey Grammer, MD
National Intrepid Center of Excellence
Walter Reed National Military
   Medical Center
Bethesda, MD

Joseph M. Helms, MD
Helms Medical Institute
Berkeley, CA

Julia E. Hoffman, PsyD
Mental Health Services
U.S. Department of Veterans Affairs
National Center for PTSD
VA Palo Alto Healthcare System
Menlo Park, CA

Marina Khusid, MD, ND, MSA
Department of Defense Deployment
   Health Clinical Center
Defense Centers of Excellence for
   Psychological Health and Traumatic
   Brain Injury
Bethesda, MD

Robert Koffman, MD
National Intrepid Center of Excellence
Walter Reed National Military
   Medical Center
Bethesda, MD

Eric Kuhn, PhD
National Center for PTSD
Dissemination & Training Division
VA Palo Alto Health Care System
Menlo Park, CA

Ariel J. Lang, MD
VA San Diego Center of Excellence
   for Stress and Mental Health
University of California
San Diego, CA

Robert N. McLay, MD, PhD
Naval Medical Center San Diego
San Diego, CA

Derek M. Miletich, MD
Naval Medical Center San Diego
San Diego, CA

Megan Olden, MD
Department of Psychiatry
Weill Cornell Medical College
New York, NY

Meg Daley Olmert
Warrior Canine Connection
Brookeville, MD

Jason E. Owen, PhD, MPH
National Center for PTSD
Dissemination & Training Division
VA Palo Alto Health Care System
Menlo Park, CA

Melissa Peskin, MD
Department of Psychiatry
Weill Cornell Medical College
New York, NY

Brian Pilecki, MD
Rhode Island Hospital
Alpert Medical School of Brown
  University
Providence, RI

Holly J. Ramsawh, PhD
Center for the Study of Traumatic Stress
Department of Psychiatry
Uniformed Services University of
  the Health Science
Bethesda, MD

Elspeth Cameron Ritchie, MD, MPH
Department of Psychiatry
Uniformed Services University of
  the Health Sciences
Bethesda, MD

Albert Rizzo, PhD
Institute for Creative Technologies
Department of Psychiatry and School
  of Gerontology
University of Southern California
Marina del Rey, CA

Lesley Ross, MD
Naval Medical Center San Diego
San Diego, CA

Barbara O. Rothbaum, PhD, ABPP
Trauma and Anxiety Recovery
  Program
Emory University School
  of Medicine
Atlanta, GA

Michael J. Roy, MD, MPH
Division of Military Internal Medicine
Uniformed Services University of
  the Health Sciences
Bethesda, MD

Christina Rumayor
82nd Airborne
Fort Bragg, NC

Josef I. Ruzek, PhD
Dissemination and Training Division
National Center for PTSD
VA Palo Alto Health Care System
Menlo Park, CA

Janina Scarlet
Veterans Medical Research
  Foundation
San Diego, CA

Matthew St. Laurent
Occupational Therapy
Department of Rehabilitation
Walter Reed National Military
  Medical Center
Bethesda, MD

Robin L. Toblin, PhD
Center for Military Psychiatry and
  Neuroscience
Walter Reed Army Institute of Research
Silver Spring, MD
Commissioned Corps of the U.S. Public
  Health Service
Rockville, MD

Robyn D. Walser
National Center for PTSD
Dissemination and Training Division
University of California
Berkeley, CA

Christine Winter, DO
Department of Behavioral Health
Walter Reed National Military
  Medical Center
Bethesda, MD

Gary H. Wynn, MD, FAPA
Center for the Study of Traumatic Stress
Department of Psychiatry
Uniformed Services University of
  the Health Science
Bethesda, MD

Rick A. Yount, MS
Warrior Canine Connection
Brookeville, MD

PART
1

INTRODUCTION

ONE

Introduction

GARY H. WYNN AND DAVID M. BENEDEK

BACKGROUND

For more than 10 years complementary and alternative medicine, often referred to simply as *CAM*, has become increasingly available and used throughout the United States for a variety of medical disorders and mental health conditions. This rise in popularity can be attributed to a number of factors, but the expanded use by clinicians results from a combination of increases in perceived therapeutic benefit, patient preference, recognition of CAM's potential as an augmentation to more traditional approaches, and a growing recognition that there must be options when traditional interventions are insufficient to address a patient's suffering (Wynn, 2015). These factors overlay the variability in use by CAM modality and chronicity of disorder. For potentially grave disorders such as cancer, the role of CAM is primarily additive to treatments such as chemotherapy, radiation, and/or surgery, whereas for some mental health conditions, patients may use CAM modalities as the only form of treatment. Navigating this complex landscape can be complicated for both clinician and patient.

Not unlike CAM, posttraumatic stress disorder (PTSD) has seen a substantial increased interest by the medical community, mental health professionals, and society at large. This increased interest is a result, in part, of scientific and media attention to the conflicts in Iraq and Afghanistan, although the causes of trauma include a great deal more than just military conflict. Originally included in the *Diagnostic and Statistical Manual for Mental Disorders* (American Psychiatric Association,

1980), PTSD has seen several revisions and substantial controversy during the past 35 years. Questions surrounding the biological basis of the disorder, the efficacy of various treatments, and the validity of various diagnostic criteria have proved challenging to answer. Despite these controversies, the scientific and clinical communities have continued to make strides in understanding the foundations of the disorder as well as the means for alleviating its attendant suffering. Given ongoing conflicts around the world, the increasing frequency of natural disasters and severe weather events and their impact on human populations, and the frequency of interpersonal violence, PTSD will, unfortunately, be an ongoing issue and future concern that will require much more work across the spectrum of research—from basic science to treatment and implementation—to address this large-scale human suffering. CAM interventions present an excellent avenue for researchers, clinicians, and patients to explore other options for treatment.

The use of CAM specifically for the treatment of PTSD has also increased greatly during the past decade. The reasons for this expanded use are myriad, but high among them are the lack of sufficient effective traditional pharmacological and psychotherapeutic treatment options, continued stigma associated with participating in mental health care, and increased societal interest in options beyond traditional western medicine approaches to treatment.

WHAT IS CAM?

One difficult issue with CAM is how to define it. The struggle for definitional coherence likely stems, in part, from the breadth of treatments considered CAM. In addition, CAM is often defined as "those things not in traditional western medicine." Defining a concept by its separateness from something else also not clearly defined results in a definition that is both very broad and ambiguous. This "everything that isn't traditional western medicine" approach arguably leaves the entirety of human experience not included specifically in traditional western medicine as possible CAM. The most frequent approaches to defining CAM have been to classify it into categories of major content areas. The National Center for Complementary and Integrative Health, formerly the National Center for Complementary and Alternative Medicine, has proposed three major content areas: natural products, mind and body medicine, and other complementary approaches (see Table 1.1 for details).

The other major approach to defining CAM, and the one used in this text, is to divide the concept into its component parts: complementary medicine and alternative medicine (see Table 1.1 for details). Alternative medicine is divided further into

TABLE 1.1 Major Definitional Approaches to CAM

Approach	Description
National Center for Complementary and Integrative Health	
Natural products	Includes herbs, vitamins, and probiotics
Mind and body medicine	Includes a wide variety of procedures and techniques such as yoga, meditation, acupuncture, hypnotherapy, movement therapies, and relaxation techniques
Other complementary approaches	Includes treatments that fall outside natural products and mind and body medicine, such as traditional healing approaches and naturopathy
Component-based definition of CAM	
Complementary	Practices that, primarily, augment traditional interventions and are not likely to replace standard practices
Alternative treatments	Nonmainstream treatments that are either already being used or have the potential to be used as monotherapy within typical western medical practice
Alternative delivery method	Primarily new technologies and platforms to provide traditional interventions

CAM, complementary and alternative medicine.

alternative treatments and alternative delivery methods. Complementary treatments are those that augment more traditional approaches but are not likely to replace standard practices. Yoga and recreational therapy are good examples of complementary treatments. Many clinicians have recommended a patient consider yoga in addition to the work being done in therapy or through medication management. Some forward-thinking healthcare organizations have included yoga and other complementary modalities into treatment protocols and into staff wellness programs. It is likely, though, that the majority of providers and healthcare organizations will not recommend yoga as a stand-alone treatment option for PTSD. The probable long-term role for yoga, recreational therapy, and similar treatments will be to complement the benefits made through other more traditional clinical interventions.

Alternative treatments are nonmainstream approaches that are either already being used or have the potential to be used as "monotherapy," or the primary treatment modality within typical western medical practice. Acupuncture and neurostimulation are excellent examples. Both acupuncture and neurostimulation are provider-centric modalities with a growing body of evidence supporting use in PTSD treatment as well as other mental health and medical disorders. It is not a far stretch to see how these interventions could be prescribed as a stand-alone course of treatment for PTSD in lieu of psychotherapy or pharmacotherapy. These and other similar treatments can, and in some cases most likely will, replace current primary treatment approaches for some portion of those seeking care for PTSD. This "alternative" category, more so than "complementary," can be cause for controversy primarily because of the designation of a given treatment as *alternative* rather than *primary* or *standard*. For some well-studied treatments with solid scientific evidence, the designation of alternative rather than standard practice may be troubling to that given treatment's advocates. This perceived marginalization can be a reminder of long-standing bias and dismissal by the larger healthcare community. Those involved in the creation of this text are well aware of the marginalization of long duration experienced by many practitioners or practices considered "different," and acknowledge the role many of these early adopters played in bringing these practices and treatments to the forefront. For our purposes, any reference to a given treatment as alternative or otherwise is with the hope of bringing further understanding to the various options available to clinicians when addressing the suffering caused by PTSD.

Alternative delivery methods reference new means of delivering well-established treatments. This category encompasses primarily new technologies and platforms for the provision of existing treatments. As communication technology continues its dramatic advance, the ways in which we communicate, and thus provide treatment to our patients, continues to evolve. These new methods of delivery include smartphone applications, virtual reality, telepsychiatry, and Internet-based delivery of psychotherapies. In addition, technological advances will also spawn new treatments that fit into either the complementary or alternative category. The overlap among these three categories can be substantial and at times confusing. For providers, however, the good news is that determining which specific category a treatment might belong in is less important than understanding the clinical benefit of a given treatment.

CAM AND RESEARCH

The biggest hurdle facing CAM treatments is the lack of robust evidence regarding benefit. There are few studies that take a rigorous scientific approach to clarifying the benefit of CAM in PTSD. This problem stems from both the difficulty with research on CAM treatments and the lack of system-level interest, infrastructure, and support for completing this kind of research. With regard to the difficulty of conducting CAM research for PTSD there are a handful of major issues. These issues are described here and include ensuring a reasonable hypothesis, defining PTSD sufficiently, using standard metrics, differentiating efficacy from effectiveness, conducting manualization, and performing randomized controlled trials (RCTs) (McLay et al., 2013).

A reasonable hypothesis is the cornerstone of modern scientific inquiry, but this is often lacking in CAM research. A CAM-related research hypothesis can fall into one of three categories: (1) modalities that fit within the modern conceptualization of medical science, (2) modalities that do not fit within this conceptualization, and (3) modalities that challenge established scientific principles (McLay et al., 2013). Hypotheses that fall into category one or two can present reasonable scientific inquiry whereas the third category violates basic precepts of modern science. Hypothesizing that benefits stem from supernatural or metaphysical phenomena is unnecessary to study the benefits of a given behavior. Such hypotheses serve only to undermine the validity of otherwise valid scientific inquiry that is vitally needed to understand the clinical utility of CAM for PTSD.

Ensuring the proper definition of PTSD is critical to quality research. PTSD has specific criteria and an established definition. Using nontraditional definitions of PTSD to evaluate nontraditional treatments degrades the validity of the research and serves to further the negative perceptions of CAM and CAM research within the larger medical community.

Researchers seeking to investigate the benefits of CAM treatments for PTSD need to ensure they use standard metrics to evaluate efficacy. Metrics such as satisfaction, happiness, relaxation, and sense of well-being can be included, but should be secondary or exploratory outcomes, whereas metrics such as the Posttraumatic Checklist and Clinician-Administered PTSD Scale are used as primary outcomes.

Another complication for CAM researchers is the issue of efficacy versus effectiveness. For much of modern medical research, the critique is that lab-based study of efficacy does not translate to real-world effectiveness. For CAM, the criticism often trends in the opposite direction. The real-world effectiveness experienced by some patients undergoing CAM treatment has not been tested in a more controlled setting, raising the question of whether there is benefit beyond placebo. Lack of knowledge about efficacy in controlled conditions undercuts the limited existing knowledge about the clinical utility.

A major issue for CAM research is manualization of the treatment and, to be fair, this is no small undertaking. For some modalities, such as yoga, this could entail extremely detailed predefining of every move and position for each session or, for recreational therapy, attempting to define the specific actions and behavior of the participants over what may be a multiday experience. Outlining these methods in such detail can be a Herculean task likely overcome by events. The result is often research that allows flexibility of experience at the expense of the control necessary to evaluate more vigorously the benefit of the intervention. Other treatments, such as acupuncture, can be manualized more effectively, resulting in better scientific comparison with placebo.

The final issue for CAM treatments is the lack of RCTs. Often, research into CAM—for reasons including some already discussed here—is done as an open-label trial or similarly designed trial rather than an RCT. This lack of placebo, wait list, or active comparison control diminishes the value of research performed and adds to the long-standing stigma against CAM treatments and CAM research.

Beyond the struggles with performing research, there is a lack of system-level support for these complicated projects. Whether stemming from a lack of belief in CAM, from worries that research into CAM will not have the same return on investment as traditional lines of inquiry, or from beliefs that the complexities of CAM research decrease its competitiveness in the scientific review process, it is evident that CAM research has not received the level of funding and support necessary to understand the benefit of these modalities. The often-isolated researchers interested in CAM are at a significant disadvantage in pursuit of funding against well-established labs pursuing more traditional science through more traditional means.

THE PURPOSE OF THIS TEXTBOOK

The driving force behind this textbook was the recognition of the increasing need for more consolidated information on CAM for PTSD. During the past decade, many of the contributors to this text have seen a growing number of individuals returning from military deployment suffering from PTSD, alongside the rising use and interest in CAM. This mounting interest has led to significant increases in research, including some attention devoted to various CAM modalities. While looking across the clinical and research landscape, it was an easy decision to move forward with a project dedicated to consolidating the growing wealth of current information on CAM and PTSD. The hope is that this book provides easily digestible information that can assist clinicians, advocates, patients, and students in their pursuit of better understanding this important and growing topic.

HOW TO USE THIS TEXTBOOK

For clinicians, this textbook is a useful desktop reference to be picked up as needed to read sections pertinent to an ongoing case or other aspect of daily practice. As a complete volume, this textbook provides an excellent starting point for learning more about CAM modalities for PTSD. Whether a senior clinician is looking for further education on the topic or a student is investigating it for the first time, this book provides a solid understanding of the current knowledge surrounding the utility of CAM in PTSD. This textbook is designed for practical use whether at the bedside, on rounds, in the clinic, or in the hands of a CAM practitioner out in the community. The book is divided into four main parts: (1) introduction, (2) alternative treatments, (3) complementary treatments, and (4) alternative delivery methods.

Part 1, "Introduction," includes this introduction and an overview of PTSD in Chapter 2. This section sets the stage for the rest of the book by acknowledging current western standards of care and their limitations. Chapter 2 provides an easy-to-understand look at PTSD. As a stand-alone chapter it delivers an excellent basic overview of PTSD phenomenology, epidemiology, and standard treatment.

Part 2, "Alternative Treatments," includes the topics acceptance and commitment Therapy, meditation techniques, transcranial magnetic stimulation, and alternative pharmacology. Chapter 3, "Acceptance and Commitment Therapy for PTSD," is an excellent review of this burgeoning treatment option and includes approaches and clinical application to those suffering from PTSD. Chapter 4, "Meditation Techniques for PTSD," addresses the basics of meditation for PTSD, including a number of the major types and clinical utility of each. Chapter 5, "Transcranial Magnetic Stimulation Treatment," covers the mechanism of action and basic clinical application of neurostimulation, with a focus on transcranial magnetic stimulation. Chapter 6, "Acupuncture," is a review of the state-of-the-art approach to acupuncture for trauma. Part 2 ends with a review of alternative pharmacology in Chapter 7. This in-depth review describes concepts in selecting alternative pharmacological treatments, followed by a discussion of off-label use, synthesized natural substances, plant-based treatments, and substances of abuse.

Part 3, "Complementary Treatments," includes the topics canines as assistive therapy, family-focused interventions, recreational therapy, yoga, and resilience training. Chapter 8, Canines as Assistive Therapy for Treatment of PTSD in the U.S. Military," addresses the compelling approach to PTSD during which the individual suffering from PTSD is partnered with a specially trained service dog. Family-focused interventions are reviewed in detail in Chapter 9. Chapter 10, "Recreational Therapy for PTSD," describes a variety of recreational activities that have been investigated for use in PTSD, including equine-related therapy, adventure/wilderness therapy, and therapeutic fly-fishing, as well as a discussion of possible mechanisms of benefit. Chapter 11 reviews yoga and yoga-related practices, such as yoga breath, followed by a discussion of the benefits in PTSD and the potential mechanisms of action. Part 3 ends with a review, in Chapter 12, of resilience training as a complementary treatment for PTSD.

Part 4, "Alternative Delivery Methods," includes the topics virtual reality, Internet and computer-based treatments, and mobile applications. This section is

followed by a brief conclusion and recap of the major concepts covered throughout this book. Chapter 13, "Virtual Reality Exposure Therapy for PTSD," addresses the basics of using virtual reality as a treatment for PTSD and includes
an in-depth discussion of a couple of the virtual worlds created for this work.
Chapter 14, "Internet and Computer-Based Treatments for the Management
of PTSD," reviews a variety of telehealth applications for PTSD, along with
a number of computer-aided and -delivered treatments. Chapter 15, "Mobile
Apps to Improve Outreach, Engagement, Self-management, and Treatment for
Posttraumatic Stress Disorder," covers the burgeoning area of smartphone and
tablet applications developed or being developed for the treatment of PTSD.
A brief conclusion, Chapter 16, simply summarize the main points of the preceding chapters.

Beyond describing specific types and applications of CAM to PTSD, the chapter authors provide a review of the evidence basis to date for the various modalities
highlighted in this volume. Perhaps an assessment of the gaps in existing understanding will inspire additional research. More important, we hope this review helps
clinicians and their patients make informed decisions as they explore comprehensive
approaches to the management of the symptoms, distress, and dysfunction associated with PTSD.

REFERENCES

American Psychiatric Association. (1980). *Diagnostic and Statistical Manual of Mental Disorders*, 3rd ed. Washington, DC: American Psychiatric Press.

McLay, R. N., Loeffler, G. H., & Wynn, G. H. (2013). Research Methodology for the Study of Complementary and Alternative Medicine in the Treatment of Military PTSD. *Psychiatric Annals*, 43:1.

Wynn, G. H. (2015). Complementary and Alternative Medicine Approaches in the Treatment of PTSD. *Curr Psychiatry Rep*, 17:62.

TWO

Posttraumatic Stress Disorder

An Overview

DAVID M. BENEDEK AND GARY H. WYNN

POSTTRAUMATIC STRESS DISORDER (PTSD) MAY DEVELOP AFTER EXPOSURE TO A traumatic event (or events) such as interpersonal violence, disasters, war, or terrorism. PTSD is characterized by specific symptoms organized into core clusters, including reexperience, hyperarousal, avoidance, and negative alterations in mood and cognition. Although these symptoms may resolve without any intervention, they may also progress to a chronic and debilitating state. The characteristics of the disorder are described in the "Core Clinical Features" section of this chapter. "Epidemiology" describes the incidence and prevalence of PTSD and subgroups that may be at greater risk. The fact that many persons exposed to traumatic events do not develop lasting symptoms of PTSD (or PTSD at all) is explained in a discussion of risk and protective factors. The last sections of this chapter review briefly the diagnostic assessment and current (i.e., noncomplementary/nonalternative) treatments supported by practice guidelines and clinical consensus.

CORE CLINICAL FEATURES

PTSD is distinguished from most other mental disorders by its requirement for exposure to an extreme environmental stressor as part a part of its diagnostic criteria.

TABLE 2.1 Diagnostic criteria for PTSD

A. Exposure to actual/threatened death, serious injury or sexual violence in at least one of the following ways:

    1. Direct experience of the traumatic event(s)

    2. Witnessing event(s) occurring to others

    3. Learning that traumatic event(s) occurred to a close family member/close friend (in close friends or family members actual or threatened death as might be anticipated due to prolonged or acute medical illness does not qualify—it must be sudden, violent, unexpected)

    4. Experiencing repeated or extreme exposure to aversive details of the traumatic event(s) via direct personal exposure (not through electronic media, television, movies, or pictures, unless work related).

B. Presence of at least one intrusion symptom:

    1. Recurrent, involuntary, and intrusive distressing memories of the traumatic event(s)

    2. Recurrent distressing dreams in which the content of the dream is related to the event(s)

    3. Dissociative reactions ("flashbacks") in which the individual feels or acts as if the traumatic event(s) were recurring.

    4. Intense or prolonged psychological distress at exposure to cues that symbolize or resemble an aspect of the traumatic event(s). Cues may be internal or external.

    5. Marked physiological reaction to cues that resemble an aspect of the traumatic event(s) Cues may be internal or external.

C. Persistent avoidance of event-related stimuli as evidenced by either or both of the following:

    1. Avoidance/efforts to avoid distressing memories, thoughts, or feelings about the traumatic event(s)

    2. Avoidance/efforts to avoid external reminders (people, places, conversations, activities, objects, situations) that arouse distressing memories, thoughts, or feelings about the traumatic event(s)

D. Negative alterations in mood and cognition associated with the traumatic event(s), as evidence by at least two of the following:

    1. Inability to remember an important aspect of the traumatic event(s) (due to dissociation and not head injury, alcohol, or drugs)

    2. Persistent and exaggerated negative beliefs or expectations about oneself.

    3. Persistent, distorted cognitions about the cause or consequences of the traumatic event(s) leading to self-blame or blame of others

    4. Persistent negative emotional state such as shame, fear or anger

    5. Markedly diminished interest/participation in significant activities

    6. Feelings of social or interpersonal detachment or estrangement

    7. Inability to experience positive emotions

(continued)

TABLE 2.1 Continued

E. Marked alterations in arousal and reactivity associated with the traumatic event(s) as evidenced by at least two of the following:
1. Irritable behavior and angry outbursts (with minimal provocation) typically in the form of verbal or physical aggression toward people or objects
2. Reckless or self-destructive behavior
3. Hypervigilance
4. Exaggerated startle response
5. Difficulty with concentration
6. Sleep disturbance (restless sleep, insomnia)

F. Duration of the symptoms of more than 1 month.

G. The symptoms result in clinically significant distress or impairment in social, occupational or other important areas of functioning

H. The disturbance is not attributable to the physiological effects of a substance or another medical condition

"With dissociative symptoms" if symptoms meet the criteria for PTSD and the individual experiences persistent or recurrent *depersonalization* or *derealization*

"With delayed expression" if the full criteria are not met until at least 6 months after the event

Source: Adapted from DSM-5.

PTSD is characterized by the onset of psychiatric symptoms linked temporally to exposure to an event that involves exposure to actual or threatened death, serious injury, or sexual violence (American Psychiatric Association, 2013). This exposure may be through direct experience, witnessing trauma to others, learning that trauma occurred to a family member or friend, or through repeated or extreme aversive exposure to the details of the traumatic event. These means of exposure, as defined by the *Diagnostic and Statistical Manual of Mental Disorders*, fifth edition (DSM-5), are a substantial broadening of the diagnostic criteria compared with the *Diagnostic and Statistical Manual of Mental Disorders*, fourth edition (DSM-IV)–text revision (American Psychiatric Association, 2000). The diagnosis no longer requires that an individual respond to an event with intense fear or horror, as required in previous editions of the DSM. At least one of five intrusion symptoms (recurrent, involuntary, and distressing memories; recurrent distressing dreams; or dissociative reactions) is required. At least one of two avoidance symptoms (avoidance of distressing memories, thoughts, or feelings about the trauma; or avoidance of external reminders of the trauma) is required. At least two of seven negative cognition/mood symptoms (inability to remember important aspects of the trauma, persistent negative beliefs about oneself, distorted cognitions about the cause or consequences of the trauma, negative

TABLE 2.2 Comparison of Diagnostic Criteria for ASD and PTSD

Description of Criteria	ASD Criterion	PTSD Criterion
Characteristics of traumatic exposure	Criterion A	Criterion A
Exposure to actual or threatened death, serious injury, or sexual violence in one (or more) of the following ways:		
1. Directly experiencing the traumatic event(s)		
2. Witnessing, in person, the event(s) as it occurred to others		
3. Learning that the traumatic event(s) occurred to a close family member or close friend		
4. Experiencing repeated or extreme exposure to aversive details of the traumatic event(s)		
Intrusion symptoms	Except for item 5, these symptoms, if present, count toward the nine or more symptoms required for ASD	Criterion B (one or more intrusion symptom)
1. Recurrent, involuntary, and intrusive distressing memories of the traumatic event(s)		
2. Recurrent distressing dreams in which the content and/or affect of the dream are related to the event(s)		
3. Dissociative reactions (e.g., flashbacks) in which the individual feels or acts as if the traumatic event(s) were recurring		
4. Intense or prolonged psychological distress at exposure to internal or external cues that symbolize or resemble an aspect of the traumatic event(s)		
5. Marked physiological reaction to internal or external cues that symbolize or resemble an aspect of the traumatic event(s)		
Avoidance symptoms	These symptoms, if present, count toward the nine or more symptoms required for ASD	Criterion C (one or more avoidance symptom)
1. Avoidance of or efforts to avoid distressing memories, thoughts, or feelings about or closely associated with the traumatic event(s)		
2. Avoidance of or efforts to avoid external reminders (people, places, conversations, activities, objects, situations) that arouse distressing memories, thoughts, or feelings about or closely associated with the traumatic event(s)		

Negative alterations in cognitions/mood

Criterion D (two or more symptoms), except for item 8

Items 1, 7, and 8, if present, count toward the nine or more symptoms required for ASD

1. Inability to remember an important aspect of the traumatic event(s) (typically a result of dissociative amnesia and not other factors such as head injury, alcohol, or drugs)

2. Persistent and exaggerated negative beliefs or expectations about oneself, others, or the world (e.g., "I am bad," "No one can be trusted," "The world is completely dangerous," "My whole nervous system is completely ruined")

3. Persistent, distorted cognitions about the cause or consequences of the traumatic event(s) that lead the individual to blame himself, herself, or others.

4. Persistent negative emotional state (e.g., fear, horror, anger, guilt, shame)

5. Markedly diminished interest or participation in significant activities

6. Feelings of detachment or estrangement from others

7. Persistent inability to experience positive emotions (e.g., inability to experience happiness, satisfaction, or loving feelings)

8. An altered sense of the reality of one's surroundings or oneself (e.g., seeing oneself from another person's perspective, being in a daze, time slowing)

Arousal and reactivity symptoms

Criterion E (two or more symptoms)

Except for item 2, these symptoms, if present, count toward the nine or more symptoms required for ASD

1. Irritable behavior and angry outbursts (with little or no provocation) typically expressed as verbal or physical aggression toward people or objects

2. Reckless or self-destructive behavior

3. Hypervigilance

4. Exaggerated startle response

5. Problems with concentration

6. Sleep disturbance (e.g., difficulty falling or staying asleep or restless sleep).

(continued)

TABLE 2.2 Continued

Description of Criteria	ASD Criterion	PTSD Criterion
Duration of disturbance	Minimum of 3 days, maximum of 1 month	More than 1 month
Temporal relationship to traumatic event	Typically begins immediately after trauma exposure	With delayed expression is specified if full criteria not met until at least 6 months after trauma
Distress or impairment in functioning: The disturbance causes clinically significant distress or impairment in social, occupational, or other important areas of functioning.	Criterion D	Criterion G
Exclusion of other conditions	Criterion E	Criterion H
The disturbance is not attributable to the physiological effects of a substance (e.g., medication or alcohol) or another medical condition	Criterion E	
Not better explained by a brief psychotic disorder	Criterion E	Not included in PTSD criteria

ASD, acute stress disorder; PTSD, posttraumatic stress disorder.

emotional state, diminished interest in pleasurable activities, feelings of detachment, or inability to experience positive emotions) are required. At least two of six arousal symptoms (irritability, self-destructive behavior, hypervigilance, exaggerated startle response, problems with concentration, or sleep disturbance) are required.

PTSD with delayed expression is specified if the full diagnostic criteria are not met until at least 6 months after the event, although some symptoms may be present before 6 months (American Psychiatric Association, 2013). Table 2.1 lists the complete diagnostic criteria for PTSD; Table 2.2 offers a summarized comparison of PTSD with its often transient precursor: acute stress disorder (ASD).

ASSOCIATED CLINICAL FEATURES

A number of additional features may be associated with PTSD, including somatic complaints, shame, impaired modulation of affect, survivor guilt, difficulties in interpersonal relationships, or changed personality. Limited seeking of mental health care has also been observed, with notable disparities based on sex, race, education, and socioeconomic status (Ghafoori et al., 2014). Although not necessarily the target of clinical trials for PTSD, this group of less clearly quantifiable symptoms contributes greatly to the total burden of social and occupational dysfunction or impairment resulting from the disorder. Associated symptoms such as shame, inappropriate guilt, or hopelessness may also be indicative of depression, which is often comorbid with PTSD. Depression may be related causally to the traumatic experience and resultant PTSD or may occur independently during the aftermath of disaster and require separate intervention (Jordan et al., 1991; Keane & Wolf, 1990; Stander et al., 2014). Somatic complaints without clear etiology are common phenomena among persons with histories of traumatic exposure and anxiety disorders including ASD and PTSD (Drossman, 1995; Salmon & Calderbank, 1996; St Cyr et al., 2014). Finally, trauma-exposed populations may experience comorbid substance-related disorders (Cross et al., 2015; Ulibarri et al., 2015; Vlahov et al., 2002). This relationship is complicated by the fact that substance intoxication may precede or precipitate traumatic experience (McFarlane, 1998).

DIFFERENTIAL DIAGNOSIS

The differential diagnosis for PTSD encompasses a range of psychiatric and physical diagnoses as well as normative responses to extremely stressful events. If sufficient symptoms (nine) occur 2 to 30 days after traumatic exposure, ASD may be diagnosed. For a single, discrete traumatic event, ASD and PTSD can be distinguished readily from one another based on the time interval that has passed since the event. For recurring traumas, as might be experienced in cases of domestic violence, multiple combat exposures, or a series of natural disasters (such as might occur during the hurricane season in certain locations), the distinction between ASD and PTSD may be less clear. No consensus exists regarding the classification of symptom episodes lasting less than 1 month but recurring during the course of repetitive trauma over months to years. However, such symptom presentation may be better conceptualized as PTSD rather than recurrent ASD. Eliminating the source of threat (e.g., physical separation from violent partner or geographic relocation from a dangerous environment) is essential to the resolution of symptoms regardless of classification.

Other disorders applicable to trauma survivors in the acute medical setting or in the context of ongoing exposures are described in Table 2.3. Individuals exposed to events that fulfill exposure criteria for PTSD often experience transient symptoms that differ from PTSD only in duration or associated level of distress or functional impairment. In some professions—particularly those associated with disaster response (such as firefighters or policemen)—exposure to criterion A events is inevitable. To the extent to which symptoms persist, result in dysfunction or distress, but do not meet full diagnostic criteria for PTSD, a diagnosis of adjustment disorder may be warranted.

EPIDEMIOLOGY

Multiple epidemiological studies have revealed the fact that traumatic exposures (i.e., to an event that would meet DSM-5 diagnostic criterion A) are very common. Although the DSM-5 has broadened the definition of traumatic exposures, the National Comorbidity Survey (Kessler et al., 1995), a large-scale ($n = 5877$), nationally representative epidemiological study of psychiatric disorders in the United States, reported a lifetime history of at least one traumatic event for 60.7% of men and 51.2% of women, with many individuals (25%–50%) experiencing two or more such traumas (by DSM-IV criterion). Other community-based samples have reported similar or even greater incidence figures (43%–92% of men and 37%–87% of women) for at least one traumatic exposure (Breslau et al., 1991, 1998; Norris, 1992; Stein et al., 1997). The most common types of trauma reported are witnessing someone being killed or injured, being involved in a natural disaster, and being involved in a life-threatening accident. Unrepresented in these surveys are persons whose traumatic exposures were limited to hearing repeated details of others who experienced significant trauma. First responders working in the immediate aftermath

TABLE 2.3 Differential Diagnosis after Traumatic Exposures

Diagnosis	Symptomatic Criteria	Functional Criteria	Time Course	Acute Care Considerations
PTSD	A. Exposure to actual or threatened death, serious injury, or sexual violence B. Persistent intrusive symptoms associated with the traumatic event(s) C. Persistent avoidance of stimuli associated with the traumatic event(s) D. Negative alterations in cognitions and mood associated with the traumatic event(s) E. Marked alterations in arousal and reactivity associated with the traumatic event(s)	Symptoms are associated with clinically significant distress or impairments in social, occupational, or other important areas of functioning.	Duration of disturbance is more than 1 month.	Patient's symptoms frequently appear before the 1-month point.
ASD	A. Exposure to actual or threatened death, serious injury, or sexual violence B. Presence of nine or more symptoms from any of the five categories of intrusion, negative mood, dissociation, avoidance, and arousal	Symptoms are associated with clinically significant distress or impairments in social, occupational, or other important areas of functioning.	Duration of the disturbance is 3 days to 1 month.	Not all injured patients with immediate distress will experience these dissociative symptoms.
Major depressive episode	Five or more of the following symptoms: depressed mood, diminished interest in pleasurable activities, weight loss or gain, insomnia or hypersomnia, agitation or retardation, fatigue or energy loss, feelings of worthlessness, poor concentration, and suicidal ideation	Symptoms cause clinically significant distress or impairment in social, occupational, or other important areas of functioning.	Symptoms must be present for 2 weeks.	Major depressive episode can be diagnosed in conjunction with ASD or PTSD. Injured trauma survivors frequently present with multiple symptoms of a depressive episode early on (i.e., before 2 weeks after the traumatic injury).

(continued)

TABLE 2.3 Continued

Diagnosis	Symptomatic Criteria	Functional Criteria	Time Course	Acute Care Considerations
Complicated grief/ persistent complex bereavement	This diagnostic "Condition for further Study" in DSM-5 is used when bereavement extends beyond normal societal expectations of intensity and duration, often after sudden, unanticipated loss. The symptoms of complicated grief often involve distressing thoughts and experiences related to reunion, longing, and searching for the deceased loved one.	The disturbance causes clinically significant impairment in social, occupational, or other important areas of functioning.	Duration of disturbance is at least 1 month (after 6 months of bereavement).	Traumatic grief is applicable to patients who have experienced the death of a significant other—particularly a child or a life partner.
Adjustment disorder	A. Development of emotional or behavioral symptoms in response to an identifiable stressor. Symptoms can include depression, anxiety, conduct disturbance, or other emotional disturbance. B. The symptoms or behaviors are clinically significant, as evidenced by marked distress.	Emotional or behavioral symptoms are associated with marked impairment in social, occupational, or other important areas of functioning, or are out of proportion to the severity of the stressor.	Onset occurs within 3 months of the stressor(s).	DSM-5 suggests the adjustment disorder diagnosis be used for patients who develop a symptom pattern not entirely consistent with the criteria for ASD/ PTSD. Nonspecific symptomatic requirements make adjustment disorder a useful diagnosis for the many patients who experience posttraumatic behavioral and emotional disturbances that include symptoms that do not fit into other diagnostic rubrics (e.g., patients who present with marked somatic symptom amplification) or do not meet the diagnostic thresholds for ASD or PTSD.

ASD, acute stress disorder; DSM-5, Diagnostic and Statistical Manual of Mental Disorders, fifth edition; PTSD, posttraumatic stress disorder.

of a disaster and clinicians working in both the short-term and long-term with disaster victims encompass others for whom the diagnosis of PTSD must be considered within the framework of the DSM-5.

A number of community-based studies have examined the prevalence of PTSD. As with the studies of traumatic exposure, estimates vary with the diagnostic criteria applied (e.g., DSM, third edition–revised vs. DSM-IV vs. DSM-5), the sample studied, the nature of the traumatic exposure, and the assessment procedure used (e.g., telephone survey vs. face-to-face interview, clinician vs. lay interviewer, structured vs. unstructured interview) (Brewin et al., 2000). In general, the point prevalence of ASD after acute traumatic exposure has been estimated at 5% to 20% (Bryant et al., 2000). However, more recent U.S. population base estimates DSM-IV criteria have reported PTSD lifetime prevalence rates of 7% to 9% (Kessler et al., 1995). Across community population studies, the lifetime prevalence rate of PTSD in women has, in general, been twice that reported for men (Breslau, 2002; Breslau et al., 1998; Kessler et al., 1995). It should be noted that, to the degree that war may be considered a subtype of disaster, prevalence of PTSD rates in populations of recent U.S. combat veterans have been demonstrably higher than other types of exposures (Hoge et al., 2004; Tanielian et al., 2008). However, the nature of exposure in combat (e.g., repeated, unpredictable exposure to life-threatening events over months to years) may account for this discrepancy.

Still, the relatively low rate of PTSD when compared with the substantially higher rate of traumatic exposure illustrates the point that, although traumatic exposure is necessary for the development of PTSD, it is not sufficient. One reason for this is that not all traumatic exposures are equally associated with the development of PTSD. In fact, some of the most commonly experienced traumatic events are least likely to be associated with PTSD. In the National Comorbidity Study, lifetime prevalence of being in a natural disaster or fire, and witnessing someone being badly injured or killed ranged from 14% to 36% (depending on specific event and gender). The prevalence of these exposures were all greater than the prevalence of being raped (less than 1% for men and approximately 9% for women). However, the prevalence of PTSD related to rape was 46% for men and 65% for women compared with less than 10% each for being in an accident, fire, or natural disaster, and witnessing someone being badly injured or killed (Kessler et al., 1995).

Also, many reactions to traumatic events are often transient and may resolve, to a great extent, relatively soon after the event. One study of rape victims evaluated weekly for the presence of PTSD symptoms found that although 94% met full symptom (but not duration) criteria 12 days after the assault, 64% met criteria 1 month after the assault at the point when PTSD could be first diagnosed. By 3 months, 47%

met criteria for chronic PTSD (Rothbaum et al., 1992). Longitudinal studies of the cohort of New York City residents south of Canal Street demonstrated a decline in PTSD from the 7.5% initially reported to 1.7% by 5 months (Galea et al., 2003a) and 0.6% by 6 to 9 months after the terrorist attacks of 9/11 (Galea et al., 2003b). Thus, the majority of persons exposed to traumatic events and who experience symptoms of PTSD experience natural recovery. A study of battle-injured American soldiers evacuated from Iraq showed that a considerable percentage of persons who failed to meet criteria at initial screening did so at the 3- or 6-month reassessment. Thus, cross-sectional studies can underestimate the overall prevalence of this condition (Grieger et al., 2006).

In addition to the type of trauma and the gender of the victim, several other risk factors have been identified as predictors of PTSD. In the National Women's Survey ($n = 4008$), fear of being killed or being injured (i.e., threat perception) as well as receipt of physical injury independently increased the likelihood of a lifetime diagnosis of PTSD (Resnick et al., 1993). Physical injury, regardless of gender, was associated with a considerably higher rate of PTSD in workers traumatically exposed to the Murrah Federal Building bombing (North et al., 1999). In a meta-analysis of risk factors, Brewin et al. (2000) found large effect sizes for severity of trauma, lack of social support after the trauma, and life stress after the trauma. Other predictors included personal psychiatric history, family psychiatric history, and personal history of childhood abuse. Biological markers identified during recent preliminary investigations appear to include low cortisol levels during the acute aftermath of traumatic exposure and an elevated resting heart rate (Delahanty et al., 2000; Shalev et al., 1998).

DIAGNOSTIC ASSESSMENT AND SCREENING

At a minimum, the assessment PTSD (or its distinction from other trauma and stressor-related disorders) requires an elaboration of the individual's trauma history to include information on both the objective features (i.e., whether the person was exposed to an event involving actual or threatened injury, death, or loss of physical integrity to self or others) and elucidation of characteristic symptoms from each of the four clusters. Because of the presumed etiologic link between traumatic exposure and PTSD, the temporal relationship between trauma and symptoms must be established. The nature and duration of symptoms, and the resulting functional impairment should be clarified to determine whether individuals meet threshold diagnostic criteria for PTSD. Finally, because PTSD is highly comorbid with other psychiatric disorders (especially anxiety disorders, mood disorders, and substance-misuse disorders), assessment should include inquiry into possible co-occurrences of other psychiatric illness. Table 2.4 summarizes clinical domains that should be assessed in a comprehensive evaluation of PTSD.

The clinical interview remains the "gold standard" for the assessment of PTSD for several reasons. An interview allows for a detailed explanation of the nature of the traumatic stressor. It permits the clearest understanding of potentially confusing symptoms (e.g., a patient may not be able to distinguish or articulate the difference between intrusive recollections and flashbacks without an interactive explanation from an interviewer). Finally, the clinical interview allows for the progressive elaboration of symptoms in a manner sensitive to the emotional needs of the patient at the time of assessment. There may be times or settings when resources are not available

TABLE 2.4 Domains of Assessment in Comprehensive Posttrauma Evaluation

Clinical Domain	Component
Trauma history	Type, age, and duration
Safety	Threat of harm from others and dangerousness to self or others
Dissociative symptoms	Necessary for diagnosis of ASD: numbing, detachment, derealization/depersonalization, dissociative amnesia in acute response to trauma
ASD/PTSD symptoms	Reexperiencing, avoidance and numbing, hyperarousal as a consequence of trauma (PTSD is diagnosed if symptom onset is more than 30 days after the traumatic event. If less than 30 days, and if dissociative symptoms are present, ASD is diagnosed.)
Military history	Prior exposure(s), training, and preparedness for exposure
Behavioral and health risks	Substance use/abuse, sexually transmitted diseases, preexisting mental illness, nonadherence to treatment, impulsivity, and potential for further exposure to violence
Personal characteristics	Coping skills, resilience, interpersonal relatedness/ attachment, history of developmental trauma or psychodynamic conflict(s), motivation for treatment
Psychosocial situation	Home environment, social support, employment status, ongoing violence (e.g., interpersonal, disaster, war), parenting/caregiver skills or burdens
Stressors	Acute and/or chronic trauma, poverty, loss, bereavement
Legal system involvement	Meaning of symptoms, compensation based on disability determination or degree of distress

ASD, acute stress disorder; PTSD, posttraumatic stress disorder.

to permit an in-depth interview of all affected persons requesting or requiring immediate mental health assistance. In disaster situations, or to augment assessment, several clinician-administered and self-report instruments can be used to obtain diagnostic information (and, in some cases, indications of the degree of severity or response to intervention). The most widely used instruments are listed in Box 2.1.

There are several reliable and valid instruments used to obtain diagnostic information (and in some cases index of severity) for PTSD (First et al., 1995). The PTSD module, the Structured Clinical Interview for DSM-5, has been developed and asks open-ended questions about each of the 20 symptoms of DSM-5 PTSD; it is currently being validated. The evaluator must judge whether each symptom and its functional criteria are either absent, subthreshold, or at/above threshold. The result leads to a determination of the presence or absence of disorder as well as a severity index of mild, moderate, or severe. The most commonly used PTSD measure in research before the recent change in diagnostic criteria was the Clinician-Administered PTSD scale (CAPS), which asks the patient about the frequency and severity of each symptom, rating each on a scale of 1 to 4 points and yielding a total score of between 0 and 136 points. A minimum score of 50 points was used as an entry criterion for PTSD research (Blake et al., 1990). The CAPS has been revised to reflect the new diagnostic criteria as a 30-item structured interview, and new scoring and threshold scores have been developed that allow a clinician to assess severity (mild, moderate, severe) as well deliver a current (past month and/or past week) or lifetime diagnosis. The PTSD Checklist for DSM-5 (PCL-5) is a self-report measure that can be completed by patients (or disaster victims) in a traditional clinical or a more austere environment. It takes approximately 5 to 10 minutes to complete, and results can easily be interpreted by clinicians according to a variety of scoring rules.

BOX 2.1
INSTRUMENTS USED IN THE ASSESSMENT
AND DIAGNOSIS OF PTSD

- The Structured Clinical Interview for DSM-5 (SCID-5)[a]
- The Clinician-Administered PTSD Scale (CAPS)[a]
- The Davidson Trauma Scale (DTS)
- The PTSD Symptom Scale Interview (PSSI)[a]
- The PTSD Symptom Scale Self-Report (PSS-SR)
- The Impact of Event Scale (IES)

---

[a]*Clinician administered.*

Adapted from its highly used predecessor (the PCL-17 for DSM-IV) and validated for DSM-5, it will likely be widely used in post disaster research, surveillance, and needs assessment for the foreseeable future. The CAPS-5 and PCL-5 are currently the most widely used clinician- and patient-administered PTSD assessments, respectively. Other instruments listed in Box 2.1 have proved useful historically—in part as a result of their brevity of administration—but it is not clear whether they will be revised to reflect DSM-5 criteria at this time.

TREATMENT AND PREVENTION

Professional organizations and institutions—including the U.S. Department of Defense (DoD) and U.S. Department of Veterans Affairs (VA), and the American Psychiatric Association—have developed and published practice guidelines for the treatment of PTSD (see Box 2.2). Practice guidelines do not define the standard of care. However, their synthesis of research and expert consensus augments clinical experience in treating patients, educating the public, guiding research, and establishing credibility for medical care delivery. In the final section of this chapter, essential recommendations of these practice guidelines are summarized. The limitations of existing guidelines are summarized in Box 2.2. Last, developments in treatment and prevention that have emerged recently are outlined as a segue to the remainder of this text.

BOX 2.2
LIMITATIONS OF PTSD PRACTICE GUIDELINES

Emphasis on published randomized controlled trials (RCTs) limits the contributions of clinical experience.

Restrictive eligibility, short treatment duration, and high dropout rates of RCTs diminish generalizability of findings to clinical populations.

Medication adherence in RCT protocol may not reflect medication adherence in clinical populations.

Negative trials are often unpublished; therefore, results are not synthesized into guideline recommendations.

Different criteria used for evaluating quality of evidence leads to disparate recommendations.

Guidelines rarely assess population-based approaches.

There is a limited evidence basis to support current early-intervention strategies.

Interest group representation on guideline committees may affect recommendations.

Clinical advances occurring during guideline development may not be included.

PSYCHOPHARMACOLOGY

Although it is hypothesized that pharmacological treatment soon after trauma exposure may prevent the development of PTSD, existing evidence is not supportive. Given the significance of noradrenergic mechanisms within the amygdala in the consolidation of memory and learning of fear in response to stressful events, it is not surprising that disruption of this process with postsynaptic beta-blocking agents has been investigated as a preventive intervention. Rigorous studies of beta-blockers, corticosteroids, and opioids administered acutely after trauma exposure have not demonstrated broad reductions in the development of PTSD (Sijbrandij et al., 2015; U.S. Department of Veterans Affairs, 2013). Selective serotonin reuptake inhibitors (SSRIs) and serotonin norepinephrine reuptake inhibitors (SNRIs) are considered the first-line medication treatment for PTSD. In both male and female patients, treatment with these antidepressants has been associated with reductions of core PTSD symptoms in all clusters. Other antidepressants, including tricyclic antidepressants, monoamine oxidase inhibitors, nefazodone, and mirtazapine are considered to have fair evidence for efficacy based on previous, and in some cases less rigorous, studies (Benedek et al., 2009). Prazosin, a centrally active alpha-1 receptor antagonist, has been shown to reduce trauma-related nightmares and overall levels of PTSD in a series of combat veterans and other trauma victims (Raskind et al., 2013). The most recent VA/DoD clinical practice guideline lists prazosin as having fair evidence in treating sleep/nightmare symptoms as well as providing a benefit for global PTSD symptoms.

Benzodiazepines appear to reduce anxiety and improve sleep. They also oppose norepinephrine's memory-potentiating activity in the amygdala (although to a lesser degree than beta-blockers). They are often used in trauma-exposed individuals, including those with PTSD. Because of observations including increased incidence of PTSD after early treatment, worsening symptoms on withdrawal, and the possibility of dependence, benzodiazepines are considered to have no benefit and are noted to be potentially harmful (U.S Department of Veterans Affairs, 2013).

Limited studies suggest that some second-generation antipsychotic medications (e.g., olanzapine and quetiapine) may be helpful in some patients with PTSD. Risperidone is considered ineffective in the treatment of PTSD (Krystal et al., 2011). Although flashbacks and intrusive symptoms are considered to be distinct from psychotic phenomena, the similarity between particularly intense flashbacks and other impairments in reality testing may provide a partial explanation for these observations. The neurophysiological kindling model suggests a theoretical basis for anticonvulsant medications (e.g., carbamazepine and lamotrigine) in terms of preventive as well as therapeutic efficacy. Although preventive effects have not been quantified, limited studies suggest therapeutic benefit, particularly in the reexperiencing symptom cluster, with these agents (Connor & Butterfield, 2003). The anticonvulsants topiramate, valproate, and tiagabine, along with guanfacine, are considered to be ineffective in treating PTSD (DoD/VA guidelines [U.S. Department of Veterans Affairs, 2013]).

PSYCHOSOCIAL INTERVENTIONS

Evidence supports the effectiveness of brief psychotherapeutic approaches (four to five sessions) immediately after trauma in preventing the development of ASD and perhaps PTSD. Cognitive–behavioral therapy (CBT) attempts to correct cognitive distortions (e.g., overgeneralization of threat levels) and reduce the frequency and symptomatology associated with traumatic memories by reexposure (imagined or in vivo) in a controlled setting. Studies of CBT with individuals who have suffered a variety of trauma types suggest that CBT delivered over a few sessions during the weeks after trauma may speed recovery and prevent the development of PTSD (U.S. Department of Veterans Affairs, 2013).

Trauma-focused psychotherapies that include components of exposure and/or cognitive restructuring, as well as stress inoculation training are listed as having the highest level of evidence and benefit in the DoD/VA guidelines (U.S. Department of Veterans Affairs, 2013). Trauma-focused therapies such as prolonged exposure, eye movement desensitization and reprocessing (EMDR), and cognitive processing therapy (CPT) share with traditional CBT the incorporation of an element of progressive and guided reexposure to traumatic recollections as part of the therapeutic process. Cognitive processing therapy has demonstrated good outcomes in a group setting with sexual assault victims. EMDR combines a reexposure element with eye movement, memory recall, and verbalization. A meta-analysis of effective treatments for PTSD found cognitive therapy, exposure therapy, and EMDR to be effective in treating PTSD from a variety of trauma types (Watts et al., 2013). Despite the benefit for PTSD, the efficacy of these treatments in the postdisaster setting has not been well established.

The idea that trauma exposure and the development of ASD or PTSD occurred simultaneously in large groups or communities was recognized long before it was confirmed in epidemiological studies of combat veterans or survivors of the 9/11 terrorist attacks. As a consequence, group-based interventions aimed at preventing PTSD have been explored. Techniques applied to groups of law enforcement personnel, emergency service providers, and civilians, and referred to collectively as *psychological debriefing*, gained popularity even before being reviewed scientifically. Although many who receive debriefing experience the process as beneficial, there is no evidence to suggest debriefings prevent PTSD, and some studies suggest the process may be harmful (Bryant, 2005). The American Psychiatric Association (2013) practice guidelines do not recommend Critical Incident Stress Debriefing (CISD) or other forms of psychological debriefing for the prevention or treatment of ASD or PTSD. Similarly, the VA/DoD guidelines list group psychological debriefing as having insufficient evidence of benefit (U.S. Department of Veterans Affairs, 2013). In light of the lack of evidence and potential harm from group psychological debriefing, there were several calls to create a population-based approach to exposure to the psychological impact of mass violence, with the goal of reducing ASD and PTSD. One such is psychological first aid (PFA). PFA (National Center for Posttraumatic Stress Disorder, 2006) is an evidence-informed modular approach for assisting people during the immediate aftermath of disaster and terrorism to reduce initial distress and to foster short- and long-term adaptive functioning. PFA covers a variety of important postdisaster issues such as safety and social engagement. A systematic literature review of PFA found insufficient evidence to determine the efficacy of PFA (Dieltjens et al., 2014).

In summary, although traditional pharmacotherapy and cognitive therapy-based approaches have sufficient evidence bases for continued use in the treatment of PTSD, the facts that medications may cause side effects, that many persons believe they should be able to recover without the use of medications, that some people refuse medications regardless of whether they believe other treatments are effective, coupled with the reality that still others refrain from seeking traditional psychotherapy as a result of stigma all result in a significant population of PTSD sufferers not receiving even minimally adequate treatment for the disorder. Although antistigma efforts and public awareness campaigns have a place, so too, must there be a place for nonpharmacological (and even nontraditional psychotherapeutic) treatment approaches seen as less stigmatizing. Such treatments will allow providers to "meet the patient where he or she is at" in terms of developing a plan in which the patient may be most likely to engage initially and remain engaged.

Complementary and alternative medicine approaches have received increasing attention during the past decade. Complementary medicine may be distinguished from alternative medicine. Complementary practices and treatments are, primarily, modalities that augment traditional interventions but are not likely ever to replace standard medical practice. Alternative modalities, such as acupuncture, are nonmainstream medical approaches that are either already being used by or have the potential to be used as "monotherapy" within the typical western meaning of this term (Wynn, 2015). Currently, these approaches are considered not to have sufficient evidence for inclusion in any of the major ASD and PTSD treatment guidelines. Nonetheless, physicians, allied health professionals, lay counselors, and concerned public partners are developing an ever-broadening experience base and research base regarding these practices.

CONCLUSION

Social scientists, historians, and psychiatrists concerned themselves with the consequences of traumatic experiences on individuals and populations for decades before the diagnosis PTSD was identified specifically. Descriptive literature, clinical experience, and case study guided the characterization and treatment of persons suffering from the aftermath of trauma before epidemiological studies and RCTs became the standards for disease classification and treatment evaluation. History and scientific investigation have refined our understanding of the highly variable range of human response to traumatic events. Such study has led to the characterization and refinement of the diagnosis of PTSD along the continuum of neuropsychological response to the terror, loss, and disruption created by events such disasters, and intrapersonal violence or combat. Research and clinical experience to date have led to the development of relatively effective pharmacological and psychosocial treatments for PTSD, but the available treatments are—for a variety of reasons—not well suited for many persons suffering from symptoms of this disorder. Moreover, these treatments may not address symptoms associated frequently with PTSD that fall outside the parameters of formal diagnosis.

This volume describes emerging treatments that have demonstrated varying degrees of promise in terms of relieving the suffering associated with PTSD— approaches that may target core symptoms or frequently associated comorbidity, or both. It is hoped that such descriptions will augment future research and encourage creative treatment approaches tailored to individual patients in the context of a growing population searching for nontraditional treatment options, and an expanding evidence basis for choosing such alternatives.

REFERENCES

American Psychiatric Association. (2000). *Diagnostic and Statistical Manual of Mental Disorders*, 4th edition, text revision. Arlington, VA: American Psychiatric Press.

American Psychiatric Association. (2013). *Diagnostic and Statistical Manual of Mental Disorders*, 5th edition. Washington, DC: American Psychiatric Press.

Benedek, D. M., Friedman, M. J., Zatzick, D., et al. (2009). *Guideline Watch (March 2009): Practice Guideline for the Treatment of Patients with Acute Stress Disorder and Posttraumatic Stress Disorder*. Arlington, VA: American Psychiatric Press.

Blake, D. D., Weathers, F. W., Nagy, L. M., et al. (1990). A clinician rating scale for current and lifetime PTSD: the CAPS-1. *Behavior Therapist*, **18**, 187–188.

Breslau, N. (2002). Gender differences in trauma and post traumatic stress disorder. *Journal of Gender Specific Medicine*, **5**, 34–40.

Breslau, N., Davis, G. C., Andreski, P., et al. (1991). Traumatic events and posttraumatic stress disorder in an urban population of young adults. *Archives of General Psychiatry*, **48**, 216–222.

Breslau, N., Kessler, R. C., Chilcoat, H. D., et al. (1998). Trauma and posttraumatic stress disorder in the community: the 1996 Detroit area survey of trauma. *Archives of General Psychiatry*, **55**, 626–632.

Brewin, C. R., Andrews, B., & Valentine, J. D. (2000). Meta-analysis of risk factors for post-traumatic stress disorder in trauma-exposed adults. *Journal of Consulting and Clinical Psychology*, **68**, 748–766.

Bryant, R. A. (2005). Psychosocial approaches to acute stress reactions. *CNS Spectrums*, **10**, 116–122.

Bryant, R. A., Moulds, M. L., & Guthrie, R. M. (2000). Acute stress disorder scale: a self-report measure of acute stress disorder. *Psychological Assessment*, **12**, 61–68.

Connor, K. M., & Butterfield, M. I. (2003). Posttraumatic stress disorder. *FOCUS*, **I**, 247–262.

Cross, D., Crow, T., Powers, A., et al. (2015). Childhood trauma, PTSD, and problematic alcohol and substance use in low-income, African-American men and women. *Child Abuse and Neglect*, **44**, 26–35.

Delahanty, D. L., Raimonde, J., & Spoonster, E. (2000). Initial post-traumatic urinary cortisol levels predict subsequent symptoms in motor vehicle accident victims. *Biological Psychiatry*, **48**, 940–947.

Dieltjens, T., Moonens, I., Van Praet, K., et al. (2014). A systematic literature search on psychological first aid: lack of evidence to develop guidelines. *PLoS One*, **9**, e113714.

Drossman, D. A. (1995). Sexual and physical abuse and gastrointestinal illness. *Scandinavian Journal of Gastroenterology*, **30** (Suppl 208), 90–96.

First, M. B., Spitzer, R. L., Gibbon, M., et al. (1995). *Structured Clinical Interview for DSM–IV Axis I Disorders–Patient Edition (SCID I/P Version 2)*. New York, NY: Biometrics Research Department, New York State Psychiatric Institute.

Galea, S., Boscarino, J., Resnick, H., et al. (2003a). Mental health in New York City after the September 11th terrorist attacks: results from two population surveys. In *Mental Health, United States, 2002*, eds. R. W. Mandersheid & M. J. Henderson. Washington, DC: US Government Printing Office.

Galea, S., Vlahov, D., Resick, H. et al. (2003b). Trends of probable post-traumatic stress disorder in New York City after the September 11th terrorist attacks. *American Journal of Epidemiology*, **158**, 514–524.

Ghafoori, B., Barragan, B., & Palinkas, L. (2014). Mental health service use among trauma-exposed adults: a mixed-methods study. *Journal of Nervous and Mental Disease*, **202**, 239–246.

Grieger, A., Cozza, S. J., Ursano, R. J., et al. (2006). Post-traumatic stress disorder and depression in battle-injured soldiers. *American Journal of Psychiatry*, **163**, 1777–1783.

Hoge, C. W., Castro, C. A., Messer, et al. (2004). Combat duty in Iraq and Afghanistan, mental health problems, and barriers to care. *New England Journal of Medicine*, **351**, 13–22.

Jordan, B. K., Schlenger, W. E., Hough, R., et al. (1991). Lifetime and current prevalence of specific psychiatric disorders among Vietnam veterans and controls. *Archives of General Psychiatry*, **48**, 207–215.

Keane, T. M., & Wolf, J. (1990). Comorbidity in posttraumatic stress disorder: an analysis of community and clinical studies. *Journal of Applied Social Psychology*, **20**, 1776–1778.

Kessler, R. C., Sonnega, A., Bromet, E., et al. (1995). Posttraumatic stress disorder in the National Comorbidity Survey. *Archives of General Psychiatry*, **52**, 1048–1060.

Krystal, J. H., Rosenheck, R. A., Cramer, J. A., et al. (2011). Adjunctive risperidone treatment for antidepressant-resistant symptoms of chronic military service-related PTSD: a randomized trial. *Journal of the American Medical Association*, **306**, 493–502.

McFarlane, A. C. (1998). Epidemiological evidence about the relationship between PTSD and alcohol abuse: the nature of the association. *Addictive Behaviors*, **23**, 813–825.

Norris, F. H. (1992). Epidemiology of trauma: frequency and impact of different potentially traumatic events on different demographic groups. *Journal of Consulting and Clinical Psychology*, **60**, 409–418.

North, C. S., Nixon, S. J., Shariat, S., et al. (1999). Psychiatric disorders among survivors of the Oklahoma City bombing. *Journal of the American Medical Association*, **282**, 755–762.

Brymer M., Jacobs A., Layne C., et al. (2006). Psychological First Aid—Field Operations Guide. National Center for PTSD, White River Junction, NH.

Raskind, M. A., Peterson, K., Williams, T., et al. (2013). A trial of prazosin for combat trauma PTSD with nightmares in active-duty soldiers returned from Iraq and Afghanistan. *American Journal of Psychiatry*, **170**, 1003–1010.

Resnick, H. S., Kilpatrick, D. G., Dansky, B. S., et al. (1993). Prevalence of civilian trauma and posttraumatic stress disorder in a representative national sample of women. *Journal of Consulting and Clinical Psychology*, **61**, 984–991.

Rothbaum, B. O., Foa, E. B., Murdock, T., et al. (1992). A prospective examination of post-traumatic stress disorder in rape victims. *Journal of Traumatic Stress*, **5**, 455–475.

Salmon, P., & Calderbank, S. (1996). The relationship of childhood physical and sexual abuse to adult illness behavior. *Journal of Psychosomatic Research*, **40**, 329–336.

Shalev, A. Y., Sahar, T., Freedman, S., et al. (1998). A prospective study of heart rate response following trauma and the subsequent development of posttraumatic stress disorder. *Archives of General Psychiatry*, **55**, 553–559.

Sijbrandij, M., Kleiboer, A., Bisson, J. I., et al. (2015). Pharmacological prevention of post-traumatic stress disorder and acute stress disorder: a systematic review and meta-analysis. *Lancet Psychiatry*, **2**(5), 413–421.

Stander, V. A., Thomsen, C. J., & Highfill-McRoy, R. M. (2014). Etiology of depression comorbidity in combat-related PTSD: a review of the literature. *Clinical Psychology Review*, **34**, 87–98.

St Cyr, K., McIntyre-Smith, A., Contractor, A. A., et al. (2014). Somatic symptoms and health-related quality of life among treatment-seeking Canadian Forces personnel with PTSD. *Psychiatry Research*, **218**, 148–152.

Stein, M. B., Walker, J. R., Hazen, A. L., et al. (1997). Full and partial posttraumatic stress disorder: findings from a community survey. *American Journal of Psychiatry*, **154**, 1114–1119.

Tanielian, T., & Jaycox L. H. (2008). *Invisible Wounds of War: Psychological and Cognitive Injuries, Their Consequences, and Services to Assist Recovery*. Santa Monica, CA: RAND Corporation.

Ulibarri, M. D., Ulloa, E. C., & Salazar, M. (2015). Associations between mental health, substance abuse, and sexual abuse experience among Latinas. *Journal of Child Sexual Abuse*, **24**, 35–54.

U.S. Department of Veterans Affairs. (2013). *VA/DoD Clinical Practice Guidelines: PTSD Pocket Guide*. Washington, DC: U.S. Dept of Veterans Affairs.

Vlahov, D., Galea, S., Resnick, H., et al. (2002). Increased use of cigarettes, alcohol, and marijuana among Manhattan, New York residents after the September 11th terrorist attacks. *American Journal of Epidemiology*, **155**, 988–996.

Watts, B. V., Schnurr, P. P., Mayo, L., et al. (2013). Meta-analysis of the efficacy of treatments for posttraumatic stress disorder. *Journal of Clinical Psychiatry*, **74**, e541–e550.

Wynn, G. H. (2015). Complementary and alternative medicine approaches in the treatment of PTSD. *Current Psychiatry Report*, **17**, 62.

PART
2

ALTERNATIVE TREATMENTS

THREE

Acceptance and Commitment Therapy for Posttraumatic Stress Disorder

JANINA SCARLET, ARIEL J. LANG, AND ROBYN D. WALSER

ACCEPTANCE AND COMMITMENT THERAPY (ACT) IS A PSYCHOTHERAPY THAT encourages the pursuit of one's values and goals even in the presence of psychological and emotional challenges that potentially interfere with healthy behavior (Hayes, Luoma, Bond, Masuda, & Lillis, 2006). Trauma and its aftermath can be one of those challenges. For those suffering with posttraumatic stress disorder (PTSD), pursuit of personal values is often disrupted, and finding meaning in life can be lost to the fear and memories that follow a traumatic event. An intervention that supports a reengagement in values-based living, such as ACT, may serve to encourage recovery and restoration of functioning.

ACT is part of the "third wave" of psychotherapy (Fletcher & Hayes, 2005). The first wave of behavior therapy consisted primarily of modification of observable behavior based on learning principles (i.e., classical and operant conditioning) with little attention to cognition or subjective experience. The second wave was prompted by the "cognitive revolution" and added change strategies based on cognitive restructuring and social learning models to produce emotional and behavioral change (Hayes, 2004). The third-wave therapies combined some of the cognitive–behavioral (second-wave) techniques with mindfulness (i.e., nonjudgmental awareness of current experience [Fletcher & Hayes, 2005]) and acceptance (i.e., openness to all experiences and psychological events [Hayes, 2004]), as well as other techniques. In addition to ACT, third-wave therapies include dialectical behavior therapy (Linehan, 1993), mindfulness-based cognitive therapy (Segal, Williams, & Teasdale, 2002), functional analytic psychotherapy (Kohlenberg & Tsai, 1991), behavioral activation (Dobson et al., 2008), Cognitive Behavioral Analysis System of Psychotherapy (McCullough, 2010), and integrative behavioral couples therapy (Jacobson & Christensen, 1998). Most of these therapies are grounded in behavioral theory. One of the distinguishing features of these therapies, and the reason why they are considered "third wave," is related to their movement away from a focus on cognition, and instead toward a functional analytic understanding of behavior and the context in which it occurs. In line with this tradition, ACT is considered a behavioral intervention that focuses on the *function* of behavior rather than its form. ACT incorporates a behavioral understanding of cognition and emotion with a focus on acceptance, mindfulness, and taking meaningful actions in the service of one's personal values (Smout, Hayes, Atkins, Klausen, & Duguid, 2012). Furthermore, although ACT falls under the umbrella of cognitive–behavioral therapies (Hayes, 2004, 2008), it diverges from traditional cognitive therapy (CT). Although CT focuses on changing the *content* or structure of problematic thoughts (e.g., questioning how likely a predicted outcome might be to create a more realistic appraisal), ACT focuses on changing the function of the thought or the *context* in which thoughts occur (e.g., a thought can be viewed as an inherently meaningless momentary experience [Fletcher & Hayes, 2005]).

MECHANISMS OF ACTION

In ACT, psychological *in*flexibility is the target of change. Psychological inflexibility is a maladaptive state characterized by six pathological processes: (1) experiential avoidance (avoidance of thoughts, feelings, behaviors, and sensations), (2) cognitive fusion (excessive attachment to thoughts), (3) lack of clearly defined values or inaction, (4) attachment to the conceptualized self (seeing oneself in an overly narrow way), (5) excessive focus on past or future events (lack of present-moment mindfulness, lack of self-knowledge), and (6) lack of action and/or impulsivity. The goal of ACT is to increase psychological flexibility through six core processes developed to counter the pathological processes: (1) acceptance, (2) cognitive defusion, (3) clearly defined values, (4) a developed sense of self as larger than the content of events experienced (e.g., emotions and thoughts), (5) mindfulness/present-moment

TABLE 3.1 Pathological and Psychological Flexibility Processes

Pathological Processes	Psychological Flexibility
Experiential avoidance	Acceptance
Cognitive fusion	Cognitive defusion
Lack of clearly defined values or inaction	Clearly defined values
Attachment to the conceptualized self	A developed sense of self
Excessive focus on past or future events	Mindfulness/present moment awareness
Lack of action and/or impulsivity	Committed action

awareness, and (6) commitment to action (Hayes & Smith, 2005; Hayes et al., 2006; Luoma, Hayes, & Walser, 2007). The following text focuses on the empirical evidence supporting each of these processes (Table 3.1).

Many researchers have tried to evaluate whether change in these six core processes is, in fact, responsible for outcomes observed when using ACT. *Experiential avoidance*, which refers to the avoidance of unwanted internal experiences, such as emotions, physical sensations, and cognitions (Hayes, Wilson, Gifford, Follette, & Strosahl, 1996), has probably received the most attention. Such avoidance, along with negative evaluation of these cognitions and sensations, has been suggested to be a major contributor to human suffering (Fletcher & Hayes, 2005; Hayes et al., 1996) and increases risk of PTSD and anxiety (Kumpula, Orcutt, Bardeen, & Varkovitzky, 2011; Meyer, Morissette, Kimbrel, Kruse, & Gulliver, 2013; Tull, Gratz, Salters, & Roemer, 2004), in particular for patients who tend to have heightened sensitivity to anxiety (Forsyth, Parker, & Finlay, 2003). Furthermore, experiential avoidance has been linked to several clinical disorders, including addiction (Gifford et al., 2011; Hayes et al., 1996; Litvin, Kovacs, Hayes, & Brandon, 2012; Petersen & Zettle, 2009), panic (Levitt, Brown, Orsillo, & Barlow, 2004), anxiety and depression (Forman, Herbert, Moitra, Yeomans, & Geller, 2007), suicide (Luoma & Villatte, 2012), social anxiety disorder (Kashdan, Morina, & Priebe, 2009), and PTSD (Twohig, 2009; Walser & Hayes, 2006). Research suggests experiential avoidance can increase anticipatory anxiety (Braams, Blechert, Boden, & Gross, 2012) and symptom severity (Tull et al., 2004), whereas acceptance (i.e., being open both to positively and negatively evaluated internal experiences without changing them) can facilitate better recovery after distress (Campbell-Sills, Barlow, Brown, & Hofmann, 2006). Indeed, less thought suppression (an avoidance strategy) has been associated with improvement in PTSD symptoms (Walser, Sears, Young, Wagner, & Young, 2013). Thus, one of the main goals of ACT is to reduce experiential avoidance by assisting the patient with facing the difficult experiences while accepting the discomfort they create (Hayes et al., 1996).

The degree of avoidance/acceptance experienced by the individual is usually measured using the Acceptance and Action Questionnaire (AAQ [Bond et al., 2011]). The AAQ, and the newer AAQ-II, are validated, brief self-report measures. The AAQ has also been found to be a good predictor of depression and anxiety disorders, as well as PTSD (Kashdan, Barrios, Forsyth, & Steger, 2006; Kumpula et al., 2011; Meyer et al., 2013). For example, a recent study with veterans from Iraq and Afghanistan found the AAQ-II had sufficient predictive validity, such that higher AAQ-II scores (demonstrating a greater degree of psychological *in*flexibility) were associated with all three *Diagnostics and Statistical Manual of Mental disorders*—fourth edition clusters of PTSD symptoms: reexperiencing, hyperarousal, and avoidance (Meyer et al., 2013). These results can be interpreted to mean that the greater degree of experiential avoidance can potentially increase the likelihood of developing or maintaining PTSD, and that the AAQ-II can be used to predict it. To further this point, a recent case study demonstrated that when a participant with PTSD received an ACT intervention focused on reducing avoidance and increasing her acceptance (as measured by the AAQ-II), her PTSD symptoms reduced as well (Burrows, 2013). It remains unclear, however, whether change in experiential avoidance can be separated from general clinical improvement. For example, change in AAQ scores are associated with change related to psychotherapies that do not target experiential avoidance specifically (Arch et al., 2012; Lang et al., 2015).

Furthermore, experiential avoidance may lead to treatment discontinuation; attrition tends to be high in exposure-based treatments for PTSD (approximately 27% [Zayfert et al., 2005]). In fact, a recent study found that in interventions that use exposure components, as many as 76% of the participants who dropped out of PTSD studies did so to avoid imaginal exposure (Zayfert et al., 2005). Thus, a treatment approach, such as ACT, which focuses directly on reducing experiential avoidance, might lower attrition rates and promote motivation and commitment to treatment. A recent article examined the possibility of using ACT to promote patients' willingness in undergoing exposure (Thompson, Luoma, & LeJeune, 2013). Two case studies demonstrated the feasibility of implementing ACT in the treatment of PTSD and, in both cases, the patients were able to engage with the treatment, including the exposure and demonstrated reductions in their trauma symptoms (Burrows, 2013; Twohig, 2009).

Mindfulness is another strategy used in ACT to target experiential avoidance, as well as the psychological dominance of past and/or future events, attachment to the conceptualized self, and cognitive fusion (Hayes et al., 2006; Luoma & Villatte, 2012). Mindfulness can be defined as present-moment awareness and nonjudgmental response to the observer's internal experience (Roemer & Orsillo, 2012).

Key experiences that tend to be most problematic for patients with PTSD might potentially be improved by increasing mindfulness. For instance, several studies show that low scores on the Mindful Attention Awareness Scale (MAAS [Brown & Ryan, 2003]) or the Five Facet Mindfulness Questionnaire (Baer, Smith, Hopkins, Krietemeyer, & Toney, 2006) are associated with increases in depression, anxiety, negative affect, neuroticism, suicidality, and stress (Brown & Ryan, 2003; Brown, Ryan, & Creswell, 2007; Luoma & Villatte, 2012; McCracken, Gauntlett-Gilbert, & Vowles, 2007; Walser, Karlin, Trockel, Mazina, & Taylor, 2013). In addition, McCracken, et al. (2007) found that low levels of mindfulness on the MAAS predict pain-related anxiety, disability, and depression, whereas higher levels of mindfulness predict improved emotional health. Other studies demonstrated that changes in anxiety and depression symptoms are associated with or can be mediated by mindfulness training (Coffey & Hartman, 2008; Ma & Teasdale, 2004; Sears & Kraus, 2009; Vøllestad, Sivertsen, & Nielsen, 2011; Walser, Karlin, et al., 2013). Finally, mindfulness (as measured by the MAAS) can also predict the development of depression, anxiety, and PTSD in recently deployed members of the National Guard, in whom higher degrees of mindfulness were associated with lower risk of the development of these disorders (Call, Pitcock, & Pyne, 2015).

Several recent studies have investigated the use of mindfulness in the treatment of PTSD and have found positive outcomes (Boden et al., 2012; Hankey, 2007; Kimbrough, Magyari, Langenberg, Chesney, & Berman, 2010; Niles et al., 2012; Simpson et al., 2007; Thompson & Waltz, 2010; Woidneck, Morrison, & Twohig, 2014). One of these was an uncontrolled pilot study that analyzed the effects of mindfulness training through Mindfulness-based stress reduction (MBSR) on depression and PTSD in childhood sexual abuse survivors. In this study, it was found that improvements in mindfulness (as measured by the MAAS) were related to significant reductions in PTSD and depressive symptoms (Kimbrough et al., 2010). Because mindfulness promotes present-focused awareness, it likely operates through reducing the focus on and the impact of negative evaluations of past experiences or future worries, moving individuals into the "here and now" and out of unhelpful rumination (e.g., unwarranted guilt and self-blame), as well as its associated dysphoria (Luoma & Villatte, 2012).

Less research has been conducted to evaluate the hypothesized relationship between *cognitive defusion* and change in outcomes. Briefly, the function of a thought refers to how a particular thought operates in an individual's life (see Hayes, Strosahl, & Wilson, 2012). For instance, the thought "I'm a failure," held as personally valid, can function to prevent an individual from engaging in certain activities (e.g., refusal to participate in projects or social events). The thought

itself seems to be causing the problem; it is functioning to keep the patient isolated. An ACT-oriented therapist would work with the patient to change the function of the thought. This would be done by teaching the patient to observe that a
thought occurred, and to notice that, although the thought was experienced, the
patient does not need to react to it or allow it to influence behavior. From this
perspective, there is no need to change the thought. It can simply be witnessed as
part of the ongoing process of thinking. The thought is allowed to "pass" through
the mind, just as other thoughts do. Indeed, from the ACT perspective, thoughts
are viewed as highly associated with behaviors and feelings, but they need not
cause either.

In one recent example, ACT was compared with pharmacotherapy in patients diagnosed with psychotic disorders (Gaudiano, Herbert, & Hayes, 2010). The results of
the study revealed that the reduced believability of psychotic thoughts (i.e., defusion)
and reduction of experiential avoidance (rather than frequency of hallucinations) mediated the reduction of hallucination-related distress. This finding underlines ACT's
emphasis on producing a meaningful and functional change in the relationship patients have with their symptoms, rather than on the symptoms themselves. Another
study examined the efficacy of cognitive defusion training on depression, distress, and
cognitive flexibility (Hinton & Gaynor, 2008). The results of this study suggest that,
compared with the wait-list control group, the participants in the cognitive defusion
training group demonstrated significant improvements in depression (as evidenced by
the Beck Depression Inventory), distress, cognitive flexibility, and self-esteem. These
effects were maintained after a 1-month follow-up. Given the fact that similar types of
negative affect can co-occur with PTSD, it is not unreasonable to suppose that these
mechanisms can also be applied to PTSD.

The concept of *self-as-context* (i.e., developing a sense of self that is broader than
thoughts and experiences, rather a sense of a self that is an observer of them [Levin,
Hildebrandt, Lillis, & Hayes, 2012]) has not received much empirical attention as
an independent concept. Nonetheless, it is theorized to be an important component
of ACT because it teaches patients about the importance of nonattachment (Hayes
et al., 2006), which has been shown to be involved in distress regulation (Coffey &
Hartman, 2008). One randomized controlled trial evaluated self-as-context as an important component of ACT with Vietnam veterans diagnosed with PTSD (Williams,
2006). This study compared two groups: ACT with self-as-context and ACT with
the self-as-context component removed. It was found that, although both groups
improved on symptoms of PTSD, the ACT group that received self-as-context in the
treatment package faired significantly better than the group that did not receive this
component (Williams, 2006).

The remaining two components of ACT include *values* and *committed action*, where the concept of values refers to personally selected life directions (e.g., belonging, love, compassion) across the various domains (e.g., relationships, career, personal growth), whereas the concept of committed action refers to the development of behaviors that are in line with those selected directions (Hayes et al., 2006). Another key goal of ACT, then, is to promote values-driven actions to improve the patient's quality of life as defined by the patient. This work is designed to promote recovery and reengagement in the patient's life. Indeed, the previous core concepts, such as acceptance and mindfulness, serve to assist patients in taking values-based actions (Hayes et al., 2006). For example, a patient who is suffering from PTSD might engage in experiential avoidance (e.g., he might avoid family functions or going to public places) to escape from painful experiences, such as anxiety. Increasing acceptance and mindfulness would allow the patient to relate to thoughts, sensations, and emotions differently, freeing the patient from being controlled by the perceived "dangerousness" that these thoughts seem to have. This can function to reduce experiential avoidance, allowing the patient to begin engaging in values-based actions, such as connecting with loved ones or engaging in social activities. In PTSD, changing one's relationship to the memory of the event through acceptance and mindfulness may help the individual to be aware of the process more fully—observing a memory arose, but choosing to engage in values-based actions regardless of that experience.

The concepts of values and values-based actions have been studied using the Valued Living Questionnaire (Wilson, Sandoz, & Kitchens, 2010), the Chronic Pain Values Inventory (McCracken & Yang, 2006), and, more recently, the Valuing Questionnaire (Davies & Smout, 2011). A recent study found that an ACT-based intervention with a values core concept increased pain tolerance significantly in participants compared with an ACT-based intervention without the values core concept (Branstetter-Rost, Cushing, & Douleh, 2009). In this study, healthy participants received an acceptance-only training, acceptance-plus-values training, or no training (control group). After the training, participants were asked to submerge their hands into a cold pressor for up to 10 minutes to induce an acute state of pain. Although all three groups reported experiencing the pain sensation at approximately the same time after the immersion, the acceptance-plus-values group demonstrated significantly greater pain tolerance than the other two groups. These results suggest that personal values can affect tolerance of difficult sensations, such as physical pain. Another study also found significant reductions in depression, disability, and pain-related anxiety from pretreatment to posttreatment and 3-months of follow-up in acceptance and values-based action groups (Vowles & McCracken, 2008). Finally, the use of ACT in patients diagnosed with depression has been associated with improvement on the World Health Organization quality-of-life measure (Walser, Karlin, et al., 2013; Folke, Parling, & Melin, 2012), suggesting the work done in ACT impacts the patient's experience of improved life quality, which is in agreement with making values-driven life choices.

THE ROLE OF LANGUAGE IN PTSD

ACT is based on a behavioral understanding of language known as relational frame theory (a behavioral analysis of language), which lays out the critical role that language plays in human suffering (Hayes, Barnes-Holmes, & Roche, 2001). Relational frame theory postulates that language allows human beings to form cognitive and semantic relations (i.e., relational frames) between different objects and events, and that these relations are transferable (i.e., can be related) to other situations and events (for further explanation see Hayes et al. [2001, 2012] and Hayes and Hayes [1992]). In other words, humans need not have direct experience with an object or situation, but rather can derive relationships based on prior learning, bringing any relationship to bear in the current context. For instance, the word *apple* is enough to elicit the image of an apple, as well as its taste, smell, and texture. If you learn that the word *apple* is the same as the word *pomme*, you now know the taste, smell, and texture of a *pomme*, although you may have never had direct training between a physical apple and the word *pomme*. This kind of derived relational responding becomes a behavior itself; and, soon enough, through learning, verbal humans can derive verbal relationships in infinite ways. The link between this kind of verbal relating and PTSD can be made clear with a simple example. If a woman who was raped by a man wearing a red shirt, she could conclude that all people who wear red shirts are dangerous and, indeed, she may come to react to red shirts as if they, themselves, are dangerous. These verbal relationships may come to dominate her thoughts in such a way that they function to promote avoidance (e.g., she cannot be anywhere near people who wear red shirts).

In general, the ability to derive verbal relationships has many positive qualities. It allows us to understand the modern world more fully, improves communication with others, and promotes better survival strategies. This process has contributed to growth in knowledge and greater control as it is applied to much of the world around us. Unfortunately, this ability has a cost. As growth in knowledge has instantiated our ability to control the external world, it has led us falsely to believe we can apply the same rules of control to the internal world. However, when control is applied excessively and inappropriately to inner experiences, it can create problems. Patients with

PTSD might expect to be able to apply the control techniques used in the external environment to their emotions about the trauma. For example, if one is not satisfied with the color of paint on his walls, he can repaint the walls to a preferable color. However, if that individual is struggling with anxiety, the same technique cannot be applied to "fix it." In fact, the very control used to suppress an emotion or forget a specific memory can strengthen the memory that one wishes to forget by causing it to be recalled more frequently. Moreover, if one absorbs the conventional ideas that certain states are better than others (e.g., it is better to be happy than sad), this can lead to distress from finding oneself in the less preferred state (Hayes & Smith, 2005). The distress in this case is not necessarily the result of one's actual experience of the state, but rather because of one's expectation. Furthermore, verbal messages suggesting one should be in control of his or her emotions can reinforce these inflexible rules further.

EVIDENCE FOR ACT FOR PTSD

Although ACT was developed during the 1980s, it has generated considerable public and professional interest more recently and has been recognized as an evidence-based psychotherapeutic approach (American Psychiatric Association, 2013; Substance Abuse and Mental Health Services Administration, 2013). Earlier studies have suggested that ACT may be as effective as CT for patients diagnosed with depressive disorders (Zettle & Hayes, 1986; Zettle & Rains, 1989). More recent evidence of ACT's efficacy has been established for a number of mental and physical health conditions, including depression (Cuijpers, Van Straten, Andersson, & Van Oppen, 2008; Forman et al., 2007; Karlin et al., 2013; Petersen & Zettle, 2009; Wetherell et al., 2011), generalized anxiety disorder (Roemer & Orsillo, 2007, 2012; Wetherell et al., 2011), substance abuse (Hayes et al., 2004), chronic pain (Gutiérrez, Luciano, Rodríguez, & Fink, 2004; Wetherell et al., 2011), psychosis (Gaudiano & Herbert, 2006), obsessive compulsive disorder (Twohig et al., 2010), social anxiety (Block & Wulfert, 2000), and weight control (Forman et al., 2013), and other research is promising for PTSD (Orsillo & Batten, 2005; Twohig, 2009; Walser, Sears, et al., 2013), but further evaluation is needed.

A recent randomized controlled study with veterans who were previously deployed to Iraq or Afghanistan (Operations Enduring Freedom [OEF], Operation Iraqi Freedom [OIF], and Operation New Dawn [OND]) compared the effects of a 2-hour ACT workshop with a wait-list control for assistance with reintegration (Blevins, Roca, & Spencer, 2011). Veterans who participated in the ACT workshop showed significant reductions in depression and greater relationship satisfaction.

Three uncontrolled pilot studies have also suggested that ACT may be an effective treatment for those suffering from PTSD (Sears, Mazina, Wagner & Walser, 2012; Walser, Sears, et al., 2013). Walser, Sears, et al. (2013) found reductions in PTSD symptoms experienced by veterans in pilot investigations of ACT in group ($n = 6$ [Walser, Sears, et al., 2013]) and individual therapy ($n = 9$ [Sears et al., 2012]). Each of the two pilot studies followed a structured protocol that lasted 10 to 14 sessions, delivered once per week. Four of six participants in the group study and eight of nine participants in the individual study reported reductions in PTSD symptoms from pre- to postintervention ($d = 0.77$ and $d = 0.71$, respectively) as measured by the Posttraumatic Checklist (Weathers, Litz, Herman, Huska, & Keane, 1993). A third pilot study ($n = 8$), focused on protocol development for the treatment of comorbid substance use and PTSD (Hermann et al., 2012), also found reductions in PTSD symptoms (five of seven treatment completers) as measured by the Posttraumatic Checklist from pre- to postintervention ($d = 0.87$). Although the findings in these studies generally show reductions in PTSD symptoms, they have a number of limitations, most notably small sample size and lack of control comparisons. A recent, large randomized controlled trial ($n = 160$) of ACT for a transdiagnostic group of OEF/OIF/OND veterans examined its impact on the subgroup with PTSD ($n = 131$). In that study, ACT did not outperform a supportive psychotherapeutic approach and was associated with a moderate effect size ($d = 0.68$ [Lang et al., 2015]), which is similar to other studies of ACT for PTSD, but on the low end of observed effect sizes for empirically supported PTSD interventions (Bradley, Greene, Russ, Dutra, & Westen, 2005). Thus, more studies need to be conducted and possible protocol refinement may need to take place before it can be used as a first-line approach to treat PTSD.

ACT IN PRACTICE

Introducing ACT

To cope with painful thoughts and experiences after a traumatic event, many patients try to avoid these feelings. They may engage in various avoidance behaviors, including behaving impulsively, withdrawing from regular activities, avoiding social or romantic relationships, or engaging in substance abuse. These behaviors are reinforced negatively by producing short-term relief but creating long-term suffering. For example, OIF/OEF/OND veterans may drive erratically after returning home to avoid "roadside bombs," a manager of a bank may stop going to work after a "takeover" robbery, whereas a survivor of sexual assault might stop having intercourse with her partner to avoid painful memories. Most of the time, however, these strategies pave the way to additional feelings of hopelessness and anxiety, often leading these individuals to engage in more avoidance behaviors. Hence, the short-term escape creates long-term suffering.

In addition, these patterns are often maintained through verbal relationships, which can come to dominate experience (e.g., what the "mind" says is more important than what experience says). That is, a person engaging in avoidance behaviors may have learned these kinds of internal events (feeling anxious while driving, having thoughts about dying, or experiencing fears of intimacy) are negative and problematic and, indeed, suggest that something is "wrong" and "needs to fixed." This logical approach (e.g., find the problem and solve the problem) to negatively evaluated experiences takes the person out of the relationship of seeing these experiences for what they are (anxiety while driving, having thoughts, and so on) and places them into a relationship of being the things experienced (e.g., I am anxiety, I am dying). Thus, thoughts and feelings about the trauma (and related internal experiences) become problems that "need to be solved." The solution in which most individuals engage involves attempting to take *control* of the problem (i.e., efforts are made to eliminate or reduce trauma-related thoughts and feelings). In most cases, however, this worsens the problem. In addition to feeling sad and hopeless when efforts to control fail, individuals may begin to feel ashamed or feel sad and hopeless about feeling sad and hopeless. Moreover, the very control strategies themselves are potentially problematic (e.g., substance use).

To target these problematic patterns in therapy, ACT often starts with a process called "creative hopelessness"—a mechanism designed to undermine the dominance of control. This process begins by surveying all the strategies (both positive and negative) patients have used in the past to reduce their distress about the trauma. Examples of negative strategies were just discussed; examples of positive strategies include coping skills, relaxation exercises, support groups, bibliotherapy, and psychotherapy. Therapist and patient gather all the implemented strategies and determine their usefulness in terms of short- and long-term effects (Walser & Hayes, 2006; Walser & Westrup, 2007).

During the process of creative hopelessness, most patients find the strategies they have implemented in the past have only worked short term and have not been helpful in the long term (Walser & Westrup, 2007). At this point, the patient and therapist explore the utility of control as it is it applies to internal experience. This is not only based solely on a verbal understanding of how well the strategies have worked, but also it is based on an experiential understanding. Patients are asked to notice how successful, in their own experience, these strategies have been at eliminating the difficult memories, thoughts, and feelings. Indeed, patients often recognize during this part of the therapy that experiential avoidance, more often than not, leads to additional suffering (e.g., being away from loved ones, not working, remaining intoxicated). When efforts at excessive and misapplied control of thoughts and feelings are recognized as part of the problem, the rest of the core components of ACT are introduced.

Acceptance

Willingness or acceptance is offered as an alternative to control of internal events. As noted, after a painful or traumatic experience many people attempt to control their emotions and thought content (i.e., their internal state). Although learning to control the external environment can prove to be adaptive and useful, it is not helpful universally when dealing with an internal struggle (Walser & Westrup, 2007). In fact, avoidance of one's painful thoughts and feelings, as well as avoidance of actions that can lead to such thoughts and feelings are recognized as problematic across multiple modalities of psychotherapy, including cognitive–behavioral therapy, dialectical behavior therapy, and couples therapy (Hayes et al., 1996).

ACT presents the notion that avoidance, paradoxically, creates an increased awareness of the traumatic experience. Avoidance, in all its forms and all its effects, is explored with the patient—for instance, the paradox of how trying not to think of a memory actually brings the memory to mind or how trying not to have anxiety can lead to the experience of having fear of one's own anxiety. A common exercise in ACT is to illustrate this process using the Anxiety Detection Machine Exercise (Hayes, Strosahl, & Wilson, 2012). The therapist asks the patient to imagine being connected to a perfect anxiety detection machine and, while connected, to remain perfectly calm. As a point of motivation to remain calm, the therapist notes that if the patient experiences any anxiety, it will lead to negative consequence (e.g., the patient will be thrown into a shark tank). The goal of this exercise is to demonstrate that struggling to control and avoid experiencing a painful emotion, such as anxiety, often results in the opposite (see Hayes and Smith [2005] or Walser and Westrup [2007] for a full description of the exercise). In real life, the shark tank represents something rather important, such as self-worth (e.g., if I get anxious, I am broken, bad, incompetent). The alternative to avoidance and control is acceptance, or a willingness to experience both positively and negatively evaluated thoughts and feelings.

Acceptance of internal experience is designed to increase psychological flexibility by reducing the struggle present in trying *not* to experience certain internal or private events. Patients are supported in freeing themselves from the suffering created by this struggle. Throughout the course of the therapy, patients are invited to practice acceptance by remaining open to and by observing thoughts and emotions as they occur. In addition, acceptance is couched as a stance taken; it is an active and open process rather than one of resignation or tolerance. A number of different exercises are applied during the session to help establish acceptance as an alternative to control.

On occasion, patients can misinterpret acceptance, believing that it means that what they endured (e.g., sexual assault) is acceptable or they need to somehow learn to be OK with what happened. In fact, this is not the case, because acceptance does not refer to condoning or "getting over" the painful event; rather, it refers to an openness to experiencing the internal events that have arisen from the trauma. It is very important to clarify this distinction early in therapy and throughout treatment as needed. Individuals who no longer need to try and control their PTSD symptoms often experience the freedom to engage in values-driven actions (Hayes et al., 2006; Walser & Westrup, 2007).

Present Moment

Being present in the here and now, or mindfulness, assists in building acceptance further. When one is focusing, without judgment, on the present moment, one is free from dwelling on the past or worrying about the future. After a traumatic event, many patients become "stuck" in the past by replaying the traumatic experience (e.g., re-membering the loss of a life) or becoming overwhelmed with worry about the future, (e.g., wondering if these symptoms will persist). As a result, the "if-only" and "what-if" scenarios are played frequently, over and over again. This kind of activity can result in increased suffering because the struggling becomes about what was or what might be. This lack of awareness of the moment is part of the suffering (Walser & Westrup, 2007). Being aware of the moment can be the antidote to being overly focused on the past or future. Practicing awareness teaches patients to observe their experiences in the here and now. Thoughts, sensations, emotions, and urges can be all be experienced without any need to make them different. All experience is en-countered as an ongoing process, rather than an outcome.

Mindfulness, as part of present-moment awareness and defusion work, is consid-ered an essential process of ACT. Patients are typically asked to practice mindful-ness on a routine basis. Many kinds of mindfulness can be used, including mindful breathing and body scans, mindful working, or simply observing the ongoing flow of experience. Other mindfulness exercises include mindful eating, mindful walk-ing, mindful tea drinking, and mindful listening to music (Hayes & Smith, 2005).

Therapists should feel free to use different types of media for awareness practice. However, they should also review any material recommended to the patient to be sure it is ACT consistent. Some mindfulness exercises are about becoming relaxed, which is not necessarily the goal in ACT. Mindfulness in ACT is about becoming aware. Many therapists using ACT start each session with some form of mindfulness exercise, many of which are designed to assist patients in contacting all five sensory experiences (i.e., sight, sound, touch, taste, smell) to connect more fully to what is present. Although not necessary for recovery, a potential and welcomed by-product of mindfulness is the reduction in distress, often prominent in those suffering from PTSD (Jain et al., 2007).

Cognitive Defusion

Cognitive defusion is the core process designed to support patients in recognizing they tend to "look through" thoughts rather than "look at" them. Patients fuse with the content of their mind, believing they are their thoughts or their thoughts reflect reality. The work done during this process involves helping patients to see thinking as an ongoing process, assisting them in "defusing" from their thoughts. Patients are encouraged to change their relationship to their thoughts through engaging in a number of exercises, (e.g., words are noticed as sounds and sequences of sounds, words are repeated until they no longer make sense, and the programming of the mind is observed). The key goal is to unlink the connection between thinker and thought. Patients observe, label, and experience thinking for what it is, thereby changing their relationship to cognition (Hayes & Smith, 2005). For instance, rather than having a PTSD patient define himself by the thought "I am broken," the therapist assists the patient in noticing the experience and process of having this thought—for instance, "In this moment I am having the thought that I am broken among other thoughts that pass through my mind." These kinds of exercises are meant to reduce attachment to any particular thought, allowing patients to experience freedom from intrusive or problematic thoughts. Patients are then able to engage in behaviors consistent with their values and thus decrease the impact of experiential avoidance (Hayes et al., 2006; Luoma et al., 2007; Walser & Westrup, 2007).

Self-as-Context

Self-as-context (rather than content) is the core process that assists patients in recognizing a sense of self that is larger than thoughts, feelings, sensations, memories, labels, and roles (e.g., husband/wife, parent, friend). During the self-as-context work, the patient and therapist explore awareness itself. The place where these experiences are held is contacted. The patient is the context for the content. The patient is assisted in observing himself as one who is experiencing these events. He is supported in taking the perspective of being aware of experience. For instance, traumatic events can elicit many internal experiences such as thoughts about being broken, being a failure, and being a victim, or they can elicit feelings of anxiety or fear. All these events can affect how the patient behaves if this content is held as the person himself. These thoughts and emotions do not, however, make the totality of the person, and the patient is taught to look at these self- or socially attributed thoughts and emotions, and instead to notice these experiences, as well as the ongoing flow of experience (whatever thoughts, feelings, memories, and sensations they may be), as an active observer.

Helping the patient to take the observer perspective is accomplished through a number of exercises and metaphors. For instance, the chessboard metaphor suggests the pieces on the board are the thoughts, feelings, roles, and sensations, and the chessboard is the patient. The board is unchanged by the arrangement of the pieces just as the fundamental aspect of the observer perspective is unchanged by the situation or momentary experience (e.g., trauma memory) (Hayes et al., 2012; Walser & Westrup, 2007).

Self-as-context is thought to be fundamental in treating PTSD. Many people who experience trauma get "stuck" in memories and thoughts about the trauma while losing contact with the multitude of experiences that make up their lives. Self-as-context helps patients to reconnect to a sense of being—awareness itself—that is beyond individual memories and identities. It is a stable and felt sense, not a logically experienced place. Recognizing self-as-context can be incredibly freeing for patients; they come to see themselves as more than any event or events, and this lends itself well to creating flexible responding because the patient is not locked into any particular identity (e.g., victim or survivor).

Values and Commitment to Action

Values refer to the patient's chosen life directions that give purpose and meaning, including such things as honor, love, loyalty, belonging, compassion, helping others, and courage. Values are distinguished from committed actions (i.e., behavioral goals) in that goals are finite behaviors that can be attained and have an outcome or completion point. Values, however, are meaningful directions patients wish to instantiate in their life. Values are explored, defined, and engaged in by making and keeping commitments to engage in behaviors (i.e., actions) consistent with personal values. Patients are encouraged to live a values-based life, rather than a life shaped by symptom elimination.

People who have experienced trauma may lose contact with their values for a number of reasons. First, they may believe they need to "fix what is broken" as a result of the trauma (i.e., their thoughts and feelings) before they can move forward with values-based behavior. Values are abandoned in the service of symptom relief. Second, during trauma, people might experience an event that is in direct conflict with their personal values. For example, if a veteran killed another human being in combat, this event might be directly counter to his or her values of compassion and love of humanity. This conflict might lead to feelings of guilt and shame—markers of problematic trauma experiences. Patients might then evaluate themselves as "evil" and not deserving of happiness or a rich life. They, consequently, might work to eliminate the thoughts and feelings associated with this experience and begin to withdraw from others or even consider suicide. Working with veterans to reconnect with their value of love of humanity may assist them on the path to recovery.

While participating in ACT, patients are reconnected to their values in a number of different ways. They can participate in values card-sorts, engage in exercises designed to explore values, or complete questionnaires that assess values. When the patient identifies her values (e.g., being loving) and the domains in which she would like to apply these values (e.g., mother–daughter relationship), she is assisted in identifying specific actions and/or goals she can undertake or pursue during the service of those values (e.g., attending her daughter's dance recital [Hayes & Smith, 2005; Walser & Westrup, 2007]). For patients with a trauma history, identifying values and living according to them can, potentially, be a powerful and healing experience (Walser & Westrup, 2007).

Summary

ACT is an exciting new alternative to existing therapies, many of which, although effective, do not meet all the needs of patients with PTSD. ACT provides an alternative to the narrow focus on symptom elimination. Through its six core processes, ACT explores acceptance and an openness to internal events as an alternative to experiential avoidance. Willingness to experience in turn frees the patient to act on personally chosen values. The ultimate goal is to live mindfully while remaining actively engaged in creating a vital life. Initial research is promising, but further investigation of this intervention for this particular population is warranted. That said, ACT can be used as a preintervention, postintervention, or adjunct to trauma-based therapies and is quite complementary to prolonged exposure and other exposure-based interventions. ACT can also be used to address comorbidities to PTSD and other life problems not captured in the diagnostic system, but relevant to survivors of trauma. For instance, ACT is currently being disseminated nationally throughout the Department of Veterans Affairs to treat depression in veterans. Initial evaluation of clinicians' training in ACT resulted in significant improvements in patients' depression and quality of life, as well as the patient–therapist alliance and therapist self-efficacy (Walser, Karlin, et al., 2013). It has been hypothesized that using ACT for PTSD would lead to similar results. At this point, there are only small open trials and case studies to support this conjecture (Hermann et al., 2012; Orsillo & Batten, 2005; Petersen & Zettle, 2009; Twohig, 2009).

OBTAINING TRAINING IN ACT

It is recommended one receive proper training and supervision before implementing ACT. Although learning a new modality of treatment can sometimes be intimidating, evidence suggests that obtaining training in ACT is beneficial both to the patient and to the therapist, (Walser, Karlin, et al., 2013). Because ACT uses many skills found in other therapies, and because it is manualized (e.g., Harris, 2011; Hayes & Smith, 2005; Hayes et al., 2012; Roemer & Orsillo, 2010; Walser & Westrup, 2007), it is taught readily and can be used for a variety of different diagnoses. Training in ACT is available worldwide. In addition, the Association for Contextual Behavioral Science website provides an array of training materials and worksheets, as do many of the previously mentioned manuals. In addition, a vast variety of metaphors for ACT can be found in the *Big Book of ACT Metaphors* (Stoddard & Afari, 2014). Therapists are invited to engage in the same processes in ACT they are learning and exploring with their patients—living a life that is open, aware, and active.

KEY POINTS

- ACT is a behavioral intervention that focuses on the pursuit of valued goals despite uncomfortable internal experiences that may arise.
- ACT is comprised of six primary change processes: (1) acceptance, (2) cognitive defusion (recognition of the limited ability of language to capture true experience), (3) clearly defined values, (4) a broadly developed sense of self, (5) present-moment awareness, and (6) commitment to action.
- A major difference between ACT and cognitive behavioral therapies is its focus on the process rather than the content of thoughts.

• The current evidence base supports the use of ACT for depression and for management of some physical health conditions.

• Experimental work suggests ACT may address pathological processes that maintain PTSD.

• Efficacy of ACT for PTSD has yet to be established; additional research is recommended to address limitations in the current evidence base.

REFERENCES

American Psychological Association (APA), Division 12. (2013). *Psychological Treatments.* Retrieved from http://www.div12.org/PsychologicalTreatments/treatments.html

American Psychiatric Association (2000). *Diagnostic and statistical manual of mental disorders* (DSM-4-TR) (4th ed.) Washington, D.C.: American Psychiatric Association.

Arch, J. J., Eifert, G. H., Davies, C., Vilardaga, J. P., Rose, R. D., & Craske, M. G. (2012). Randomized clinical trial of cognitive behavioral therapy (CBT) versus acceptance and commitment therapy (ACT) for mixed anxiety disorders. *Journal of Consulting And Clinical Psychology*, **80**(5), 750–765. doi:10.1037/a0028310

Association for Contextual Behavioral Science. *Resources.* Retrieved from http://contextualscience.org/resources.

Baer, R. A, Smith, G. T., Hopkins, J., Krietemeyer, J., & Toney, L. (2006). Using self-report assessment methods to explore facets of mindfulness. *Assessment*, **13**(1), 27–45. doi:10.1177/1073191105283504

Blevins, D., Roca, J. V., & Spencer, T. (2011). Life Guard: Evaluation of an ACT-based workshop to facilitate reintegration of OIF/OEF veterans. *Professional Psychology: Research and Practice*, **42**(1), 32–39. doi:10.1037/a0022321

Block, J. A., & Wulfert, E. (2000). Acceptance or change: Treating socially anxious college students with ACT or CBGT. *The Behavior Analyst Today*, **1**(2), 1–55.

Boden, M. T., Bernstein, A., Walser, R. D., Bui, L., Alvarez, J., & Bonn-Miller, M. O. (2012). Changes in facets of mindfulness and posttraumatic stress disorder treatment outcome. *Psychiatry Research*, **200**(2-3), 609–613.

Bond, F. W., Hayes, S. C., Baer, R. A, Carpenter, K. M., Guenole, N., Orcutt, H. K., . . . Zettle, R. (2011). Preliminary psychometric properties of the Acceptance and Action Questionnaire-II: a revised measure of psychological inflexibility and experiential avoidance. *Behavior Therapy*, **42**(4), 676–688. doi:10.1016/j.beth.2011.03.007

Braams, B. R., Blechert, J., Boden, M. T., & Gross, J. J. (2012). The effects of acceptance and suppression on anticipation and receipt of painful stimulation. *Journal of Behavior Therapy and Experimental Psychiatry*, **43**(4), 1014–1018. doi:10.1016/j.jbtep.2012.04.001

Bradley, R., Greene, J., Russ, E., Dutra, L., & Westen, D. (2005). Reviews and overviews: A multidimensional meta-analysis of psychotherapy for PTSD. *American Journal of Psychiatry*, **162**(February), 214–227.

Branstetter-Rost, A., Cushing, C., & Douleh, T. (2009). Personal values and pain tolerance: does a values intervention add to acceptance? *The journal of pain: Official Journal of the American Pain Society*, **10**(8), 887–892. doi:10.1016/j.jpain.2009.01.001

Brown, K. W., & Ryan, R. M. (2003). The benefits of being present: Mindfulness and its role in psychological well-being. *Journal of Personality and Social Psychology*, **84**(4), 822–848. doi:10.1037/0022-3514.84.4.822

Brown, K. W., Ryan, R. M., & Creswell, J. D. (2007). Mindfulness: Theoretical foundations and evidence for its salutary effects. *Psychological Inquiry*, **18**(4), 211–237. doi:10.1080/10478400701598298

Burrows, C. J. (2013). Acceptance and commitment therapy with survivors of adult sexual assault: A case study. *Clinical Case Studies*, **12**(3), 246–259.

Call, D., Pitcock, J., & Pyne, J. (2015). Longitudinal Evaluation of the Relationship Between Mindfulness, General Distress, Anxiety, and PTSD in a Recently Deployed National Guard Sample. *Mindfulness*, **6**(6), 1303–1312.

Campbell-Sills, L., Barlow, D. H., Brown, T. A., & Hofmann, S. G. (2006). Effects of emotional suppression and acceptance in individuals with anxiety and mood disorders. *Behaviour Research and Therapy*, **44**, 1251–1263.

Coffey, K. A., & Hartman, M. (2008). Mechanisms of action in the inverse relationship between mindfulness and psychological distress. *Complementary Health Practice Review*, **13**(2), 79–91.

Cuijpers, P., Van Straten, A., Andersson, G., & Van Oppen, P. (2008). Psychotherapy for depression in adults: a meta-analysis of comparative outcome studies. *Journal of Consulting and Clinical Psychology*, **76**(6), 909–922. doi:10.1037/a0013075

Davies, M., & Smout, M. (2011). *Development of the Valuing Questionnaire*. Association for Contextual Behavioral Science World Conference IX, Parma, Italy.

Dobson, K. S., Hollon, S. D., Dimidjian, S., Schmaling, K. B., Kohlenberg, R. J., Gallop, R., . . . Jacobson, N. S. (2008). Randomized trial of behavioral activation, cognitive therapy, and antidepressant medication in the prevention of relapse and recurrence in major depression. *Journal of Consulting and Clinical Psychology*, **76**, 468–477. doi:10.1037/0022-006X.76.3.468

Fletcher, L., & Hayes, S. C. (2005). Relational frame theory, acceptance and commitment therapy, and a functional analytic definition of mindfulness. *Journal of Rational-Emotive & Cognitive-Behavior Therapy*, **23**(4), 315–336. doi:10.1007/s10942-005-0017-7

Folke, F., Parling, T., & Melin, L. (2012). Acceptance and commitment therapy for depression: A preliminary randomized clinical trial for unemployed on long-term sick leave. *Cognitive and Behavioral Practice*, **19**(4), 583–594. doi:10.1016/j.cbpra.2012.01.002

Forman, E. M., Butryn, M. L., Juarascio, A. S., Bradley, L. E., Lowe, M. R., Herbert, J. D., & Shaw, J. A. (2013). The mind your health project: A randomized controlled trial of an innovative behavioral treatment for obesity. *Obesity*, **21**, 1119–1126. doi:10.1002/oby.20169

Forman, E. M., Herbert, J. D., Moitra, E., Yeomans, P. D., & Geller, P. A. (2007). A randomized controlled effectiveness trial of acceptance and commitment therapy and cognitive therapy for anxiety and depression. *Behavior Modification*, **31**(6), 772–799. doi:10.1177/0145445507302202

Forsyth, J. P., Parker, J., & Finlay, C. G. (2003). Anxiety sensitivity, controllability, and experiential avoidance and their relation to drug of choice and addiction severity in a residential sample of substance abusing veterans. *Addictive Behaviors*, **28**, 851–870.

Gaudiano, B. A., & Herbert, J. D. (2006). Believability of hallucinations as a potential mediator of their frequency and associated distress in psychotic inpatients. *Behavioural and Cognitive Psychotherapy*, **34**, 497–502.

Gaudiano, B. A., Herbert, J. D., & Hayes, S. C. (2010). Is it the symptom or the relation to it? Investigating potential mediators of change in Acceptance and Commitment Therapy for psychosis. *Behavior Therapy*, **41**(4), 543–554. doi:10.1016/j.beth.2010.03.001

Gifford, E. V, Kohlenberg, B. S., Hayes, S. C., Pierson, H. M., Piasecki, M. P., Antonuccio, D. O., & Palm, K. M. (2011). Does acceptance and relationship focused behavior therapy contribute to bupropion outcomes? A randomized controlled trial of functional analytic psychotherapy and acceptance and commitment therapy for smoking cessation. *Behavior Therapy*, **42**(4), 700–715. doi:10.1016/j.beth.2011.03.002

Gutiérrez, O., Luciano, C., Rodríguez, M., & Fink, B. C. (2004). Comparison between an acceptance-based and a cognitive-control-based protocol for coping with pain. *Behavior therapy*, **35**(4), 767–783.

Hankey, A. (2007). CAM and Post-Traumatic Stress Disorder. *Evidence-based complementary and alternative medicine: eCAM*, **4**(1), 131–132. doi:10.1093/ecam/nel041

Hayes, S. C. (2004). Acceptance and Commitment Therapy, Relational Frame Theory, and the third wave of behavioral and cognitive therapies the waves of behavior therapy. *Behavior Therapy*, **35**, 639–665.

Hayes, S. C. (2008). Climbing our hills: A beginning conversation on the comparison of Acceptance and Commitment Therapy and traditional Cognitive Behavioral Therapy. *Clinical Psychology: Science and Practice*, **15**(4), 286–295. doi:10.1111/j.1468-2850.2008.00139.x

Hayes, S. C., Barnes-Holmes, D., & Roche, B. (2001). *Relational frame theory: A post-Skinnerian account of human language and cognition*. New York, NY: Plenum Press.

Hayes, S. C., & Hayes, L. J. (1992). Verbal relations and the evolution of behavior analysis. *American Psychologist*, **47**, 1383–1395.

Hayes, S. C., Luoma, J. B., Bond, F. W., Masuda, A., & Lillis, J. (2006). Acceptance and Commitment Therapy: Model, processes and outcomes. *Behaviour Research and Therapy*, **44**(1), 1–25. doi:10.1016/j.brat.2005.06.006

Hayes, S. C., & Smith, S. (2005). *Get out of your mind and into your life: The new acceptance and commitment therapy*. Oakland, CA US: New Harbinger Publications.

Hayes, S. C., Strosahl, K. D., & Wilson, K. G. (2012). *Acceptance and Commitment Therapy: The process and practice of mindful change (2nd ed.)*. New York, NY US: Guilford Press.

Hayes, S. C., Wilson, K. G., Gifford, E. V, Follette, V. M., & Strosahl, K. (1996). Experiential avoidance and behavioral disorders: A functional dimensional approach to diagnosis and treatment. *Journal of Consulting and Clinical Psychology*, **64**(6), 1152–1168.

Harris, R. (2011). *The happiness trap: How to stop struggling and start living*. Boston, MA: Trumpeter Books.

Hermann, B., Meyer, E., Schnurr, P., Batten, S., Seim, R., Walser, R., Klocek, J., & Gulliver, S.B. (2012). *Acceptance and Commitment Therapy: Mindfulness and values in the treatment of PTSD*. Presentation at the 28th Annual Meeting of the International Society for Traumatic Stress Studies (ISTSS), Los Angeles, California.

Hinton, M. J., & Gaynor, S. T. (2008). Cognitive defusion for psychological distress, dysphoria, and low self-esteem: A randomized technique evaluation trial of vocalizing strategies. *International Journal of Behavioral Consultation and Therapy*, **6**(3), 164–186.

Jacobson, N. S., & Christensen, A. (1998). *Acceptance and change in couple therapy: A therapist's guide to transforming relationships*. New York: Norton & Company.

Jain, S., Shapiro, S. L., Swanick, S., Roesch, S. C., Mills, P. J., Bell, I., & Schwartz, G. E. (2007). A randomized controlled trial of mindfulness meditation versus relaxation training: effects on distress, positive states of mind, rumination, and distraction. *Annals of behavioral medicine*, **33**(1), 11–21.

Karlin, B. E., Walser, R. D., Yesavage, J., Zhang, A., Trockel, M., & Taylor, C. B. (2013). Effectiveness of acceptance and commitment therapy for depression: Comparison among older and younger veterans. *Aging & mental health*, **17**(5), 555–563. doi:10.1080/13607863.2013.789002

Kashdan, T. B., Barrios, V., Forsyth, J. P., & Steger, M. F. (2006). Experiential avoidance as a generalized psychological vulnerability: comparisons with coping and emotion regulation strategies. *Behaviour Research and Therapy*, **44**(9), 1301–1320. doi:10.1016/j.brat.2005.10.003

Kashdan, T. B., Morina, N., & Priebe, S. (2009). Post-traumatic stress disorder, social anxiety disorder, and depression in survivors of the Kosovo War: experiential avoidance as a contributor to distress and quality of life. *Journal of Anxiety Disorders*, **23**(2), 185–196. doi:10.1016/j.janxdis.2008.06.006

Kimbrough, E., Magyari, T., Langenberg, P., Chesney, M., & Berman, B. (2010). Mindfulness Intervention for Child Abuse Survivors. *Journal of Clinical Psychology*, **66**(1), 17–33. doi:10.1002/jclp

Kohlenberg, R. J., & Tsai, M. (1991). *Functional analytic psychotherapy: Creating intense and curative therapeutic relationships*. New York: Plenum Press.

Kumpula, M. J., Orcutt, H. K., Bardeen, J. R., & Varkovitzky, R. L. (2011). Peritraumatic dissociation and experiential avoidance as prospective predictors of posttraumatic stress symptoms. *Journal of Abnormal Psychology*, **120**(3), 617–627. doi:10.1037/a0023927

Levin, M. E., Hildebrandt, M. J., Lillis, J., & Hayes, S. C. (2012). The impact of treatment components suggested by the psychological flexibility model: a meta-analysis of laboratory-based component studies. *Behavior Therapy*, **43**(4), 741–756. doi:10.1016/j.beth.2012.05.003

Levitt, J. T., Brown, T. A., Orsillo, S. M., & Barlow, D. H. (2004). The effects of acceptance versus suppression of emotion on subjective and psychophysiological response to carbon dioxide challenge in patients with panic disorder. *Behavior Therapy,* **35**, 747–766. doi:10.1016/S0005-7894(04)80018-2

Linehan, M. M. (1993). *Cognitive-behavioral treatment of borderline personality disorder.* New York: Guilford Press.

Litvin, E. B., Kovacs, M. A., Hayes, P. L., & Brandon, T. H. (2012). Responding to tobacco craving: experimental test of acceptance versus suppression. *Psychology of Addictive Behaviors: Journal of the Society of Psychologists in Addictive Behaviors,* **26**(4), 830–837. doi:10.1037/a0030351

Luoma, J. B., Hayes, S. C., & Walser, R. D. (2007). *Learning ACT: An acceptance and commitment therapy skills-training manual for therapists.* Oakland, CA US: New Harbinger Publications.

Luoma, J. B., & Villatte, J. L. (2012). Mindfulness in the treatment of suicidal individuals. *Cognitive and behavioral practice,* **19**(2), 265–276. doi:10.1016/j.cbpra.2010.12.003

Ma, S. H., & Teasdale, J. D. (2004). Mindfulness-based cognitive therapy for depression: replication and exploration of differential relapse prevention effects. *Journal of Consulting and Clinical Psychology,* **72**(1), 31–40. doi:10.1037/0022-006X.72.1.31

McCracken, L. M., Gauntlett-Gilbert, J., & Vowles, K. E. (2007). The role of mindfulness in a contextual cognitive-behavioral analysis of chronic pain-related suffering and disability. *Pain,* **131**(1-2), 63–69. doi:10.1016/j.pain.2006.12.013

McCracken, L. M., & Yang, S. (2006). The role of values in a contextual cognitive-behavioral approach to chronic pain. *Pain,* **123**, 137–145.

McCullough, J. P. (2010). CBASP, the third wave and the treatment of chronic depression. *European Psychotherapy,* **9**, 169–190.

Meyer, E. C., Morissette, S. B., Kimbrel, N. A., Kruse, M. I., & Gulliver, S. B. (2013). Acceptance and Action Questionnaire—II scores as a predictor of posttraumatic stress disorder symptoms among war veterans. *Psychological Trauma: Theory, Research, Practice, and Policy.* doi:10.1037/a0030178

Niles, B. L., Klunk-Gillis, J., Ryngala, D. J., Silberbogen, A. K., Paysnick, A., & Wolf, E. J. (2012). Comparing mindfulness and psychoeducation treatments for combat-related PTSD using a telehealth approach. *Psychological Trauma: Theory, Research, Practice, and Policy,* **4**(5), 538–547. doi:10.1037/a0026161

Orsillo, S. M., & Batten, S. V. (2005). Acceptance and commitment therapy in the treatment of posttraumatic stress disorder. *Behavior Modification,* **29**(1), 95–129. doi:10.1177/0145445504270876

Petersen, C. L., & Zettle, R. D. (2009). Treating inpatients with comorbid depression and alcohol use disorders: Comparison of acceptance and commitment therapy versus treatment as usual. *The Psychological Record,* **59**, 521–536.

Roemer, L., & Orsillo, S. M. (2010). *Mindfulness- and acceptance-based behavioral therapies in practice.* New York, NY: Guilford Press.

Roemer, L., & Orsillo, S. M. (2012). An acceptance-based behavioral treatment for generalized anxiety disorder. *Directions in Psychiatry,* **32**(4), 211–224. US: The Hatherleigh Company, Ltd.

Sears, S., & Kraus, S. (2009). I think therefore I om: Cognitive distortions and coping style as mediators for the effects of mindfulness meditation on anxiety, positive and negative affect, and hope. *Journal of Clinical Psychology,* **65**(6), 561–574. doi:10.1002/jclp

Sears, K.C., Mazina, V., Wagner, A., & Walser, R.D. (2012). *Acceptance and Commitment Therapy as an Alternative to Exposure: A Pilot Study in the Treatment of Veterans Diagnosed with PTSD.* Poster presented at the Association for Contextual Behavioral Science Annual World Conference 10, Washington, D.C.

Segal, Z. V.,Williams, J. M. G., & Teasdale, J. D. (2002). *Mindfulness-based cognitive therapy for depression: A new approach to preventing relapse.* New York: Guilford Press.

Simpson, T. L., Kaysen, D., Bowen, S., Chawla, N., Blume, A., Marlatt, G. A., & Larimer, M. (2007). PTSD Symptoms, Substance Use, and Vipassana Meditation among Incarcerated Individuals. **20**(3), 239–249. doi:10.1002/jts

Smout, M. F., Hayes, L., Atkins, P. W. B., Klausen, J., & Duguid, J. E. (2012). The empirically supported status of acceptance and commitment therapy: An update. *Clinical Psychologist*, **16**(3), 97–109. doi:10.1111/j.1742-9552.2012.00051.x

Stoddard, J. A., & Afari, N. (2014). *The big book of ACT metaphors: A clinician's guide to experiential exercises and metaphors in acceptance and commitment therapy.* New Harbinger Publications: Oakland, CA.

Substance Abuse and Mental Health Services Administration (SAMHSA). (2013). *National Registry of Evidence based Programs and Practices (NREPP: Acceptance and Commitment Therapy.* Retrieved from http://nrepp.samhsa.gov/ViewIntervention.aspx?id=191

Thompson, B. L., Luoma, J. B., & LeJeune, J. T. (2013). Using acceptance and commitment therapy to guide exposure-based interventions for posttraumatic stress disorder. *Journal of Contemporary Psychotherapy*, **43**(3), 133–140. doi:10.1007/s10879-013-9233-0

Thompson, B. L., & Waltz, J. (2010). Mindfulness and experiential avoidance as predictors of posttraumatic stress disorder avoidance symptom severity. *Journal of anxiety disorders*, **24**(4), 409–415. doi:10.1016/j.janxdis.2010.02.005

Tull, M. T., Gratz, K. L., Salters, K., & Roemer, L. (2004). The role of experiential avoidance in posttraumatic stress symptoms and symptoms of depression, anxiety, and somatization. *Journal of Nervous and Mental Disease*, **192**(11), 754–761.

Twohig, M. P. (2009). Acceptance and Commitment Therapy for treatment-resistant posttraumatic stress disorder: A case study. *Cognitive and Behavioral Practice*, **16**(3), 243–252. doi:10.1016/j.cbpra.2008.10.002

Twohig, M. P., Hayes, S. C., Plumb, J. C., Pruitt, L. D., Collins, A. B., Hazlett-Stevens, H., & Woidneck, M. R. (2010). A randomized clinical trial of acceptance and commitment therapy vs. progressive relaxation training for obsessive compulsive disorder. *Journal of Consulting and Clinical Psychology*, **78**, 705–716.

Vøllestad, J., Sivertsen, B., & Nielsen, G. H. (2011). Mindfulness-based stress reduction for patients with anxiety disorders: evaluation in a randomized controlled trial. *Behaviour Research and Therapy*, **49**(4), 281–288. doi:10.1016/j.brat.2011.01.007

Vowles, K. E., & McCracken, L. M. (2008). Acceptance and values-based action in chronic pain: a study of treatment effectiveness and process. *Journal of Consulting and Clinical Psychology*, **76**(3), 397–407. doi:10.1037/0022-006X.76.3.397

Walser, R. D., & Hayes, S. C. (2006). Acceptance and Commitment Therapy in the treatment of posttraumatic stress disorder: Theoretical and applied issues. In V. M. Follette & J. I. Ruzek (Eds.), *Cognitive-behavioral therapies for trauma (2nd ed.).* (pp. 146–172). New York, NY US: Guilford Press.

Walser, R. D., Karlin, B. E., Trockel, M., Mazina, B., & Taylor, C. B. (2013). Training in and implementation of Acceptance and Commitment Therapy for depression in the Veterans Health Administration: Therapist and patient outcomes. *Behaviour Research and Therapy*, **51**, 555–563. doi:http://dx.doi.org/10.1016/j.brat.2013.05.009

Walser, R. D., Sears, K. C., Young, K., Wagner, A. & Young, H. (2013) Acceptance and commitment therapy in the treatment of PTSD: Two pilot investigations. Manuscript in preparation. National Center for PTSD, Menlo Park, CA.

Walser, R. D., & Westrup, D. (2007). *Acceptance & commitment therapy for the treatment of posttraumatic stress disorder and trauma-related problems: A practitioner's guide to using mindfulness and acceptance strategies.* Oakland, CA US: New Harbinger Publications.

Weathers, F., Litz, B., Herman, D., Huska, J., & Keane, T. (1993). The PTSD Checklist (PCL): Reliability, Validity, and Diagnostic Utility. Paper presented at the Annual Convention of the International Society for Traumatic Stress Studies, San Antonio, TX.

Wetherell, J. L., Afari, N., Ayers, C. R., Stoddard, J. A, Ruberg, J., Sorrell, J. T., . . . Patterson, T. L. (2011). Acceptance and Commitment Therapy for generalized anxiety disorder in older adults: a preliminary report. *Behavior Therapy*, **42**(1), 127–134. doi:10.1016/j.beth.2010.07.002

Williams, L. M. (2006). Acceptance and commitment therapy: An example of third-wave therapy as a treatment for Australian Vietnam War veterans with posttraumatic stress disorder. Unpublished dissertation, Charles Stuart University, Bathurst, New South Wales.

Wilson, K. G., Sandoz, K., & Kitchens, J. (2010). The Valued Living Questionnaire: Defining and measuring valued action within a behavioral framework. *The Psychological Record*, **60**, 249–272.

Woidneck, M. R., Morrison, K. L., & Twohig, M. P. (2014). Acceptance and commitment therapy for the treatment of posttraumatic stress among adolescents. *Behavior Modification*, **38**(4), 451–476. doi:10.1177/0145445513510527

Zayfert, C., Deviva, J. C., Becker, C. B., Pike, J. L., Gillock, K. L., & Hayes, S. A. (2005). Exposure utilization and completion of cognitive behavioral therapy for PTSD in a "real world" clinical practice. *Journal of Traumatic Stress*, **18**(6), 637–645. doi:10.1002/jts.20072

Zettle, R. D., & Hayes, S. C. (1986). Dysfunctional control by client verbal behavior: The context of reason-giving. *The Analysis of Verbal Behavior*, **4**, 30–38.

Zettle, R. D., & Rains, J. C. (1989). Group cognitive and contextual therapies in treatment of depression. *Journal of clinical psychology*, **45**(3), 436–445.

FOUR

Meditation Techniques for Posttraumatic Stress Disorder

MARINA KHUSID

ALTHOUGH CURRENTLY THERE IS INSUFFICIENT EVIDENCE TO SUPPORT MEDITATION as a first-line treatment for posttraumatic stress disorder (PTSD), the evidence base for meditation used adjunctively in the management of PTSD and related psychiatric comorbidities is expanding rapidly. The 2010 Veterans Administration (VA)/Department of Defense (DoD) clinical practice guideline for the management of PTSD states that mind–body approaches may be considered as adjunctive treatment for hyperarousal symptoms through activation of a relaxation response by addressing some comorbid conditions and facilitating engagement in medical care (The Management of Post-Traumatic Stress Working Group, 2010). Although several reviews (Strauss, Coeytaux, McDuffie, Nagi & Williams, 2011; Kim, Schneider, Kravitz, Mermier & Burge, 2013) support the conclusions reflected in the 2010 VA/DoD clinical practice guideline, others suggest that meditation interventions may be more useful in the management of PTSD than originally speculated. Meditation may help reduce intrusive memories, avoidance, and anger; and may increase self-esteem, pain tolerance, energy and ability to relax, and the ability to cope with stress (Bränström, Kvillemo, Brandberg & Moskowitz, 2010; Strauss, 2012; Kim, Schneider, Kravitz, Mermier & Burge, 2013). Goyal et al. (2014), in their comparative effectiveness review, concluded that mindfulness meditation is beneficial in reducing psychological stress consequences such as depression and pain, and in increasing mental health-related quality of life.

In addition to emerging evidence, meditation is safe, portable, easy to learn, and affordable. Among various mind–body approaches, meditation is one of the most accepted among veterans, and is being widely implemented across the VA and DoD (Libby, Pilver & Desai, 2012; Libby, Reddy, Pilver & Desai, 2012). A 2012 survey of 125 VA-specialized PTSD treatment programs indicated that 88% offered sitting meditation practices or movement meditation practices such as yoga. The self-care quality of meditation is particularly valuable. It allows patients to feel more in control of their symptoms, and empowers them to take charge of their healing process. Finally, because of the self-management nature of meditation, it is very cost-effective and may help reduce long-term personal and societal costs.

Meditation is a form of mental training aimed at cultivating well-being and effective emotion regulation (Lutz, Slagter, Dunne & Davidson, 2008). It has been

---

BOX 4.1

MEDITATION CLASSIFICATION ACCORDING TO POSTURE AND FOCUS

1. Movement meditations (e.g., yoga, Tai Chi)
2. Sitting meditations with different focus
   2A. Focus on breathing
      - Traditional Buddhist mindfulness meditations (e.g., Shambhala, Zen, and Vipassana)
      - Mindfulness-based group interventions (e.g., mindfulness-based stress reduction)
   2B. Focus on specific body sensation or use of special senses
      - Focus on sensations in different body parts (e.g., progressive muscle relaxation, body scan)
      - Focus on energy centers described in various eastern healing traditions (e.g., central channel meditation, chakra meditation, qigong with focus on dantian, and kundalini meditation)
      - Focus on a physical source of emotion (e.g., focusing on a physical space occupied by heart during some forms of compassion meditation)
      - Visual focus on a specific object (e.g., mandala meditation, one-point concentration)
      - Using sound to focus (e.g., Mantram Repetition Program, chanting, and transcendental meditation use sound and the vibration it produces to focus and clear the mind)
   2C. Multiple focus
      - For example, relaxation response training uses breath, mantra, and progressive muscle relaxation to guide focus and physiological relaxation

practiced in different cultures and traditions since antiquity. Each meditative practice is rooted in the spiritual and health beliefs of its unique culture of origin. Although meditation may take different shapes and forms, the common denominator is that each practice represents a form of mental training. A recent quantitative meta-analysis of 10 neuroimaging studies illustrates that different meditative traditions share the same central process underlying this phenomenon of emotion regulation and attention training, and involve activation of the basal ganglia (caudate body), limbic system, and medial prefrontal cortex (Sperduti, Martinelli & Piolino, 2012). The aim of such training is to reduce or eliminate maladaptive thought processes, leading to physical and mental relaxation, stress reduction, psychoemotional stability, and enhanced concentration (Rubia, 2009). The distinctness usually lies in the body position assumed during practice (sitting or movement) and an object of focus (e.g., breath, sensation), as described in Box 4.1.

Three meditation traditions that have the most emerging scientific evidence for PTSD to date are mantram repetition, mindfulness meditation, and compassion meditation. Their practice, mechanisms, and relevant clinical research are summarized in this chapter, and each section concludes with an outline of key therapeutic features and clinical applications. The criteria for inclusion of studies to evaluate the effectiveness of each intervention are summarized in Box 4.2, and the literature search was completed on October 1, 2015. Simple instructions, evidence tables, and the key

---

BOX 4.2
CLINICAL TRIAL INCLUSION CRITERIA

1. *Participants*: Subjects included civilian, active-duty, and veteran adults with documented or reported diagnosis of posttraumatic stress disorder.
2. *Intervention*: Interventions included Mantram Repetition Program, mindfulness meditation, group mindfulness-based interventions, and compassion meditation.
3. *Comparator*: Studies that use an active comparator consistent with the current standard of care were prioritized, but in their absence, studies with a wait-list control were also included.
4. *Outcomes*: Outcomes included change in symptom severity, mental health-related quality of life, use of standard pharmacotherapy, functional status, and mindfulness.
5. *Timing and setting*: Inclusion criteria were not limited by timing or setting.
6. *Study design*: Systematic reviews, meta-analyses, and randomized clinical trials were prioritized. Other designs were considered only in the absence of randomized clinical trials.

benefits these techniques offer in PTSD management are provided with the purpose of guiding providers, and allowing them to custom-tailor treatment to each unique case to achieve the most therapeutic benefit. Patients are encouraged to choose a technique that resonates with them, and that they are most likely to adopt as regular practice and a life-long health behavior change.

MANTRAM REPETITION PROGRAM

Definition

The Mantram Repetition Program (MRP) belongs to a group of mantra meditations. In Sanskrit, *mantra* means "to cross the mind." A practice of using mantra is present in all major spiritual traditions, and it has a purpose of bringing inner peace and clarity. Two other well-known practices in this group are transcendental meditation (TM) and relaxation response training, and both use similar techniques of repeating a word, phrase or sound silently or aloud to create a sense of calm and relaxation (Ospina et al., 2007). The term *mantram*, rather than mantra, is used to differentiate MRP from TM and to acknowledge its originator, Eknath Easwaran (Easwaran, 2008).

MRP is a practice of meditation during which the individual chooses a spiritually significant word or phrase (i.e., mantram) and repeats it silently or out loud (Bormann et al., 2005). A mantram is meant to be a source of comfort, inner truth, inspiration, and peace. It can be used intermittently when symptoms arise to interrupt intrusive ruminating thoughts or emotions common in PTSD, and to improve concentration and attention. MRP redirects the person's attention from maladaptive thought patterns, and allows time to slow down and make decisions (Vujanovic, Niles, Pietrefesa, Schmertz & Potter, 2011). Patients report an increase in spiritual well-being and a decrease of hyperarousal symptoms, anxiousness, and fear through the facilitation of a physiological relaxation response (Bormann, 2005; Bormann, Thorp, Wetherell & Golshan, 2008). MRP is powerful in eliciting feelings of well-being (Bormann, Liu, Thorp & Lang, 2012; Lang et al., 2012) and self-efficacy (Oman & Bormann, 2015), and mitigating self-reported feelings of guilt and shame so critical in the process of reintegration and PTSD recovery.

Clinical Research

Several randomized trials of MRP have been conducted by Bormann et al. in combat veterans with PTSD (Bormann, Thorp, Wetherell & Golshan, 2008; Bormann, Thorp,

Wetherell, Golshan & Lang, 2013; Bormann, Oman, Walter & Johnson, 2014; Oman & Bormann, 2015). These randomized controlled trials (RCTs) are summarized in Table 4.1 and suggest that those who completed six group sessions of MRP in addition to usual care compared with control subjects receiving usual care demonstrated a significantly greater reduction of self-reported and clinician-assessed PTSD symptoms and depressive symptoms, and an improvement in mental health-related quality of life and mindful attention. Changes in these clinical outcomes were mediated through two mechanisms: (1) self-efficacy (Oman & Bormann, 2015), which is recognized as a predictor of recovery from trauma, and (2) levels of spiritual well-being (Bormann, Liu, Thorp & Lang, 2012), highlighting the importance of the spiritual aspect of the practice. All studies report very few dropouts, good satisfaction, acceptability among veterans, and no safety concerns with MRP use.

The concept of self-efficacy is described by Benight and Bandura (2004) as improved coping with benefits such as gains in positive health behavior (e.g., exercise) and reductions in substance abuse or other maladaptive coping strategies, as well as improvement in physical health related to decreased distress (Benight & Bandura, 2004). Oman and Bormann (2015) conclude that MRP fosters self-efficacy for managing PTSD symptoms, favorably affecting diverse facets of well-being (Oman & Bormann, 2015). Such gain in self-efficacy that promotes better coping, reintegration, and patient engagement could be a valuable tool in PTSD management; current evidence-based pharmacotherapy or trauma-focused psychotherapy do not emphasize this aspect of recovery sufficiently (Table 4.1).

Although preliminary results are promising, additional studies that establish reproducibility by other researchers are necessary. Future study designs should include testing MRP's effectiveness as monotherapy, an active comparison group consistent with first-line treatment (e.g., trauma-focused psychotherapy), and parallel investigation of underlying neural mechanisms. At this time, using mantram repetition adjunctively with standard care and regular follow-up visits seems most appropriate. Its advantages include the fact that it may be an empowering self-management strategy that is highly practical, free, portable, immediate, safe, easy to use, and private, and allows for creating individual spiritual meaning (Bormann et al., 2005). Box 4.3 summarizes key therapeutic benefits of MRP. Box 4.4 and Table 4.2 offer simple mantram repetition instructions and a list of common mantrams from six different spiritual traditions.

A Word on Transcendental Meditation

Although TM belongs to the same group of meditations as MRP and has been publicized widely in the media, it does not have sufficient evidence of efficacy for PTSD

TABLE 4.1 Evidence Table: Mantram Repetition Program for Combat PTSD

Reference, Study Design, Size, and Aims	Population, Intervention, Comparator, and Outcome	Conclusions	Strengths and Limitations
Reference: Bormann et al. (2013, 2014) and Oman and Bormann (2015) *Design:* RCT *Size:* N = 146 *Aims:* 1) To evaluate effects of adjunctive MRP on PTSD and depressive symptom severity, MHRQL, and spiritual well-being 2) To evaluate effects of adjunctive MRP on mindful attention as a mediator of PTSD symptom improvement 3) To evaluate effects of MRP on self-efficacy for managing PTSD symptoms	*Population:* veterans with PTSD *Intervention:* MRP and TAU *Comparator:* TAU (i.e., medication and case management) *Outcome:* CAPS, PCL-C, BSI-18, SF-12v2, MAAS, FACIT-Sp, novel self-efficacy 1-item tool	Compared with control: 1. Adjunctive MRP shows better reduction in PTSD, hyperarousal, and depressive symptoms; improved MHRQL; and enhanced spiritual well-being. 2. Adjunctive MRP results in increased mindful attention that, in turn, mediates a decrease in PTSD and depression symptoms. Frequency of MRP practice is correlated positively with an increase in mindful attention. 3. Adjunctive MRP results in a significant increase in self-efficacy that partially mediates improvement in PTSD and depressive symptoms, and physical and mental health satisfaction.	*Strengths:* RCT, sample size, intent-to-treat analysis, allocation concealment, low dropout (7%), validated measures, both CAPS and PCL were used *Limitations:* not controlled for nonspecific effects of weekly meetings, self-selected male veteran sample limits generalizability
Reference: Bormann et al. (2008) *Study design:* RCT pilot *Size:* N = 33 *Aim:* To evaluate effects of adjunctive MRP on PTSD and depressive symptom severity, MHRQL, and well-being	*Population:* veterans with combat PTSD *Intervention:* MRP and TAU *Comparator:* wait list and TAU *Outcome:* CAPS, PCL, BSI-18, STAXI-2, Q-LES-Q-SF, FACIT-Sp	Compared with control: 1. Adjunctive MRP shows significant reduction in PTSD symptom severity and psychological distress, and increased quality of life. 2. Results suggest high patient satisfaction and acceptability of MRP.	*Strengths:* RCT, both CAPS and PCL were used *Limitations:* small size, no active control other than TAU, self-selected male veteran sample limits generalizability

BSI-18, *Brief Symptom Inventory-18 Depression Scale;* CAPS, *Clinician-administered PTSD Scale;* FACIT-Sp, *Functional Assessment of Chronic Illness Therapy–Spiritual Well-being Scale;* MAAS, *Mindfulness Attention Awareness Scale;* MHRQL, *mental health-related quality of life;* MRP, *Mantram Repetition Program;* PCL, *PTSD Checklist;* PCL-C, *PTSD Checklist—Civilian Version;* PTSD, *posttraumatic stress disorder;* Q-LES-Q-SF, *Quality-of-Life Enjoyment and Satisfaction Questionnaire–Short Form;* RCT, *randomized controlled trial;* SF-12v2, *Short Form Health Survey-12v2;* STAXI-2, *State–Trait Anger Expression Inventory 2;* TAU, *treatment as usual.*

BOX 4.3
KEY BENEFITS OF ADJUNCTIVE MANTRAM REPETITION PROGRAM

- Reduces symptoms of posttraumatic stress disorder
  - Facilitates relaxation and reduces hyperarousal
  - May help mitigate guilt, and shame, and encourages forgiveness
  - Reduces depressive symptoms
- Improves coping, reintegration, and life satisfaction
  - Increases self-efficacy
  - Improves spiritual well-being
  - Improves mindfulness
  - Improves mental health-related quality of life

---

at this time. There are three very small ($N = 11$, $N = 18$, and $N = 29$) uncontrolled poorly designed studies and one small RCT ($N = 42$) that looked at change in posttraumatic symptoms without established diagnosis of PTSD and did not use allocation concealment, active control, or intent-to-treat analysis (Rosenthal, Grosswald, Ross & Rosenthal, 2011; Barnes, Rigg & Williams, 2013; Rees, Travis, Shapiro & Chant, 2013; Rees, Travis, Shapiro & Chant, 2014). Therefore, evidence is lacking for drawing any meaningful and clinically relevant conclusions at this time.

BOX 4.4
MANTRAM REPETITION INSTRUCTIONS

1. Choose your mantram that carries a spiritual significance for you and has a positive feeling or even sound. A mantram is a spiritual word, phrase, or brief prayer we repeat silently to calm the body, quiet the mind, and improve concentration to restore the spirit. If you do not have one in mind, you can try examples from Table 4.2.
2. Use a mantram simply by repeating it to yourself as often as you can—silently, aloud, or in writing.
3. At first, use it at times when you are calm and relaxed, before sleep, while walking, and so on. Later, you can repeat your mantram when symptoms of distress arise—anytime, anyplace, and intermittently throughout the day.
4. Make using your mantram a daily habit. With practice and persistence, you will feel less stress, be able to interrupt intrusive thoughts and emotions more quickly, and improve your quality of life and add a sense of well-being. The more you use your mantram, the better you'll feel, think, and be.

TABLE 4.2 List of Common Religious Mantrams (Bormann et al., 2005)

Mantrams	Meaning
Buddhist	
Om Mane Padme Hum (Ohm mah-nee pod-may-hume)	An invocation to the jewel (Self) in the lotus of the heart
Namo Butsaya (Nah-mo boot-sie-yah)	I bow to the Buddha
Christian	
My God and My All	St. Francis of Assisi's mantra
Maranatha (Mar-uh-naw-tha)	Lord of the Heart (Aramaic)
Kyrie Eleison (Kir-ee-ay Ee-lay-ee-sone)	Lord have mercy
Christe Eleison (Kreest-ay Ee-lay-ee-sone)	Christ have mercy
Jesus, Jesus	Son of God
Hail Mary or Ave Maria	Mother of Jesus
Hindu/Indian	
Rama (Rah-mah)	Eternal joy within
Ram Ram Sri Ram (Rahm rahm shree rahm)	Gandhi's mantra (variation on Rama)
Om Namah Shivaya (Ohm Nah-mah Shee-vy-yah)	An invocation to beauty and fearlessness
Om Prema (Ohm Pray-Mah)	A call for universal love
Om Shanti (Ohm Shawn-tee)	An invocation to eternal peace
So Hum (So hum)	I am that Self within
Jewish	
Barukh Atah Adonoi (Bah-ruke Ah-tah Ah-don-aye)	Blessed are Thou O Lord
Ribono Shel Olam (Ree-boh-noh Shel Oh-lahm)	Lord of the Universe
Shalom	Peace
Sheheena (Sha Hee-nah)	Feminine aspect of God
Muslim	
Allah	
Bismallah Ir-rahman Ir-rahim (Beese-mah-lah ir-rah-mun ir-rah-heem)	In the name of Allah, the merciful, the compassionate
Native American	
O Wakan Tanka	Oh, Great Spirit

Source: Bormann, J., Smith, T., Becker, S., Gershwin, M., Pada, L., Grudzinski, A., et al. (2005). Efficacy of frequent mantram repetition on stress, quality of life, and spiritual well-being in veterans: a pilot study. J Holist Nurs., 23(4), 401.

Just like MRP, TM involves the repetition of a phrase. However, in TM, a mantra is assigned by a certified TM teacher instead of being chosen by patients themselves. The TM technique is a registered trademark and can be learned only at specialized centers at a substantial cost, which limits patient access to this intervention. Because

TM is a registered trademark, and all materials are proprietary, most published trials do not use training manuals and are not able to describe interventions in sufficient detail. This presents a unique research reproducibility challenge.

MINDFULNESS MEDITATION

Definition

Jon Kabat-Zinn, the pioneer of the clinical application of mindfulness in the West, defines mindfulness as "the ability to maintain moment by moment, open, acceptant, non-judgmental awareness" (Kabat-Zinn, 2005 p. 22). Segal (2008), whose research focuses on adopting mindfulness meditation to mental health, further describes four characteristics of this type of attention to the present experience: curiosity, openness, acceptance, and love (Segal, 2008). He suggests that curiosity and the ability simply to observe our feelings, thoughts, and reactions with openness lie at the heart of mindfulness and help generate self-acceptance and self-love. Neuroimaging studies by Farb et al. (2007) further show how mindfulness practice engages the medial prefrontal cortex and results in cognitive control of negative emotions. Such voluntary regulation of the prefrontal cortex and directing attention toward the transitory nature of a present somatosensory experience provides an alternative to cognitive efforts to control negative emotion, and cultivates a conscious open and receptive attitude rooted in the now (Chiesa & Serretti, 2010; Farb et al., 2010).

Mindfulness Meditation and Mindfulness-Based Group Interventions

Various types of mindfulness meditation originated from different Buddhist monastic traditions, such as Zen, Vipassana, and Shambhala meditations (Chiesa & Malinowski, 2011). These types differ slightly on details such as posture, but all involve sitting still and observing one's breathing. When thoughts inevitably arise, the meditator acknowledges and accepts them without judgment, and then brings attention back to the sensation of air going in and out of the body in a natural and relaxed way. This practice of returning one's attention repeatedly to the process of respiration is simple and takes only 15 to 20 minutes a day. Yet, over time, it trains the brain in the art of staying in the present and offers significant benefits of controlling one's otherwise automatic stress response to negative emotions or thoughts and intrusive memories of trauma (Lang et al., 2012; Khusid, 2013).

In addition to the traditional Buddhist techniques mentioned here, which can be practiced at home or at community meditation centers, several group mindfulness-based therapeutic techniques have been developed and adopted in clinical environments. These methods have been studied in people facing mental health challenges such as depression or PTSD. Each combines group training in mindfulness techniques with daily mindfulness meditation practice tailored to a specific clinical condition, with various forms of follow-up. The instructions for daily mindfulness meditation practice are well documented in research by Richard J. Davidson, one of the most prominent scientists investigating the neurobiological basis of meditation (Davidson & Begley, 2012). The three most common mindfulness-based group protocols are described in the following sections.

Mindfulness-Based Stress Reduction

Mindfulness-based stress reduction (MBSR) was developed originally by Jon Kabat-Zinn at the University of Massachusetts Medical School to help individuals manage chronic pain and psychological concerns related to chronic illness (Kabat-Zinn, 1982). The MBSR groups usually meet for 2 hours once a week for 8 weeks, followed by a day-long retreat (Kearney, McDermott, Malte, Martinez & Simpson, 2013). MBSR instruction emphasizes bringing a curious, kind, and nonjudgmental attitude to the present moment and to any difficult or unpleasant thoughts, sensations, or experiences.

During each class, participants receive instruction in mindfulness meditation, have an opportunity to ask questions, and practice newly learned skills. Training includes developing the ability to focus and maintain attention on the breath and learning flexibility of attention (that is, to let go of ruminative cycles of thought and return attention to the breath). Two additional exercises are the "body scan," during which attention is directed systematically to each part of the body, and gentle yoga. Homework assignments include daily meditation or yoga for 45 minutes per day and bringing mindful attention to experiences in daily life. During the day-long, mostly silent retreat, participants practice mindfulness exercises more intensively.

Mindfulness-Based Cognitive Therapy

Mindfulness-based cognitive therapy (MBCT) is a group program that integrates cognitive behavioral techniques and mindfulness meditation. Initially developed by Teasdale, Segal, and Williams to prevent relapses of depression currently in remission (Teasdale et al., 2000), the program teaches individuals to become more aware of negative emotions and thoughts, and to view them as mental "events" rather than accurate reflections of self or reality. Adopting this mode of neutral, nonjudgmental observation empowers patients to recognize and disengage from counterproductive ruminative thought patterns that may trigger habitual negative emotions. Increasing awareness of these patterns provides the meditator with the freedom to choose an emotional response, instead of falling into the habitual negative pattern of feeling overwhelmed that is so characteristic of depression (Teasdale et al., 2000).

MBCT instructors lead participants in eight weekly, 2-hour group training sessions, with daily homework exercises. Homework consists of awareness exercises directed at increasing moment-by-moment, nonjudgmental awareness of bodily sensations, thoughts, and feelings. Participants also practice integrating awareness skills into daily life. Specific strategies to prevent depression relapses are also explored. Most MBCT programs also offer up to four monthly follow-up meetings, thus extending guided support for this therapeutic intervention for up to 6 months.

Mindfulness-Based Relapse Prevention

Mindfulness-based relapse prevention (MBRP) was designed to treat substance use disorder. Because substance use disorders are highly comorbid with PTSD, MBRP may provide a more targeted approach for clinical cases in which both conditions are present. MBRP integrates mindfulness meditation and cognitive behavior skills to help meditators avoid relapses into substrance misuse. An effective combination of these two strategies teaches nonjudgmental, open, and acceptant observation of cravings as a mental "event," decoupling the negative thoughts and emotions associated with cravings. The meditator gains space to choose a reaction, instead of turning reflexively to an addictive substance. Like the other therapeutic program, MBRP is usually delivered by an instructor in eight weekly, 2-hour group training sessions, with daily mindfulness meditation as homework.

Mindfulness Meditation Mechanism

There is a shared neuropathological pattern present in PTSD, depression, poor impulse control in addictions, and aggressive outbursts. In all four clinical situations, the prefrontal cortex is underresponsive and therefore generates insufficient negative feedback on the hyperactive amygdala. Because the amygdala is responsible for negative emotion processing, an overactive amygdala, common in those with PTSD, can manifest as persistent fear, phobic avoidance, hyperarousal, and reexperiencing of painful memories. In patients with depression, the same mechanism manifests as increased negative rumination and emotional reactivity. Individuals may also have difficulty controlling their impulses to misuse substances, or may react aggressively or violently. Neuroimaging research shows that mindfulness meditation can reverse this neural pattern shared by several psychiatric pathologies through prefrontal cortex activation resulting in amygdala inhibition (Creswell, Way, Eisenberger & Lieberman, 2007; Chiesa & Serretti, 2010; Bränström, Kvillemo & Akerstedt, 2013).

In a landmark study, anatomic magnetic resonance imaging was conducted before and after an 8-week MBSR program ($N = 26$) and illustrated that reported reduction in perceived stress correlated positively with a decrease in right basolateral amygdala gray matter density. By decreasing amygdala activity, these MBSR-mediated neuroplastic changes can help decrease the negative consequence of chronic stress (Hölzel et al., 2010). MBSR also increased gray matter volume in areas of learning, attention and memory processing, and emotion regulation (Hölzel et al., 2011). MBSR has been shown to increase positive mood and reduce distractive ruminative thoughts and behaviors (Nakamura, Lipschitz, Kuhn, Kinney & Donaldson, 2013), reduce emotional reactivity (Barnhofer, Duggan & Griffith, 2011; Taylor et al., 2011), and improve impulse control (Kozasa et al., 2012). One study showed that MBSR may influence the hypothalamic–pituitary–adrenocortical axis, resulting in an adjustment of cortisol levels (Creswell, Way, Eisenberger & Lieberman, 2007). Higher plasma melatonin levels were also shown in advanced meditators, which may be helpful in mitigating PTSD-related sleep difficulties (Solberg et al., 2004). These multifaceted neural, endocrine, and psychological effects of mindfulness meditation suggest the treatment has versatile, wide-spectrum therapeutic potential for PTSD and commonly co-occurring conditions.

Clinical Research

A limited number of clinical trials of mindfulness meditation for combat PTSD exist to date and they are summarized in Table 4.3. The largest and most rigorous RCT ($N = 116$) was completed by Polusny et al. (2015). It compared adjunctive MBSR and present-centered group psychotherapy in veterans with a PTSD diagnosis or subthreshold PTSD. Study participants did not use any other psychotherapy during the study, but some were on psychoactive medications used at doses stable for at least 2 months before the beginning of the study. MBSR resulted in a greater decrease of PTSD and depressive symptoms, and showed improvement in mindfulness and quality of life. This therapeutic gain was sustained during the 9-week intervention administration and at the 2-month follow-up.

In 2013, Kearney, Malte, et al. conducted an RCT ($N = 47$) to assess outcomes associated with an 8-week MBSR program for veterans with PTSD. They randomized participants to treatment as usual or to MBSR plus treatment as usual (Kearney, McDermott, Malte, Martinez & Simpson, 2013). Although no difference was noted immediately after intervention, veterans in the adjunctive MBSR group showed a clinically significant change in PTSD symptoms, mental health-related quality of life, and mindfulness skills. Two RCTs in Iranian combat veterans with PTSD ($N = 62$,

$N = 28$) showed adjunctive MBSR was more effective than treatment as usual alone in regulating depressive and anxious moods, and improving health-related quality of life (Omidi, Mohammadi, Zargar & Akbari, 2013; Azad & Hashemi, 2014).

In nonveteran populations and in individuals with noncombat PTSD, the evidence is insufficient to recommend mindfulness meditation at this time. A few studies that are published are a challenge to interpret because some use subjects who do not have a documented PTSD diagnosis and others do not use an RCT design, are limited by a small sample size, or contain other significant methodological limitations. For example, a mindfulness meditation intervention was used in a nonrandomized pilot of mental health workers with PTSD who, 10 weeks after Hurricane Katrina, received 4 hours of mindfulness training, followed by an 8-week home study (Waelde et al., 2008). Participants reported good treatment adherence, significant improvements in well-being, and a decrease in PTSD and anxiety symptoms. Another example is two consequent RCTs in cancer patients ($N = 71$) with PTSD-like symptoms related to cancer prognosis and treatment, but no established PTSD diagnosis (Bränström, Kvillemo, Brandberg & Moskowitz, 2010; Bränström, Kvillemo & Akerstedt, 2013). These results suggested that an 8-week MBSR training course decreased perceived stress and post- traumatic avoidance symptoms significantly, and increased positive affect and mindfulness compared with a wait-list control group immediately postintervention and at the 6-month follow-up (Bränström, Kvillemo, Brandberg & Moskowitz, 2010; Bränström, Kvillemo & Akerstedt, 2013).Despite positive results in both studies, it would be premature to draw clinically relevant conclusions for populations with noncombat PTSD. Further replications of rigorous randomized controlled studies in diverse populations are needed.

To summarize, preliminary findings suggest that, in veterans with combat PTSD, adjunctive MBSR is effective at decreasing PTSD and depressive symptoms, and improving mental health-related quality of life and mindfulness. In cases when first-line psychotherapy (e.g., prolonged exposure) is not accessible or acceptable to patients, MBSR may be tried as monotherapy or in conjunction with stable pharmacotherapy (Polusny et al., 2015). MBSR is safe and well accepted by veterans, and shows good treatment adherence and meditation practice compliance at up to 6 months of follow-up (Table 4.3).

Mindfulness Meditation for Conditions Commonly Co-occurring with PTSD

Mindfulness-based interventions have been studied for conditions that co-occur commonly with PTSD, such as depression, substance use disorder, insomnia, and

TABLE 4.3 Evidence Table: Mindfulness-Based Stress Reduction for Combat PTSD

Reference, Study Design, Size, and Aims	Population, Intervention, Comparator, and Outcomes	Conclusions	Strengths and Limitations
Reference: Polusny et al. (2015) *Study design:* RCT *Size: N* = 116 *Aim:* To evaluate comparative effectiveness of MBSR and PCGT for PTSD	*Population:* veterans with PTSD or subthreshold PTSD (mostly male, mostly Vietnam veterans) *Intervention:* adjunctive* MBSR *Comparator:* adjunctive* PCGT *Outcome:* PCL, CAPS, PHQ-9, FFMQ, WHOQL-BREF, LEC	1. Both treatments were effective; however, MBSR compared with PCGT resulted in a greater decrease in PTSD and depressive symptom severity after treatment and at the 2-month follow-up. 2. MBSR was more effective at improving quality of life and mindfulness after treatment and at the 2-month follow-up. 3. Greater mindfulness was associated with better outcomes across the board. 4. MBSR had greater dropout than PCGT, but less than in first-line treatments.	*Strengths:* RCT, intent-to-treat analysis, allocation concealment, blinded outcome assessors, active evidence-based control; both CAPS and PCL were used *Limitations:* short follow-up, mostly male participants limit generalizability
Reference: Azad and Hashemi (2014) *Study design:* RCT *Size: N* = 32 *Aim:* To evaluate MBSR effect on QOL	*Population:* Iranian veterans with PTSD *Intervention:* MBSR *Comparator:* no treatment *Outcome:* WHOQOL-26	Compared with no treatment, the MBSR group showed a statistically significant increase in QOL scores.	*Strengths:* RCT, single blind *Limitations:* small size, no intent-to-treat analysis, validated scales for PTSD symptoms were not used, results are not generalizable to patients with noncombat PTSD

Reference: Omidi et al. (2013) *Study design:* RCT *Size:* N = 62 *Aim:* To evaluate the effect of adjunctive MBSR for mood symptoms and anger in veterans with PTSD	*Population:* Iranian veterans with PTSD *Interventions:* MBSR and TAU (psychotherapy) *Comparator:* TAU (psychotherapy) *Outcome:* BRUMS	1. Compared with TAU alone, the adjunctive MBSR group showed statistically significant improvement on scales of depression, tension, dizziness, and fatigue. 2. There was no statistically significant difference in the anger and vitality scales between the two groups.	*Strength:* RCT *Limitations:* small sample size, no intent-to-treat analysis, validated scales for PTSD symptoms were not used, results are not generalizable to patients with noncombat PTSD
Reference: Kearney et al. (2013) *Study design:* RCT *Size:* N = 47 *Aim:* To evaluate the effectiveness of adjunctive MBSR for PTSD management	*Population:* veterans with combat PTSD *Interventions:* MBSR and TAU *Comparator:* TAU *Outcome:* PCL, LEC, PHQ9, SF-8, mindfulness	1. No group difference on PTSD and depressive symptoms after treatment and at the 4-month follow-up. 2. Adjunctive MBSR improved mental health-related QOL after treatment that was not maintained at the 4-month follow-up. 3. Adjunctive MBSR improved physical health-related QOL at the 4-month follow-up, but there was no difference immediately after treatment.	*Strengths:* RCT, intent-to-treat analysis, allocation concealment *Limitations:* small sample size, CAPS were not used, results are not generalizable to patients with noncombat PTSD

BRUMS, inventory of mood status; CAPS, Clinician-administered PTSD Scale; FFMQ, Five Facet Mindfulness Questionnaire; LEC, Life Events Checklist; MBSR, mindfulness-based stress reduction; PCGT, present-centered group therapy; PCL, PTSD Checklist; PHQ-9, Patient Health Questionnaire 9; PTSD, posttraumatic stress disorder; QOL = quality of life; RCT, randomized controlled trial; SF-8, Short Form Health Survey 8; TAU, treatment as usual; WHOQL-BREF, World Health Organization Quality of Life–Brief; WHOQL-26, World Health Organization Quality of Life-26.

*Participants continued pharmacotherapy if their doses were stable for 2 months before the study, but did not use any other behavioral interventions.

chronic pain. There are two systematic reviews on MBCT for major depressive disorder. A 2015 systematic review by Sorbero et al. ($N = 17$ RCTs) demonstrated that MBCT plus treatment as usual resulted in a greater reduction of depressive symptoms than treatment as usual alone in high-risk patient populations who had two or more major depressive episodes. Five RCTs addressed adverse events and reported that none occurred as a result of MBCT. Another 2015 systematic review and meta-analysis by Clarke, Mayo-Wilson, Kenny, and Pilling ($N = 29$ RCTs) showed the MBCT group had a 21% reduction in the average risk of developing a new episode of major depressive disorder by 12 months. Several individual RCTs focused on demonstrating that adjunctive MBCT reliably reduces depression relapse rates in recovered patients with a prior history of three or more episodes of recurrent depression (Ma & Teasdale, 2004; Kuyken et al., 2008; Segal et al., 2010). MBCT also reduced residual depressive symptoms significantly and showed an added benefit in reducing psychiatric comorbidity and antidepressant use (Kuyken et al., 2008).

Two systematic reviews of small limited-quality trials showed that adjunctive MBRP is efficacious in reducing cravings and substance use rates when used as "aftercare" in individuals who completed intensive inpatient or outpatient substance use disorders (SUD) treatment (Zgierska et al., 2009; Chiesa & Serretti, 2014). In another systematic review and meta-analysis by Grant et al. (2015) ($N = 6$ RCTs), adjunctive MBRP showed improved quality of life and a decrease in legal problems in one study. However, it did not show that MBRP was more effective than any comparator (e.g., treatment as usual, cognitive–behavioral therapy, standard relapse prevention) when used adjunctively or as monotherapy for reducing relapse rate, frequency and quantity of substance use, cravings, or adverse events. Because the number and quality of studies is limited, with evidence of heterogeneity, future RCTs are needed to provide firm conclusions about the efficacy and safety of MBRP for individual substance use disorders and polysubstance abuse.

A recent systematic review by de Souza et al. (2015) ($N = 13$ RCTs) evaluated the effectiveness of mindfulness-based interventions on smoking cessation. The sample size of included RCTs ranged from 48 to 198 participants, and follow-up lasted up to 6 months. Despite methodological limitations, all included trials reported promising results for smoking cessation; a decrease in cravings, negative emotions, and number of cigarettes smoked; and relapse prevention. Many studies found that improvement in quality of life and a decrease in negative emotions helped shorten treatment duration, decreased the probability of a relapse in response to triggers, and strengthened subjects' motivation to continue treatment and maintain abstinence.

In a 2007 systematic review ($N = 4$ trials), Winbush, Gross, and Kreitzer demonstrated that mindfulness meditation interventions improved sleep duration and

---

BOX 4.5
KEY BENEFITS OF ADJUNCTIVE MINDFULNESS MEDITATION

- Decreases symptoms of posttraumatic stress disorder
  - Interrupts the stream of intrusive thoughts and memories of the past trauma
  - Improves emotion regulation and decreases emotional reactivity
  - Reduces negative affect
  - Reduces rumination and avoidance
  - Improves impulse control
- Improves coping, reintegration, and life satisfaction
  - Trains an open, nonjudgmental focus on the present and decreases maladaptive cognitive interpretation of the traumatic events
  - Allows for a more effective access and processing of emotions
  - Increases mental health-related quality of life
- Effective for several common posttraumatic stress disorder comorbidities
  - Major depressive disorder
  - Smoking cessation
  - Chronic pain

---

quality, and decreased sleep-interfering cognitive processes such as worry or racing thoughts. However, the included trials were small and had significant methodological challenges. Several RCTs have been published since. Gross et al. (2011) ($N = 30$) demonstrated that MBSR was comparable with eszopiclone in reducing the time to fall asleep and improving the quality and duration of sleep. Ong et al. (2014) ($N = 54$) showed that both MBSR and mindfulness-based treatment for insomnia

---

BOX 4.6
MINDFULNESS MEDITATION INSTRUCTIONS

1. Sit upright on the floor or a chair, keeping the spine straight and maintaining a relaxed but erect posture. Depending on your comfort level, you can keep your eyes open or closed during this practice.
2. Focus on your breathing, on the sensations it triggers throughout your body. Notice how your abdomen moves with each inhalation and exhalation, and the sensation of the air through your nostrils.
3. When you notice you have been distracted by unrelated thoughts or feelings that arise, simply return your focus to your breathing.
4. Try this for 5 to 20 minutes at a sitting, once a day.

---

were more effective than self-monitoring in treatment of chronic insomnia during the study and at the 3- and 6-month follow-up.

Finally, mindfulness meditation practitioners report better pain management compared with control subjects, with a reduction in pain intensity between 22% and 50% (Kabat-Zinn, 1982; Gard et al., 2011; Zeidan et al., 2011); a decrease in pain unpleasantness by 57% (Zeidan et al., 2011); and a decrease in anticipatory anxiety by 29% (Gard et al., 2011). In their 2011 systematic review ($N = 10$ RCTs), Chiesa and Serretti showed that mindfulness-based interventions (e.g., MBSR) were effective at reducing chronic pain and associated depressive symptoms (Box 4.5 and 4.6).

COMPASSION MEDITATION

Definition

Compassion meditation takes roots in Buddhism, and is designed to enhance the feelings of kindness and compassion for self and others. (Davidson & Begley, 2012) With continued practice, these feelings arise more readily and effortlessly, and are accompanied by a desire to act to benefit others (Lang et al., 2012). There are several variations of this practice: the two original Buddhist practices are *metta* and *tonglen*. The terms commonly used in the West include compassion, self-compassion, loving–kindness meditation, and a structured program called cognitively-based compassion training. The techniques used by various schools to enhance compassion also differ. For example, *metta* and loving-kindness meditation involve a repetition of phrases of positive intention for self and others, and *tonglen* uses visualization to release suffering, transforming it and replacing it with compassion. Box 4.7 lists key benefits of compassion meditation, and Boxes 4.8 and 4.9 provide sample instructions for tonglen and self-compassion meditations.

Mechanistic and Clinical Research

There are no published RCTs evaluating compassion meditation for PTSD, and there is only one open-label, uncontrolled pilot (Kearney et al., 2013), which is summarized in Table 4.4. However, several RCTs in veterans with PTSD are currently registered at clninicaltrials.gov (e.g., NCT02372396, NCT01347749) and they are investigating the efficacy of compassion meditation on PTSD and depressive symptoms. This newly sparked interest is a result of preliminary neuroimaging and empirical findings related to stress response, positive emotions, and social connectedness. Compassion training elicits activity in a distinct

---

BOX 4.7

KEY BENEFITS OF ADJUNCTIVE COMPASSION MEDITATION

- Improves symptoms of posttraumatic stress disorder:
  - Reduces symptom severity through enhancing self-compassion, a hypothesized predictor of posttraumatic stress disorder severity
  - Reduces negative feelings of fear, anger, shame, depression, dysphoria, and anhedonia
  - Increases positive emotions such as motivation, hope, sense of life purpose, and life-satisfaction
- Improves coping, reintegration, and life satisfaction
  - Increases social connectedness
    - Addresses symptoms of social avoidance and isolation
    - Facilitates positive relations important for recovery
  - Improves functional psychological well-being and decreases functional disability
    - Improves environmental mastery
    - Improves self-acceptance
    - Improves personal growth
  - Enhance both mindfulness and self-compassion

---

neural network, including the medial orbitofrontal cortex, putamen, pallidum, and ventral tegmental area—brain regions associated previously with positive affect (Klimecki, Leiberg, Lamm & Singer, 2012).

Both clinical and neuroimaging studies have shown that compassion meditation increases positive emotions and decreases negative emotions (Fredrickson, Cohn,

---

BOX 4.8

INSTRUCTIONS FOR *TONGLEN*

1. Visualize someone who is suffering. It can be yourself, a friend or relative who is ill, a colleague who is struggling at work, or a neighbor whose marriage is ending, to name a few examples.
2. On each inhalation, imagine the suffering leaving her, his, or your own body like fog dissipating under a bright sun.
3. On each exhalation, imagine that suffering is transformed into compassion. Direct this compassion toward her, him, or yourself—a gift of loving kindness that envelops and relieves pain.
4. Try this exercise for 5 to 10 minutes up to five times a week.

BOX 4.9
INSTRUCTIONS FOR SELF-COMPASSION MEDITATION

1. Sit comfortably with your body relaxed, and your mind and heart in open stillness.
2. Choose a phrase that represents your intention of being kind, loving, forgiving, and gentle to yourself. Create the intention that is true for you at this moment and that best opens your heart. Some examples may include the following:
   • May I be at peace and happy.
   • May I be well in body and mind.
   • May I be safe from inner and outer dangers.
   • May I be filled with loving kindness.
3. Breathe gently and recite your intention inwardly. As you repeat these phrases, picture yourself and hold that image in your accepting, loving heart. Repeat these phrases over and over again, letting the feelings permeate your body and mind.
4. Practice this meditation for 5 to 10 minutes a day for a number of weeks, until the sense of compassion for yourself grows.

Coffey, Pek & Finkel, 2008; Hutcherson, Seppala & Gross, 2008). It activates specific areas of the brain associated with positive affect and empathy, and strengthens their connections to the left medial prefrontal cortex (Lutz, Brefczynski-Lewis, Johnstone & Davidson, 2008; Lutz, Greischar, Perlman & Davidson, 2009; Engström & Söderfeldt, 2010; Davidson & Begley, 2012; Klimecki, Leiberg, Lamm & Singer, 2012; Lang et al., 2012). Fostering positive emotions and outlook may result in a profound clinical benefit by decreasing a whole cluster of negative emotions of PTSD (i.e., fear, anger, guilt, shame, depression, dysphoria), building resilience (Cohn, Fredrickson, Brown, Mikels & Conway, 2009), reducing symptoms of autonomic hyperarousal, and increasing coping (Lang et al., 2012). Compassion meditation also encourages prosocial behavior and social connectedness (Hutcherson, Seppala & Gross, 2008; Leiberg, Klimecki & Singer, 2011; Lang et al., 2012), which are essential for building social support, family relationships, resilience, and reintegration during the recovery process in individuals with PTSD (Davidson & Begley, 2012; Lang et al., 2012).

Self-compassion, in particular, has been getting a lot of attention in PTSD research. According to Neff (2003), self-compassion entails three distinct components: (1) self-kindness (being kind and understanding toward oneself in instances of pain or failure, instead of being self-critical), (2) common humanity (perceiving one's experiences as part of the larger human experience, instead of seeing them as separating or isolating), and (3) mindfulness (holding painful thoughts and feelings

TABLE 4.4 Evidence Table: Compassion Meditation for Combat PTSD

Reference, Study Design, Size, and Aims	Population, Intervention, Comparator, and Outcomes	Conclusions	Strengths and Limitations
Reference: Kearney et al. (2013, 2014) *Study design:* Open pilot trial *Size:* N = 42 *Aims:* To evaluate LKM effectiveness for PTSD and to assess whether LKM is associated with increased positive emotions and personal resources	*Population:* veterans with combat PTSD (40% female) *Interventions:* 12-week LKM and TAU *Comparator:* none *Outcome:* PSS-I, LEC, PROMIS-Depression, mindfulness, SCS, CME, decentering via EQ, ANT, SSS-21, FFMQ, psychological well-being scale	1. There was a decrease of PTSD and depressive symptoms by enhanced self-compassion after treatment and at the 3-month follow-up. 2. There was an increase in both mindfulness and self-compassion after treatment and at the 3-month follow-up. 3. There was an increase in positive emotions and a decrease in negative emotions. 4. There was an increase in environmental mastery, personal growth, purpose in life, self-acceptance, and decentering during the 12-week trial and at the 3-month follow-up. 5. There was high attendance and acceptance among veterans.	*Strength:* male and female veteran participants *Limitations:* not randomized, not controlled, small size

ANT, Attention Network Test; CME, Circumplex Measure of Emotion; EQ, Experiences Questionnaire; FFMQ, Five Facet Mindfulness Questionnaire; LEC, Life Event Checklist; LKM, loving-kindness meditation; PROMIS-Depression, Patient-Reported Outcomes Measurement Information System–Depression subsystem; PSS-I, PTSD Symptom Scale Interview; PTSD, posttraumatic stress disorder; SCS, Self-compassion Scale; SSS-21, 21-Item Sense of Support Scale; TAU, treatment as usual.

in open nonjudgmental awareness, instead of overidentifying with them). The association between self-compassion and PTSD symptom severity and functional disability has been studied in U.S. Iraq and Afghanistan war veterans (Neff, 2003; Hiraoka et al., 2015). One study, which involved 115 veterans who were monitored for 12 months, concluded that self-compassion is associated negatively with functional disability, and predicted 12-month PTSD symptom severity after accounting for combat exposure and baseline PTSD severity. In conclusion, preliminary data suggest that compassion meditation may offer a valuable adjunct to standard PTSD care aimed at enhancing positive emotions and self-compassion, and decreasing functional disability and PTSD symptom severity. Future research in this field is desperately needed.

CONCLUSION

Clinical Pearls

The evidence of the meditation effectiveness as an adjunct to standard PTSD care or self-management strategy is growing rapidly. Table 4.5 summarizes the effects of mantram, mindfulness, and compassion meditations on different aspects of PTSD care. As we can see by looking at the table, each of the three meditation practices used adjunctively have a potential to reduce PTSD and depressive symptoms, improve quality of life, and increase mindfulness. In addition, each meditation technique also has its unique therapeutic feature highlighted in right column of the table and may help guide providers in their treatment decisions. For example, mindfulness meditation could be a great choice for a patient with comorbid PTSD, chronic pain, and depression, who has difficulty with impulse and emotional control. Self-compassion meditation may be a worthwhile self-care strategy for someone who responds well to prolonged exposure, but continues to have persistent feelings of shame, guilt, and difficulty experiencing positive emotions.

The physician's role is to educate patients about the potential benefits of each meditation technique and to empower them to choose the one that resonates for adoption as a life-long practice. As the benefits of meditation accrue over time, selecting a method that motivates sustained practice is a critical factor in achieving sustained therapeutic effects (Burke, 2012). It is important to emphasize continued compliance with medications and psychotherapy while using meditation adjunctively, and to schedule regular follow-up visits. Patients should be advised not to discontinue their usual care without consulting a physician.

TABLE 4.5 Comparison of Effects on Different Aspects of PTSD Care

Meditation Intervention (Duration, Format)	Decrease in PTSD Symptoms (Effect present (+) or not (−), Outcome Measures Used)	Decrease in Depressive Symptoms (Effect present (+) or not (−), Outcome Measures Used)	Improvement in Quality of Life (Effect present (+) or not (−), Outcome Measures Used)	Improvement in Mindfulness (Change presence, Outcome Measures Used)	Unique Effects That Facilitate Coping, Reintegration, or Recovery (Effect present (+) or not (−), unique features)
Adjunctive MRP (6 weeks, group)	+ (CAPS, PCL)	+ (BSI-18)	+ (SF-12)	+ (MAAS)	+ Increases self-efficacy, and improves spiritual well-being
Adjunctive MBSR (8 weeks, group)	+ (CAPS, PCL)	+ (PHQ-9)	+ (SF-8)	+ (FFMQ)	+ Improves emotion regulation and impulse control, effective for several co-occurring conditions (e.g., MDD, smoking cessation, insomnia, pain)
Adjunctive LKM* (12 weeks, group)	+ (PSS-I)	+ (PROMIS-Depression)	Not studied	+ (FFMQ)	+ Increases positive emotions and social connectedness; improves self-compassion, well-being, and functional status (e.g., environmental mastery, life purpose)

+, Effect indicated in the title of the column present; BSI-18, Brief Symptom Inventory-18 Depression Scale; CAPS, Clinician-administered PTSD Scale; FFMQ, Five Facet Mindfulness Questionnaire; MAAS, Mindfulness Attention Awareness Scale; MBSR, mindfulness-based stress reduction; MDD, major depressive disorder MRP, Mantram Repetition Program; PCL, PTSD Checklist; PROMIS-Depression, Patient-Reported Outcomes Measurement Information System–Depression subsystem; PHQ-9, Patient Health Questionnaire 9; PSS-I, PTSD Symptom Scale Interview; SF-8, Short Form Health Survey 8; SF-12, Short Form Health Survey 12.

*Please note that the loving-kindness meditation findings summarized here are based on a nonrandomized, uncontrolled trial and mechanistic research, whereas MBSR and MRP findings are based on randomized controlled trials.

Research Limitations and Future Directions

The majority of meditation trials were limited by methodological challenges. Many had a small sample size; did not use active, specific control subjects and intent-to-treat analysis; did not blind outcome assessors; nor reported on allocation concealment and adverse events. Most trials did not report consistently the frequency and duration of meditation practiced by participants during the intervention period and during the follow-up period. Therefore, it is hard to make conclusions about the effective dose of meditation interventions, or whether consistent practice is required to maintain therapeutic gain.

Future research directions should focus on replication of high-quality RCTs in diverse populations that are powered adequately; should use specific, active control subjects; should use concealed randomization, and should include an intention-to-treat analysis with sufficient follow-up. The amount of meditation instruction and home practice needs to be reported accurately to define the effective dose. Comparative effectiveness studies between standard care alone versus standard care plus meditation versus meditation alone will help to distinguish between meditation effectiveness as monotherapy or adjunctive therapy. Last, future comparison of group, home practice, or telehealth approaches in helping individuals to learn meditation skills and to maintain consistent practice will help in selecting the most cost-effective route of administration (i.e., training) of these therapeutic techniques.

KEY POINTS

1. The self-care quality of meditation practice encourages individuals to take central stage in their pursuit of psychological health, reintegration, and rehabilitation.

2. When used adjunctively with the first-line treatment, meditation is a safe, easy-to-learn, portable, and cost-effective self-management approach for individuals with PTSD.

3. Two meditations that have been shown to reduce PTSD symptoms on both CAPS and the PCL are MRP and MBSR. They also reduce depressive symptoms, improve quality of life, and increase mindfulness.

4. Adjunctive mindfulness meditation has been shown to be effective for several PTSD comorbidities, such as tobacco use, chronic pain, and major depressive disorder.

5. The body of evidence for compassion meditation for PTSD currently lacks RCTs. However, the unique effect of compassion meditation on increasing

positive emotions, self-compassion, and social connectedness may be a great complement to the first-line treatments that do not address these concerns sufficiently.

6. Future research is needed to delineate further specific effects for each meditation intervention, their unique active ingredients, therapeutic dose (e.g., 20 minutes daily), and routes of administration (e.g., group MBSR vs. home practice vs. training via telehealth).

REFERENCES

Azad, M., & Hashemi, Z. (2014). The effectiveness of mindfulness training in improving the quality of life of the war victims with post traumatic stress disorder (PTSD). *Iran J Psychiatry., 9*(4), 228–236.

Barnes, V., Rigg, J., & Williams, J. (2013). Clinical case series: treatment of PTSD with transcendental meditation in active duty military personnel. *Mil Med., 178*(7), e836–e840.

Barnhofer, T., Duggan, D., & Griffith, J. (2011). Dispositional mindfulness moderates the relation between neuroticism and depressive symptoms. *Pers Individ Dif., 51*(8), 958–962.

Benight, C. C., & Bandura, A. (2004). Social cognitive theory of posttraumatic recovery: the role of perceived self-efficacy. *Behav Res Ther., 42*(10), 1129–1148.

Bormann, J. (2005). Frequent, silent mantram repetition: a Jacuzzi for the mind. *Top Emerg Med., 27*(2), 163–166.

Bormann, J., Liu, L., Thorp, S., & Lang, A. (2012). Spiritual well-being mediates PTSD change in veterans with military-related PTSD. *Int J Behav Med., 19*(4), 496–502.

Bormann, J., Oman, D., Walter, K., & Johnson, B. (2014). Mindful attention increases and mediates psychological outcomes following mantram repetition practice in veterans with posttraumatic stress disorder. *Med Care., 52*(12 Suppl 5), S13–S18.

Bormann, J., Smith, T., Becker, S., Gershwin, M., Pada, L., Grudzinski, A., et al. (2005). Efficacy of frequent mantram repetition on stress, quality of life, and spiritual well-being in veterans: a pilot study. *J Holist Nurs., 23*(4), 395–414.

Bormann, J., Thorp, S., Wetherell, J., & Golshan, S. (2008). A spiritually based group intervention for combat veterans with posttraumatic stress disorder: feasibility study. *J Holist Nurs., 26*(2), 109–116.

Bormann, J. E., Thorp, S. R., Wetherell, J. L., Golshan, S., & Lang, A. J. (2013). Meditation-based mantram intervention for veterans with posttraumatic stress disorder: a randomized trial. *Psychological Trauma: Theory, Research, Practice, and Policy, 5*(3), 259–267.

Bränström, R., Kvillemo, P., & Akerstedt, T. (2013). Effects of mindfulness training on levels of cortisol in cancer patients. *Psychosomatics., 54*(2), 158–164.

Bränström, R., Kvillemo, P., Brandberg, Y., & Moskowitz, J. (2010). Self-report mindfulness as a mediator of psychological well-being in a stress reduction intervention for cancer patients: a randomized study. *Ann Behav Med., 39*(2), 151–161.

Burke, A. (2012). Comparing individual preferences for four meditation techniques: Zen, Vipassana (mindfulness), qigong, and mantra. *Explore (NY)., 8*(4), 237–242.

Chiesa, A., & Malinowski, P. (2011). Mindfulness-based approaches: are they all the same? *J Clin Psychol., 67*(4), 404–424.

Chiesa, A., & Serretti, A. (2010). A systematic review of neurobiological and clinical features of mindfulness meditations. *Psychol Med., 40*(8), 1239–1252.

Chiesa, A., & Serretti, A. (2014). Are mindfulness-based interventions effective for substance use disorders? A systematic review of the evidence. *Subst Use Misuse., 49*(5), 492–512.

Clarke, K., Mayo-Wilson, E., Kenny, J., & Pilling, S. (2015). Can non-pharmacological interventions prevent relapse in adults who have recovered from depression? A systematic review and meta-analysis of randomised controlled trials. *Clin Psychol Rev., 39*, 58–70.

Cohn, M., Fredrickson, B., Brown, S., Mikels, J., & Conway, A. (2009). Happiness unpacked: positive emotions increase life satisfaction by building resilience. *Emotion., 9*(3), 361–368.

Creswell, J., Way, B., Eisenberger, N., & Lieberman, M. (2007). Neural correlates of dispositional mindfulness during affect labeling. *Psychosom Med., 69*(6), 560–565.

Davidson, R. J., & Begley, S. (2012). *The emotional life of your brain: how its unique patterns affect the way you think, feel, and live—and how you can change them.* Plume, Penguin Group, New York, NY.

de Souza, B., Gomide, H., Miranda, T., Menezes, V., Kozasa, E., Noto, A. R. (2015). Mindfulness-based interventions for the treatment of smoking: a systematic literature review. *J Altern Complement Med., 21*(3), 129–140.

Easwaran, E. (2008). *The mantram handbook* (5th ed.). Tomales, CA: Nilgiri Press.

Engström, M., & Söderfeldt, B. (2010). Brain activation during compassion meditation: a case study. *J Altern Complement Med., 16*(5), 597–599.

Farb, N., Anderson, A., Mayberg, H., Bean, J., McKeon, D., Segal, Z., et al. (2010). Minding one's emotions: mindfulness training alters the neural expression of sadness. *Emotion., 10*(1), 25–33.

Farb, N., Segal, Z., Mayberg, H., Bean, J., McKeon, D., Fatima, Z., et al. (2007). Attending to the present: mindfulness meditation reveals distinct neural modes of self-reference. *Soc Cogn Affect Neurosci., 2*(4), 313–322.

Fredrickson, B., Cohn, M., Coffey, K., Pek, J., & Finkel, S. (2008). Open hearts build lives: positive emotions, induced through loving–kindness meditation, build consequential personal resources. *J Pers Soc Psychol., 95*(5), 1045–1062.

Gard, T., Hölzel, B. K., Sack, A. T., Hempel, H., Lazar, S. W., Vaitl, D., et al. (2011). Pain attenuation through mindfulness is associated with decreased cognitive control and increased sensory processing in the brain. *Cereb Cortex., 22*(11), 2692–2702.

Goyal, M., Singh, S., Sibinga, E., Gould, N., Rowland-Seymour, A., Sharma, R., & Berger, Z. (Eds.). (2014). *Meditation programs for psychological stress and well-being: comparative effectiveness review.* Report no. 13(14)-EHC116-EF. Rockville, MD: Agency for Healthcare Research and Quality.

Grant, S., Hempel, S., Cplaiaco, B., Motala, A., Shanman, R., Booth, M., & Sorbero, M. (2015). *Mindfulness-based relapse prevention for substance use disorders: a systematic review.* From: http://www.rand.org/pubs/research_reports/RR1031.html.

Gross, C., Kreitzer, M., Reilly-Spong, M., Wall, M., Winbush, N., Patterson, R., et al. (2011). Mindfulness-based stress reduction versus pharmacotherapy for chronic primary insomnia: a randomized controlled clinical trial. *Explore (NY)., 7*(2), 76–87.

Hiraoka, R., Meyer, E., Kimbrel, N., DeBeer, B., Gulliver, S., Morissette, S., et al. (2015). Self-compassion as a prospective predictor of PTSD symptom severity among trauma-exposed U.S. Iraq and Afghanistan war veterans. *J Trauma Stress., 28*(2), 127–133.

Hölzel, B., Carmody, J., Evans, K., Hoge, E., Dusek, J., Morgan, L., et al. (2010). Stress reduction correlates with structural changes in the amygdala. *Soc Cogn Affect Neurosci., 5*(1), 11–17.

Hölzel, B., Carmody, J., Vangel, M., Congleton, C., Yerramsetti, S., Gard, T., et al. (2011). Mindfulness practice leads to increases in regional brain gray matter density. *Psychiatry Res., 191*(1), 36–43.

Hutcherson, C., Seppala, E., & Gross, J. (2008). Loving-kindness meditation increases social connectedness. *Emotion., 8*(5), 720–724.

Kabat-Zinn, J. (1982). An outpatient program in behavioral medicine for chronic pain patients based on the practice of mindfulness meditation: theoretical considerations and preliminary results. *Gen Hosp Psychiatry., 4*(1), 33–47.

Kabat-Zinn, J. (2005). Bringing mindfulness to medicine: an interview with Jon Kabat-Zinn, PhD; interview by Karolyn Gazella. *Adv Mind Body Med., 21*(2), 22–27.

Kearney, D., Malte, C., McManus, C., Martinez, M., Felleman, B., Simpson, T., et al. (2013). Loving-kindness meditation for posttraumatic stress disorder: a pilot study. *J Trauma Stress., 26*(4), 426–434.

Kearney, D., McDermott, K., Malte, C., Martinez, M., & Simpson, T. (2013). Effects of participation in a mindfulness program for veterans with posttraumatic stress disorder: a randomized controlled pilot study. *J Clin Psychol., 69*(1), 14–27.

Khusid, M. (2013). Self-care mindfulness approaches for refractory posttraumatic stress disorder. *Psychiatr Ann., 43*(7), 340–344.

Kim, S., Schneider, S., Kravitz, L., Mermier, C., & Burge, M. (2013). Mind–body practices for post-traumatic stress disorder. *J Invest Med., 61*(5), 827–834.

Klimecki, O., Leiberg, S., Lamm, C., & Singer, T. (2012). Functional neural plasticity and associated changes in positive affect after compassion training. *Cereb Cortex., 23*(7), 1552–1561.

Kozasa, E., Sato, J., Lacerda, S., Barreiros, M., Radvany, J., Russell, T., et al. (2012). Meditation training increases brain efficiency in an attention task. *Neuroimage., 59*(1), 745–749.

Kuyken, W., Byford, S., Taylor, R., Watkins, E., Holden, E., White, K., et al. (2008). Mindfulness-based cognitive therapy to prevent relapse in recurrent depression. *J Consult Clin Psychol., 76*(6), 966–978.

Lang, A., Strauss, J., Bomyea, J., Bormann, J., Hickman, S., Good, R., et al. (2012). The theoretical and empirical basis for meditation as an intervention for PTSD. *Behav Modif., 36*(6), 759–786.

Leiberg, S., Klimecki, O., & Singer, T. (2011). Short-term compassion training increases prosocial behavior in a newly developed prosocial game. *PLoS One., 6*(3), 1–10.

Libby, D., Pilver, C., & Desai, R. (2012). Complementary and alternative medicine in VA specialized PTSD treatment programs. *Psychiatr Serv., 63*(11), 1134–1136.

Libby, D., Reddy, F., Pilver, C., & Desai, R. (2012). The use of yoga in specialized VA PTSD treatment programs. *Int J Yoga Ther., 22*, 79–87.

Lutz, A., Brefczynski-Lewis, J., Johnstone, T., & Davidson, R. (2008). Regulation of the neural circuitry of emotion by compassion meditation: effects of meditative expertise. *PLoS One., 3*(3), 10.

Lutz, A., Greischar, L., Perlman, D., & Davidson, R. (2009). BOLD signal in insula is differentially related to cardiac function during compassion meditation in experts vs. novices. *Neuroimage., 47*(3), 1038–1046.

Lutz, A., Slagter, H., Dunne, J., & Davidson, R. (2008). Attention regulation and monitoring in meditation. *Trends Cogn Sci., 12*(4), 163–169.

Ma, S., & Teasdale, J. (2004). Mindfulness-based cognitive therapy for depression: replication and exploration of differential relapse prevention effects. *J Consult Clin Psychol., 72*(1), 31–40.

Nakamura, Y., Lipschitz, D., Kuhn, R., Kinney, A., & Donaldson, G. (2013). Investigating efficacy of two brief mind-body intervention programs for managing sleep disturbance in cancer survivors: a pilot randomized controlled trial. *J Cancer Surviv., 7*(2), 165–182.

Neff, K. (2003). The development and validation of a scale to measure self-compassion. *Self and Identity: the journal of the International Society for Self and Identity, 3*, 223–250.

Oman, D., & Bormann, J. (2015). Mantram repetition fosters self-efficacy in veterans for managing PTSD: a randomized trial. *Psychol Relig Spirit., 7*(1), 34–35.

Omidi, A., Mohammadi, A., Zargar, F., & Akbari, H. (2013). Efficacy of mindfulness-based stress reduction on mood states of veterans with post-traumatic stress disorder. *Arch Trauma Res., 1*(4), 151–154.

Ong, J., Manber, R., Segal, Z., Xia, Y., Shapiro, S., Wyatt, J., et al. (2014). A randomized controlled trial of mindfulness meditation for chronic insomnia. *Sleep., 37*(9), 1553–1563.

Ospina, M., Bond, K., Karkhaneh, M., Tjosvold, L., Vandermeer, B., Liang, Y., et al. (2007). Meditation practices for health: state of the research. *Evid Rep Technol Assess., 155*, 1–263.

Polusny, M., Erbes, C., Thuras, P., Moran, A., Lamberty, G., Collins, R., et al. (2015). Mindfulness-based stress reduction for posttraumatic stress disorder among veterans: a randomized clinical trial. *JAMA., 314*(5), 456–465.

Rees, B., Travis, F., Shapiro, D., & Chant, R. (2013). Reduction in posttraumatic stress symptoms in Congolese refugees practicing transcendental meditation. *J Trauma Stress., 26*(2), 295–298.

Rees, B., Travis, F., Shapiro, D., & Chant, R. (2014). Significant reductions in posttraumatic stress symptoms in Congolese refugees within 10 days of transcendental meditation practice. *J Trauma Stress., 27*(1), 112–115.

Rosenthal, J., Grosswald, S., Ross, R., & Rosenthal, N. (2011). Effects of transcendental meditation in veterans of Operation Enduring Freedom and Operation Iraqi Freedom with posttraumatic stress disorder: a pilot study. *Mil Med., 176*(6), 626–630.

Rubia, K. (2009). The neurobiology of meditation and its clinical effectiveness in psychiatric disorders. *Biol Psychol., 82*(1), 1–11.

Segal, Z. (2008). Finding daylight: mindful recovery from depression. *Psychother Networker. Jan/Feb: 1–6.* http://www.mbct.com/images/Psychotherapy_Networker.pdf

Segal, Z., Bieling, P., Young, T., MacQueen, G., Cooke, R., Martin, L., et al. (2010). Antidepressant monotherapy vs sequential pharmacotherapy and mindfulness-based cognitive therapy, or placebo, for relapse prophylaxis in recurrent depression. *Arch Gen Psychiatry., 67*(12), 1256–1264.

Solberg, E., Holen, A., Ekeberg, Ø., Østerud, B., Halvorsen, R., Sandvik, L., et al. (2004). The effects of long meditation on plasma melatonin and blood serotonin. *Med Sci Monit., 10*(3), CR96–101.

Sorbero, M., Ahluwalia, C., Reynolds, K., Lovejoy, S., Farris, C., Sloan, J., et al. (2015). *Meditation for depression: a systematic review of mindfulness-based cognitive therapy for major depressive disorder.* RAND Corporation. From: www.rand.org/pubs/research_reports/RR1138.html.

Sperduti, M., Martinelli, P., & Piolino, P. (2012). A neurocognitive model of meditation based on activation likelihood estimation (ALE) meta-analysis. *Conscious Cogn., 21*(1), 269–276.

Strauss, J. L., Lang, A. J. (2012). Complementary and alternative treatments for PTSD. *PTSD Res Q., 23*(2), 1–7.

Strauss, J., Coeytaux, R., McDuffie, J., Nagi, A., & Williams, J. J. (2011). Efficacy of complementary and alternative medicine therapies for posttraumatic stress disorder. *VA-ESP Project., 090*(010), 1–79.

Taylor, V., Grant, J., Daneault, V., Scavone, G., Breton, E., Roffe-Vidal, S., et al. (2011). Impact of mindfulness on the neural responses to emotional pictures in experienced and beginner meditators. *Neuroimage., 57*(4), 1524–1533.

Teasdale, J., Segal, Z., Williams, J., Ridgeway, V., Soulsby, J., Lau, M., et al. (2000). Prevention of relapse/recurrence in major depression by mindfulness-based cognitive therapy. *J Consult Clin Psychol., 68*(4), 615–623.

The Management of Post-Traumatic Stress Working Group. (2010). *Veterans Affairs and Department of Defense clinical practice guideline for the management of post-traumatic stress.* From: www.healthquality.va.gov/guidelines/MH/ptsd/cpg_PTSD-FULL-201011612.pdf.

Vujanovic, A. A., Niles, B., Pietrefesa, A., Schmertz, S. K., & Potter, C. M. (2011). Mindfulness in the treatment of posttraumatic stress disorder among military veterans. *Prof Psychol Res Pract., 42*(1), 24–31.

Waelde, L., Uddo, M., Marquett, R., Ropelato, M., Freightman, S., Pardo, A., et al. (2008). A pilot study of meditation for mental health workers following Hurricane Katrina. *J Trauma Stress., 21*(5), 497–500.

Winbush, N., Gross, C., & Kreitzer, M. (2007). The effects of mindfulness-based stress reduction on sleep disturbance: a systematic review. *Explore (NY)., 3*(6), 585–591.

Zeidan, F., Martucci, K., Kraft, R., Gordon, N., McHaffie, J., Coghill, R., et al. (2011). Brain mechanisms supporting the modulation of pain by mindfulness meditation. *J Neurosci., 31*(14), 5540–5548.

Zgierska, A., Rabago, D., Chawla, N., Kushner, K., Koehler, R., Marlatt, A., et al. (2009). Mindfulness meditation for substance use disorders: a systematic review. *Subst Abus., 30*(4), 266–294.

FIVE

Transcranial Magnetic Stimulation Treatment of Posttraumatic Stress Disorder

CAROLINE CLARK, JEFFREY COLE,

CHRISTINE WINTER, AND

GEOFFREY GRAMMER

POSTTRAUMATIC STRESS DISORDER (PTSD) IS A PSYCHIATRIC CONDITION IN WHICH the individual has sustained an exposure to a traumatic event and later develops symptoms from each of four criteria—intrusion, avoidance, negative alterations in cognitions and mood, or alterations in arousal and reactivity—which are the criteria included in the *Diagnostic and Statistical Manual of Mental Disorders*, fifth edition. As a result of the likelihood of experiencing traumatic events, participation in a military conflict increases the risk for PTSD. Before deployment, 5% to 9% of service members met the criteria for PTSD, and this prevalence increased to 12% to 20% and 6% to 12% after returning from Iraq and Afghanistan, respectively (Benedek & Wynn, 2011).

Current treatment options for PTSD include psychotherapy and pharmacology. Exposure therapy, a commonly used psychotherapy, helps individuals face and gain control of their distress and fear, and may therefore be beneficial for the treatment of PTSD. In this treatment modality, patients recall traumatic events with the goal of inducing extinction of the resulting negative symptoms in conjunction with relaxation exercises or techniques (Taylor, 2006). However, this therapy may trigger intense emotions that some patients are unable to tolerate, leading to early discontinuation of treatment (Taylor, 2006). Of potential pharmacological treatments, only the selective serotonin reuptake inhibitors (SSRIs) paroxetine and sertraline are Food and Drug Administration (FDA)–approved for the treatment of PTSD. SSRIs are effective in treating some patients with PTSD, but limited efficacy and poor compliance resulting from side effects constrains their utility. Because of issues of limited efficacy of traditional therapies, other off-label strategies such as mood stabilizers, benzodiazepines, antihistamines, and antipsychotics are often attempted. These agents can have significant toxicity, and data on their effectiveness for core PTSD symptoms are unclear (Group, 2010).

Neuromodulation uses medical devices to alter neuronal function. A variety of modalities have been used to treat psychiatric symptoms, including electroconvulsive therapy, cranial electrotherapy stimulation, magnetic seizure therapy, deep brain stimulation, transcranial direct-current stimulation, vagus nerve stimulation, and transcranial magnetic stimulation (TMS). An excellent review of these modalities and their use in PTSD was published recently (Novakovic et al., 2011). As a result of concerns regarding the tolerability of electroconvulsive therapy, and a lack of evidence of other modalities in patients with PTSD, TMS is the most promising of the neuromodulation therapies for this disorder. TMS is a noninvasive brain stimulation technique that has shown efficacy for neurological and psychiatric conditions, and therefore may be a potential alternative or complementary treatment option for individuals with PTSD. TMS has a low likelihood of adverse side effects in comparison with current treatment modalities, which suggests that TMS is a potential treatment option for PTSD—in particular, for military service members, who are part of a unique population with a high prevalence of PTSD.

MECHANISMS OF TRANSCRANIAL MAGNETIC STIMULATION

TMS modulates neuronal activity noninvasively in a focal area to achieve excitation or inhibition, depending on the parameters of the stimulation. In accordance with Faraday's law, when a magnetic field is pulsed over cortical neurons, a neuronal membrane action potential results, leading to firing of the neuron and release of neurotransmitters. The release of neurotransmitters from neurons modulate downstream neural network pathways. To achieve this, the TMS device creates a magnetic field by sending a variable ion current through a coil that has been placed in contact with the scalp (Horvath et al., 2011) The resulting lines of magnetic flux are perpendicular to the current and transmit through the skull to create an electrical field within the targeted neuronal area (Bolognini & Ro, 2010; Horvath et al., 2011). TMS, therefore, takes advantage of the natural electrical conductivity of the brain to induce alterations in brain activity that may improve PTSD symptoms.

Delivery of TMS incorporates several variables, including the type and configuration of the coil, the frequency of stimulus delivery, the duration of pulse sequence, interstimulation rest periods, the total number of pulses delivered, the strength of the magnetic field delivery, and the regularity of scheduled treatment delivery during the week (George et al., 2014).

TMS COIL DESIGN

The dimensions of the affected regions and power level are dependent in part on the shape of the coil. The multiple coil designs currently in use influence field depth, spatial resolution, and field strength (Hallett, 2007). Standard coil designs include figure-8, H, angular, and circular, which allows the clinician flexibility in selecting the most effective design for the desired geometric stimulation pattern. See Deng et al. (2013) for an excellent review of coil designs and the resulting magnetic fields. The characteristics of stimuli delivered by the different coil choices can be modulated further by the variables controlled by the clinician, such as pulse frequency, train length, or number of pulses per session.

STIMULI FREQUENCY

Frequency of stimuli delivery refers to the number of pulses delivered over time and, clinically, typically ranges from 1 to 20 Hz. Pulses delivered at approximately 1 Hz are considered to promote long-term inhibition; pulses delivered at greater than 5 Hz are considered to have long-term potentiating effects (O'Reardon et al., 2006). The effects of different stimulation frequencies are being explored actively in research studies. Alternative frequencies, such as theta-burst stimulation, may open additional options for neuromodulation (Bakker et al., 2015). Local stimulation, whether inhibitory or excitatory, can have far-reaching implications throughout the central nervous system by regulating downstream brain regions.

TRAINS OF STIMULI

When pulses are delivered, they are typically delivered in sequences referred to as *trains*. For example, a 10-Hz frequency might be administered over 4 seconds, for a total of 40 pulses in that train. A rest interval occurs between trains to allow for return of the neuronal resting state. Higher frequency stimulation, longer train sequences, or shorter rest intervals increase the risk of secondary generalization of the stimulation and subsequent induction of seizure activity. International guidelines exist for these parameters to ensure safe delivery of TMS (Wassermann, 1998).

The frequency of stimuli, the number of pulses in a train, and coil configuration and placement are all variables that can impact the outcome of the desired treatment significantly. The ability to select appropriate combinations of parameters offers the clinician flexibility in applying a range of treatments. As a treatment for PTSD, the number of pulses per session for the most optimal effect remains uncertain. Several factors must be considered when deciding on pulses per session, including safety, tolerability, and labor intensity. TMS has been administered up to a total of 18,000 pulses per day—a dose sixfold greater than the FDA clearance for a figure-8 coil, and was found to be safe and well tolerated (George et al., 2014).

MAGNETIC FIELD STRENGTH

The greater the strength of the magnetic field, the greater the stimulation of the neuron and thus likelihood of initiating an action potential. During repetitive TMS (rTMS), magnetic field strength is usually referenced as a percentage of motor threshold. Motor threshold is defined as a minimum magnetic field strength that depolarizes cortical neurons in the motor cortex, where 50% of the pulses elicit contraction of the abductor pollicis brevis on the targeted side. The field strength at 100% motor threshold varies by individual and can also be affected by medications and substances that impact neuronal excitability (Hallett, 2007). During treatment, pulse intensity is selected based on the desired outcome, which can be related directly to the estimated percentage of motor threshold needed. However, the neurophysiological effects of field strength when coupled with frequency remain poorly understood.

INTENSITY OF TREATMENT

Ultimately the goal of rTMS is to induce persisting neuromodulatory changes that lead to improvement in neuropsychiatric symptoms. It is unclear how often in a week treatments are required to induce the desired changes. For depression, treatments are usually given five times a week. In most PTSD trials, treatments mirrored this frequency, ranging from three to five treatments each week. It is possible that the number of pulses, stimulus intensity, and total duration of a treatment course may change this requirement. Further study is needed to determine what is most practical

for the patients and treatment facilities, while simultaneously being most facile at inducing improvement. These studies could include efforts to relate dosing parameters
to the intensity of symptoms and outcome measures, as well as to determine whether
more intensive delivery, such as multiple sessions a day, would prove beneficial.

DELIVERY OF DIFFERENT TMS REGIMENS

Several theories have helped shape rTMS techniques for PTSD. Although magnetic
flux will penetrate 2 to 3.5 cm beneath the skull, activation of neurons in the region
beneath the coil can have wider effects through brain network connectivity. For example, stimulation of the dorsolateral prefrontal cortex (DLPFC) results in changes
in the anterior cingulate, a structure well beyond the direct reach of the magnetic
field (Hernandez-Ribas et al., 2013). Activation of network connections between
brain regions that cannot typically be reached by rTMS can extend the impact of
treatment and provide more options for therapeutic intervention in individuals with
PTSD. The neuroanatomic specificity of PTSD symptoms also lends itself to more
accurate targeting of the treatment. Hyperactivity of the right hemisphere suggests
that low-frequency inhibitory stimulation may play a role in regulating PTSD symptomatology. It may be possible to use rTMS stimulation to generate secondary modulatory effects within the mood regulatory network. The medial prefrontal cortex
(mPFC) is, therefore, a particularly attractive target given its modulatory effects on
the amygdala and its role in the fear response, which is hyperresponsive in individuals with PTSD.

REGIONAL RESPONSES TO TMS

The lateralization of PTSD responses to TMS is an intriguing phenomenon that
led to additional investigations to identify more clearly, central nervous system
regionally specific responses to trauma and to determine the most efficacious locations for TMS therapy (Table 5.1). Positron emission tomographic analysis
revealed increased blood flow in right-side limbic and paralimbic regions in patients with PTSD when presented with traumatic scripts compared with neutral
scripts (Shin et al., 1997). Right-side TMS application to the DLPFC resulted in
both a global and a right-side decrease in cortical hypermetabolism, as evaluated
via fluorodeoxyglucose–positron emission tomography, and was associated with
a reduction in core PTSD symptoms (McCann et al., 1998). Using paired TMS
pulses, the interval between the two pulses results in a motor threshold stimulation dependent on γ-aminobutyric acid and glutamate tone reflected in short-latency

TABLE 5.1 Efficacious Locations for TMS Therapy

Study Reference, Type	N	Type of TMS	Trauma Type	Outcome Measure	Primary Outcomes
Figure-8 coil					
Boggio et al. (2010), randomized clinical trial	30	1. Active high-frequency to left DLPFC 2. Active high-frequency to right DLPFC 3. Sham rTMS	PTSD: 6 assaults, 5 cases of sexual abuse, 15 cases of death or severe disease of relative, 4 cases of psychological distress/perceived physical harm	TOP-8, PCL-5, HAM-A, HAM-D	Both active rTMS conditions decreased PTSD symptoms significantly, but right-side rTMS had a greater improvement compared with left. Mood scores improved for left-side treatment only ($p < .001$). Anxiety scores improved with right-side treatment only ($p < .01$). Improvement continued at 3-month follow-up.
Rosenberg et al. (2002), open label	12	1. rTMS to left DLPFC at 1 Hz 2. rTMS to left DLPRC at 5 Hz	Comorbid PTSD and major depression	SCID-C, HAM-D, POMS, USC-REMT, MISS	Both groups had improvements in depressive symptoms. Both groups had a modest improvement in PTSD symptoms 2 months after rTMS.
McCann et al. (1998), case study	2	1. Right frontal region (exact region unreported) at 1 Hz	Patient 1: more than 12 years of refractory depression and comorbid PTSD Patient 2: a 2.5-year history of PTSD secondary to a shooting incident	MPSS-SR, PET scan	Patient 1: PTSD decreased significantly during week 4 only ($p = .05$). Decreases in regional cerebral glucose metabolic rates were noted, with more prominent decreases for the right hemisphere. Patient 2: PTSD decreased significantly during weeks 2, 3, and 5 ($p < .01$). Also, the patient experienced decreases in regional cerebral glucose metabolic rates, with more prominent decreases for the right hemisphere. Both patients' symptoms returned to baseline 1 month after treatment discontinuation.

H-coil

| Isserles et al. (2013), randomized clinical trial with cross-over design | 30 | 1. EXP-STIM: DTMS on PFC after script imagery of traumatic experience followed by neutral event
2. NOEXP-STIM: DTMS on PFC after imagery of positive experience followed by a neutral event
3. EXP-SHAM: Sham DTMS on PFC after imagery of traumatic experience followed by neutral event | PTSD | CAPS, PSS-SR, HRSD-24, BDI-II, heart rate, skin conductance | EXP-STIM group had a significantly improved intrusion component of CAPS ($p < .05$).
Response was achieved by 44% ($n = 9$) of the EXP-STIM group, 12.5% ($n = 1$) of the NOEXP-STIM group, and 0% of the EXP-SHAM group.
Significant improvements on the PSS-SR, HRSD-24, and BDI-II were demonstrated only by the EXP-STIM group.
Heart rate attenuated throughout the treatment for the EXP-STIM group ($p = .042$). |

(continued)

TABLE 5.1 Continued

Study Reference, Type	N	Type of TMS	Trauma Type	Outcome Measure	Primary Outcomes
Angular shape, 14-in. diameter					
Grisaru et al. (1998), open label	10	1. Slow TMS to each side of motor cortex	PTSD: 7 accidents, 1 assault, 2 combat reactions	CGI, IES, SCL-90, background questionnaire	CGI and SCL-90 somatization subscale was lower significantly from baseline to 24 hours after TMS ($p < .05$). IES avoidance improvements continued up to 1 week after receiving TMS treatment ($p < .05$). The SCL-90 anxiety subscale showed improvements only at the 24-hour and 28-day time points ($p < .05$).

BDI-II, Beck Depression Inventory-II; CAPS, Clinician-Administered PTSD Scale; CGI, Clinical Global Impression; DLPFC, dorsolateral prefrontal cortex; DTMS, deep TMS; EXP-SHAM, Exposure-Sham; EXP-STIM, Exposure-Stimulation; HAM-A, Hamilton Anxiety Rating Scale; HAM-D, Hamilton Depression Rating Scale; HRSD-24, Hamilton Rating Scale for Depression-24 Items; IES, Impact of Event Scale; MISS, Mississippi Scale of Combat Severity; MPSS-SR, Modified PTSD Symptom Scale; NOEXP-STIM, No Exposure-Stimulation; PCL-5, PTSD Checklist for DSM-5; PET, positron emission tomography; PFC, prefrontal cortex; PSS-SR, PTSD Symptom Scale–Self-Report Version; POMS, Profile of Mood States; PTSD, posttraumatic stress disorder; rTMS, repetitive TMS; SCID-C, Structured Clinical Interview for DSM-IV Axis I Disorders–Clinician Version; SCL-90, Symptom Checklist-90; TMS, transcranial magnetic stimulation; TOP-8, Treatment Outcome PTSD Scale-8; USC-REMT, University of Southern California Repeatable Episodic Memory Test.

intracortical inhibition and long-latency intracortical inhibition, respectively. This paired pulse technique has suggested patients with PTSD have global decreases in γ-aminobutyric acid-ergic tone and increased glutamatergic tone in the right hemisphere (Rossi et al., 2006). These preliminary clinical results and functional neurological studies showed that right-side structures may be a viable target for direct modulation in patients with PTSD.

Several studies have added evidence that stimulation of the right DLPFC may be associated more closely with improvement in PTSD symptoms than the left side (Berlim & Van Den Eynde, 2014; Karsen et al., 2014) In a direct comparison, Boggio et al. (2010) established that right-side treatment was more effective at reducing core symptoms of PTSD than left-side treatment. Rosenberg et al. (2002) found little benefit in improvement of PTSD symptoms with 1-Hz or 5-Hz stimulation of the left DLPFC, but depressive symptoms did improve in both groups (Rosenberg et al., 2002). Berlim and Van Den Eynde (2014) conducted a meta-analysis of three published randomized, double-blind, and sham-controlled studies that used rTMS over the DLPFC for treatment of PTSD. Demonstrating improvement over baseline clinician-reported ($p < .001$) and self-reported ($p < .001$) PTSD symptoms, this analysis determined that right DLPFC rTMS is favored over left DLPFC rTMS. Furthermore, right DLFPC rTMS improved measures of anxiety ($p = .02$) and depression ($p = .001$) when compared with baseline values.

Karsen et al. (2014) reported a meta-analysis of the effectiveness of rTMS for the treatment of PTSD. The three studies included in the meta-analysis provided five treatment arms to be analyzed: low frequency (1 Hz, right DLPFC), high frequency (10 Hz, right DLPFC), right DLPFC, left DLPFC, and double-blind placebo (low frequency, 1 Hz on right DLPFC vs. sham). Overall, for all five treatment arms, Hedges *g* effect sizes ranged from 0.73 to 3.78, which are indicative of a large effect attributable to the treatment. All treatment arms, with the exception of the low-frequency arm, demonstrated a significant benefit for the use of rTMS as a treatment for PTSD. Depressive symptoms were also evaluated, and again the low-frequency group was the only treatment arm that did not display improvement; the Hedges *g* effect sizes ranged from 0.83 to 3.6, which are indicative of a large effect attributable to the treatment. Based on these analyses, Karsen et al. (2014) suggested that right-side treatment may be more efficacious for the treatment of PTSD than left-side treatment.

In examining the efficacy of rTMS, Wahbeh et al. (2014) conducted a systemic review of the use of complementary and alternative medicine as a treatment of PTSD, which included an evaluation of four rTMS trials. Quality assessment methodology was applied based on the Cochrane Risk of Bias Tool and the Quality Assessment Tool, with each studying being interpreted as positive, mixed, negative, or neutral based on the PTSD treatment outcomes. Based on these criteria, rTMS received a grade A, which suggests strong scientific evidence for this treatment modality for PTSD.

Although stimulation of the DLPFC appears to offer some benefit in core PTSD symptoms, neural network connectivity complicates the physiological response to treatment, and likely its effects are downstream from the target area. The DLPFC influences deeper brain structures that may be involved in many cognitive and behavioral functions relevant to PTSD (Berlim & Van Den Eynde, 2014; McNally, 2006; Moore et al., 2009). This concept of stimulating an area amenable to rTMS therapy to influence downstream neuronal regions is shared with another possible target: the mPFC.

The mPFC has demonstrated reduced activation in individuals with PTSD. Furthermore, treatments associated with activation of the mPFC, including high-frequency TMS combined with brief exposure therapy, improved PTSD symptom severity significantly, most specifically the intrusive subscale of the Clinician-Administered PTSD Scale (Isserles et al., 2013; Shin & Handwerger, 2009). This outcome may be attributable to the regulatory control exerted by the mPFC over the amygdala, for which functional neuroimaging has shown a role in acquired fear responses (Shin & Handwerger, 2009).

In summary, both the DLPFC and mPFC are potentially viable targets for rTMS stimulation. The stimulation frequency, motor threshold intensity, total number of pulses, and total treatment time require further clarification; but, despite some inconsistency in the trials, meta-analyses suggest an overall favorable benefit to PTSD symptoms.

DURATION OF RESPONSE

The duration of improvement in PTSD symptoms following treatment with rTMS is not well understood. The ultimate goal of treatment is a lasting resolution of symptoms, or perhaps a resolution that requires only occasional maintenance sessions of rTMS treatment; unfortunately, most studies have only short-term follow-up assessments performed at 4 weeks and occasionally at 8 weeks. The contradictory nature of the research published thus far suggests that further investigation is needed. Rosenberg et al. (2002) demonstrated a delayed response of a 6% reduction in PTSD symptoms at 2-month follow-up examinations. In contrast, Gisaru et al. (1998) and McCann et al. (1998) separately reported returns to baseline symptoms within 4 weeks of treatment cessation. Interpreting these disparate outcomes is difficult because the three studies of low-frequency stimulation used different courses of treatment and different treatment intensities. At this time, there is insufficient evidence to determine whether there is a lasting effect after rTMS treatment. Further research looking into longer time frames would be beneficial to determine the long-term benefits and potential long-term side effects, as well as the potential need for maintenance treatment, as is seen in electroconvulsive therapy treatment of severe depression.

RESEARCH CHALLENGES

Developing clinical recommendations from the current body of published literature is challenging. The limited number of studies with differing treatment regimens among the studies hinders a clear interpretation of the data. Although variability in treatment does allow consideration of different treatment options, it limits the amount of data that can be evaluated for one specific treatment regimen and does not allow for absolute contradictions or confirmations of results. The nature of the treatment itself also makes experimental design a challenge. For example, greater than 50% of the participants in one study were able to identify the sham or actual treatment delivery accurately (Berlim et al., 2013). Another concern is the assessment of comorbidities. Many individuals with PTSD experience depression and anxiety, but it is difficult to evaluate changes in symptoms that could in fact be attributable to comorbid conditions and not PTSD. Development of an effective treatment regimen will be limited by the current lack of knowledge about the neurobiological mechanisms of PTSD, although the use of TMS could be a valuable tool for identifying some of the mechanisms of injury. Despite these limitations, the preponderance of the evidence suggests that rTMS is effective for the treatment of PTSD.

CURRENT LIMITATIONS

TMS offers a novel treatment option for psychiatric disorders including PTSD in that its mechanism of action appears to be different than either medications or traditional psychotherapy. In addition, the likelihood of adverse side effects is low, with the most common being headaches, neck aches, or tinnitus. The largest safety concern is the very low risk of TMS treatment inducing a seizure (Hallett, 2007). The evaluation of the general clinical potential of TMS is still in its infancy, although the efficacy as a treatment for depression has been consistent and convincing. Research investigating the use of TMS as a treatment for PTSD remains limited. Advances in coil design have facilitated the stimulation of deeper regions of the brain; however, an inability to target subcortical regions specifically without affecting cortical regions limits current efforts (Taylor, 2006). In the future, the development of various coil arrangements may overcome this limitation by enabling magnetic field vector interplay.

Providers must also be aware of the limitations based on contraindications for various patient populations. People with electrical implanted devices, such as pacemakers, must be excluded because of the electromagnetic changes TMS induces. Treatment is also contraindicated in patients with metal implants in their head or neck region (Hallett, 2007).

In addition to research investigating the engineering aspects of coil design, more stimulation parameters need to be observed and explored on a large number of diverse patients, and their long-term therapeutic effects documented with controlled scales. These efforts may allow tailoring of TMS to address the specific symptoms affecting specific patient subpopulations. In time, TMS limitations will become fewer as parameters such as coil shape, frequency, intensity, periodization, stimulation site, and number of sessions are optimized for each therapy. As TMS continues to develop, it is likely to have a great impact on future noninvasive brain stimulation and neuromodulation techniques.

CONCLUSION

PTSD is a complex illness with an incompletely understood pathophysiology. It rarely occurs in isolation from other psychiatric morbidities. Furthermore, PTSD commonly fails to remit completely with standard therapies. Preliminary clinical trials investigating brain stimulation with TMS suggest a novel alternative mechanism for treatment of PTSD that may reduce the need for polypharmacy and may diminish associated systemic side effects.

There is evidence supporting the use of TMS both alone and as adjunctive therapy to exposure-based psychotherapy, but the weight of evidence and discrepancies in pulse sequences and treatment locations require further research before widespread clinical adoption. In addition, the overhead required for maintaining a TMS device and sustaining proficiency in its use support TMS treatment delivery at centers with experience using this form of neuromodulation. At the time of this writing, cost for treatment delivery and labor intensity for both the patient and provider would suggest this therapy be targeted to those with moderate to severe disease and those who have failed or chose not to pursue psychotherapy or pharmacotherapy. Any TMS treatment plan should be part of a comprehensive clinical program tailored to maximize recovery and is best implemented by providers familiar with the possible treatments for assisting patient recovery.

KEY POINTS

- Exposure therapy, a commonly used psychotherapy for the treatment of PTSD, may trigger intense emotions that some patients are unable to tolerate and may lead to early discontinuation of treatment.
- Two selective SSRIs are FDA-approved for the treatment of PTSD, although limited efficacy and poor compliance resulting from side effects constrain their utility.
- TMS is a noninvasive brain stimulation technique that has shown efficacy for neurological and psychiatric conditions, with a low likelihood of adverse side effects, and may therefore be a potential alternative or complementary treatment option for individuals with PTSD.
- TMS modulates neuronal activity in a targeted brain region to achieve excitation or inhibition, depending on the parameters of the stimulation.
- Delivery of TMS incorporates several variables, including the type and configuration of the coil, the frequency of stimulus delivery, the duration of pulse sequence, interstimulation rest periods, the total number of pulses delivered, the strength of the magnetic field delivery, and the regularity of scheduled treatment delivery in a week.
- Preliminary clinical results and functional studies showed that right-sided structures, in particular, the right DLPFC may be a viable target for direct modulation in patients with PTSD.
- The mPFC may be another target of TMS, especially when coupled with exposure-based therapy, given its modulatory effects on the amygdala and its role in the fear response.
- At this time, relative permanence of beneficial effects following a TMS treatment program is unclear and further research is required.
- Making a clear determination of the efficacy of TMS as a treatment for PTSD is limited by the use of differing treatment regimens in the few studies investigating these phenomena.
- Development of an effective treatment regimen is limited by the current lack of knowledge about the neurobiological mechanisms of PTSD.
- TMS therapy has shown some evidence for efficacy in PTSD, but optimal treatment locations and pulse sequences need further clarification before it could be considered for wide-scale clinical adoption.

DISCLAIMER

The views expressed in this article are those of the authors and do not reflect the official policy of the Departments of Army/Navy/Air Force, Department of Defense, or U.S. government. The use of trade names in this publication does not imply endorsement by the authors or the Department of Army/Navy/Air Force, Department of Defense, or U.S. government, nor does it imply criticism of similar products or devices not mentioned. This study did not receive external direct or indirect funding. The authors declare no financial, commercial, or other conflicts of interest.

REFERENCES

Bakker, N., Shahab, S., Giacobbe, P., Blumberger, D. M., Daskalakis, Z. J., Kennedy, S. H., & Downar, J. (2015). rTMS of the dorsomedial prefrontal cortex for major depression: safety, tolerability, effectiveness, and outcome predictors for 10 Hz versus intermittent theta-burst stimulation. *Brain Stimul, 8*(2), 208–215.

Benedek, D. M., Wynn, G. (2011). Epidemiology. In D. M. Benedek, Wynn, G (Eds.), *Clinical management of PTSD* (pp. 11–43). Arlington, VA: American Psychiatric Publishing.

Berlim, M. T., Broadbent, H. J., & Van den Eynde, F. (2013). Blinding integrity in randomized sham-controlled trials of repetitive transcranial magnetic stimulation for major depression: a systematic review and meta-analysis. *Int J Neuropsychopharmacology, 16*(5), 1173–1181.

Berlim, M. T., & Van Den Eynde, F. (2014). Repetitive transcranial magnetic stimulation over the dorsolateral prefrontal cortex for treating posttraumatic stress disorder: an exploratory meta-analysis of randomized, double-blind and sham-controlled trials. *Can J Psychiatry, 59*(9), 487–496.

Boggio, P. S., Rocha, M., Oliveira, M. O., Fecteau, S., Cohen, R. B., Campanha, C., . . . Fregni, F. (2010). Noninvasive brain stimulation with high-frequency and low-intensity repetitive transcranial magnetic stimulation treatment for posttraumatic stress disorder. *J Clin Psychiatry, 71*(8), 992–999.

Bolognini, N., & Ro, T. (2010). Transcranial magnetic stimulation: disrupting neural activity to alter and assess brain function. *J Neurosci, 30*(29), 9647–9650.

Deng, Z. D., Lisanby, S. H., & Peterchev, A. V. (2013). Electric field depth–focality tradeoff in transcranial magnetic stimulation: simulation comparison of 50 coil designs. *Brain Stimul, 6*(1), 1–13.

George, M. S., Raman, R., Benedek, D. M., Pelic, C. G., Grammer, G. G., Stokes, K. T., . . . Stein, M. B. (2014). A two-site pilot randomized 3 day trial of high dose left prefrontal repetitive transcranial magnetic stimulation (rTMS) for suicidal inpatients. *Brain Stimul, 7*(3), 421–431.

Grisaru, N., Amir, M., Cohen, H., & Kaplan, Z. (1998). Effect of transcranial magnetic stimulation in posttraumatic stress disorder: a preliminary study. *Biol Psychiatry, 44*(1), 52–55.

Group, T. M. o. P.-T. S. W. (2010). *VA/DoD clinical practice guideline for management of posttraumatic stress.* Washington DC.

Hallett, M. (2007). Transcranial magnetic stimulation: a primer. *Neuron, 55*(2), 187–199.

Hernandez-Ribas, R., Deus, J., Pujol, J., Segalas, C., Vallejo, J., Menchon, J. M., . . . Soriano-Mas, C. (2013). Identifying brain imaging correlates of clinical response to repetitive transcranial magnetic stimulation (rTMS) in major depression. *Brain Stimul, 6*(1), 54–61.

Horvath, J. C., Perez, J. M., Forrow, L., Fregni, F., & Pascual-Leone, A. (2011). Transcranial magnetic stimulation: a historical evaluation and future prognosis of therapeutically relevant ethical concerns. *J Med Ethics, 37*(3), 137–143.

Isserles, M., Shalev, A. Y., Roth, Y., Peri, T., Kutz, I., Zlotnick, E., & Zangen, A. (2013). Effectiveness of deep transcranial magnetic stimulation combined with a brief exposure procedure in posttraumatic stress disorder: a pilot study. *Brain Stimul, 6*(3), 377–383.

Karsen, E. F., Watts, B. V., & Holtzheimer, P. E. (2014). Review of the effectiveness of transcranial magnetic stimulation for post-traumatic stress disorder. *Brain Stimul, 7*(2), 151–157.

McCann, U. D., Kimbrell, T. A., Morgan, C. M., Anderson, T., Geraci, M., Benson, B. E., . . . Post, R. M. (1998). Repetitive transcranial magnetic stimulation for posttraumatic stress disorder. *Arch Gen Psychiatry, 55*(3), 276–279.

McNally, R. J. (2006). Cognitive abnormalities in post-traumatic stress disorder. *Trends Cogn Sci, 10*(6), 271–277.

Moore, D. F., Jerusalem, A., Nyein, M., Noels, L., Jaffee, M. S., & Radovitzky, R. A. (2009). Computational biology: modeling of primary blast effects on the central nervous system. *Neuroimage, 47*(Suppl 2), T10–T20.

Novakovic, V., Sher, L., Lapidus, K. A., Mindes, J., Golier, A. J., & Yehuda, R. (2011). Brain stimulation in posttraumatic stress disorder. *Eur J Psychotraumatol, 2*.

O'Reardon, J. P., Peshek, A. D., Romero, R., & Cristancho, P. (2006). Neuromodulation and transcranial magnetic stimulation (TMS): a 21st century paradigm for therapeutics in psychiatry. *Psychiatry (Edgmont), 3*(1), 30–40.

Rosenberg, P. B., Mehndiratta, R. B., Mehndiratta, Y. P., Wamer, A., Rosse, R. B., & Balish, M. (2002). Repetitive transcranial magnetic stimulation treatment of comorbid posttraumatic stress disorder and major depression. *J Neuropsychiatry Clin Neurosci, 14*(3), 270–276.

Rossi, S., Cappa, S. F., Ulivelli, M., De Capua, A., Bartalini, S., & Rossini, P. M. (2006). rTMS for PTSD: induced merciful oblivion or elimination of abnormal hypermnesia? *Behav Neurol, 17*(3–4), 195–199.

Shin, L. M., & Handwerger, K. (2009). Is posttraumatic stress disorder a stress-induced fear circuitry disorder? *J Trauma Stress, 22*(5), 409–415.

Shin, L. M., Kosslyn, S. M., McNally, R. J., Alpert, N. M., Thompson, W. L., Rauch, S. L., . . . Pitman, R. K. (1997). Visual imagery and perception in posttraumatic stress disorder: a positron emission tomographic investigation. *Arch Gen Psychiatry, 54*(3), 233–241.

Taylor, S. (2006). *Clinician's guide to PTSD: a cognitive–behavioral approach.* New York, NY: Guilford Press.

Wahbeh, H., Senders, A., Neuendorf, R., & Cayton, J. (2014). Complementary and alternative medicine for posttraumatic stress disorder symptoms: a systematic review. *J Evid Based Complementary Altern Med, 19*(3), 161–175.

Wassermann, E. M. (1998). Risk and safety of repetitive transcranial magnetic stimulation: report and suggested guidelines from the International Workshop on the Safety of Repetitive Transcranial Magnetic Stimulation, June 5–7, 1996. *Electroencephalogr Clin Neurophysiol, 108*(1), 1–16.

SIX

Acupuncture

DANIEL J. BALOG, ROBERT KOFFMAN,

AND JOSEPH M. HELMS

PEOPLE WHO ACQUIRE POSTTRAUMATIC STRESS DISORDER (PTSD) AFTER experiencing a traumatic event endure a constellation of debilitating symptoms, including intrusion, avoidance, negative mood alteration, and marked increases in reactivity (American Psychiatric Association, 2013). They have difficulty falling or staying asleep and often have comorbid physical and pain-related diagnoses secondary to their trauma. Despite evolving definitions and measures, estimates of prevalence of lifetime PTSD in the U.S. population have remained quite consistent since the advent of the *Diagnostic and Statistical Manual of Mental Disorders* (DSM), third edition, revised (Norris & Slone, 2013). In civilian populations, lifetime DSM, third edition, revised, PTSD prevalence rates of 9.2% (Breslau et al., 1996); DSM, fourth edition, PTSD prevalence rates of 6.8% (Kessler et al., 2008); and DSM, fifth edition, PTSD estimate rates of 5.4% (Miller, 2012) have been reported. In U.S. military populations, prevalence rates as high as 17% after combat deployments have been reported (Hoge et al., 2004). Importantly, persons with PTSD experience a greater prevalence of other psychiatric and physical comorbid conditions, including mood, substance use, and pain disorders (Wahbeh et al., 2014).

The complex psychopathology of PTSD and its frequently associated comorbid conditions result in a wide variety of clinical presentations. In addition, reductionist practices of problem-oriented medical care result in multiprong, segregated treatment paths that add further complexity to symptom constellations that may be conceptualized as unrelated by patient and care providers alike. As in many mental health disorders, one size does not fit all, and patients have unique perspectives, constitutions, and perpetuating factors that must be recognized. Many who need PTSD treatment often do not receive it secondary to embarrassment, stigma, or lack of trust in mental health providers (Hoge et al., 2004). Some patients decline exposure therapies whereas others resist psychopharmacological interventions secondary to fear of side effects or addiction. Administrative and legal processes relating to the traumatic event (e.g., disability assessments or criminal prosecutions of alleged perpetrators of an assault) may be ongoing, and patients may be coping quietly by misusing or abusing legal or illicit substances. It can be difficult to view the patient as a whole when there are so many factors involved in the treatment equation.

Acupuncture is recognized by patients and professionals to be an effective augmentor to western medical treatments for PTSD and associated symptoms (Lee et al., 2012; Pilkington et al., 2007). Although the volume of high-quality randomized trials evaluating acupuncture is sparse, and many studies have been criticized for bias, design flaws, and/or lack of placebo control (Kim et al., 2013; Vincent et al., 1995), there is increasing recognition of clinical efficacy for acupuncture. The mechanisms by which acupuncture impacts PTSD and commonly associated symptoms are not fully understood, but there are conceptual, basic science, biological, and clinical data to support treatment efficacy and to inform further avenues of research (Cabyoglu et al., 2006; Hollifield, 2011; Hui et al., 2000; Kaptchuk, 2002).

Medical acupuncture, the hybrid practice of acupuncture by physicians trained in western medicine, engages the patient as a whole and complements perfectly modern western medical treatment of PTSD and associated symptoms. Acupuncture includes a heterogeneous group of therapies, which include full-body, auricular, and scalp acupuncture, during which solid needles are inserted into select body points (Helms et al., 2001). During needling, acupuncture practitioners frequently obtain the effect of "De Qi" or "Qi" (pronounced "CHē"), which is a sensation that is described as a dull, aching, or full by patients. De Qi is not typically painful, sharp, or electrical, and when obtained, a skilled practitioner can often sense a "needle grab," indicating a point has been activated. In addition to acupuncture, traditional Chinese medicine also involves a broad range of medical practices, including herbal prescriptions (see Chapter 7, Alternative Medicine Pharmacology), massage, and cupping, which share foundational concepts.

The concept of Qi describes a vivifying force circulating through body channels to protect, nourish, and animate living beings. Although modern western medicine does not designate a term to describe this force, physicians address the outward manifestations of this dimension routinely in their patients. Physical examination entries in charts frequently describe the "brightness" of a patient's eyes, the "color" of their face, the "texture" of skin, or the "strength" of pulses. In clinical acupuncture, these observations describe the activity of Qi in a patient's constitution and presentation. The systematic qualification, quantification, and movement of Qi are central to acupuncture diagnosis and treatment planning (Helms, 2007a).

For centuries, Chinese traditional medicine has recognized an individual's constitution as an essential factor in the outward expression of illness. Modern western medicine is rooted similarly in the understanding that genetics are key to understanding illness. In medical acupuncture, treatment plans incorporate acupuncture with modern interventions to meet optimally the needs of patients. Practitioners integrate their approach and, from acupuncture perspective, view an individual's constitution through the lens of "structural biopsychotypes" that organize human characteristics along a continuum. Biopsychotypes are an outward expression of an individual's constitution as well as a specific organ and its corresponding energy channel. When a practitioner obtains De Qi during needling, a point is activated and energy in an associated channel is influenced in a way that can be beneficial (Helms, 2007b).

Patient problems, if recognized early, can often be addressed by activating the energy of channels, or meridians, that govern the organ or body region. Chronic and more complex problems often require consideration of an individual's biopsychotype to inform treatment selection and to determine how to impact energy circulation optimally in a governing meridian. Determining which meridians to target requires careful evaluation of both the presenting problem and an individual's biopsychotype. This concept is fundamental to understanding why formulaic point selection in medical acupuncture is frequently effective, and also why individually tailored treatment protocols are often needed to address patient needs comprehensively.

MECHANISMS AND TYPES OF ACUPUNCTURE

Modern practitioners of acupuncture, particularly those with medical qualifications, conceptualize acupuncture in ways that embrace both traditional and mechanistic traditions (White, 2009). Although the local and central mechanisms by which acupuncture affects anxiety, depression, acute pain, chronic pain, and even tissue repair are not fully understood, there is substantial basic and clinical science support for incorporating medical acupuncture into modern allopathic practice.

Annually, approximately 3 million Americans seek acupuncture interventions to augment medial care (Barnes, 2008), with chronic pain being the most frequent treatment target (Sherman, 2005). Acupuncture, long known to have physiological effects of analgesia (Peets, 1978; Zhang, 2004), and being increasingly recognized as a safe and effective intervention for chronic pain (Vickers et al., 2012), exerts its often lasting effects via mechanisms not yet fully understood.

In the case of psychoemotional disturbances, including anxiety, depression, and PTSD, the theoretical foundation for acupuncture is rooted similarly in tenets that embrace both modern understanding of anatomy and physiology, and principles centered in a millennia-long tradition of acupuncture in the Orient. There is an abundance of literature demonstrating biological effects of acupuncture in systems implicated in PTSD pathology (Hollifield, 2011). Neuroimaging and physiological studies, for example, have demonstrated cortical, limbic, and autonomic nervous system effects of acupuncture (Dhond, 2007; Hui et al., 2000; Kong et al., 2002). Responses in various central nervous system targets, in both animals and humans, have been shown to correlate with needle location (Haker et al., 2000), frequency of stimulation, and type of acupuncture (Kong et al., 2002; Napadow, 2005).

When treating patients with psychoemotional disturbances in general, and when clinically managing PTSD patients in particular, practitioners have their best successes when care is informed by current western medical treatment guidelines, and then augmented with acupuncture approaches that integrate patient needs and clinical responses (Helms, 2007b).

Body Acupuncture

Body acupuncture is a complex and elegant discipline that requires the professional to evaluate the patient and then implement an individualized treatment plan that combines traditional point locations, combinations, and approaches. There are a number of classic point combinations (e.g., Four Gates, Seven Dragons) that are commonly used for patients with acute and chronic psychoemotional symptoms (Helms, 2007a).

From an acupuncture perspective, an individual's constitution is impacted, and reflected, by the balance of energy that flows continually through channels coursing through muscles, and to and from organs. These channels are understood to exist as bilateral, symmetrical pairs of subcircuits. When acupuncture practitioners needle a specific acupuncture point and obtains the De Qi sensation, they activate the energy in that point and influence energy circulation in the channel where the point is located (Helms, 2007a).

One traditional point combination formula called *Four Gates*—so named because four needles are placed distally in both the upper and lower extremities—stimulates all 12 energy meridians. One of the oldest and most powerful point combinations, Four Gates is used for calming, centering, and activating homeostatic mechanisms of the body. When two midline head points are added, psychologically traumatized patients can experience rapid sense of calming and centering. This enhanced combination has been used in a multitude of clinical and military settings, including primary care clinics, hospital wards, battalion aid stations (BASs), tactical vehicles, passenger terminals, and "foxholes" (Koffman & Helms, 2013).

Another point combination, Seven Dragons, used for patients whose disturbances are deep seated or of long duration, impacts patients on a profound level. A combination of seven points, first on the back and then on the front of the body, at the same treatment, can assist in relieving the burden of traumatic images, memories, and emotions (Koffman & Helms, 2013). This treatment has provenance in the ancient lore of Chinese acupuncture in which mental illness was viewed as an invasion of malevolent entities or demons. A trusting relationship is essential when using this technique because it can catalyze an emotional release as part of the healing. As a result of this response, coauthor Koffman has invoked the phrase "Come for the needless; stay for the therapy," which describes in part why acupuncture, with its mind–body influences, integrates so well with western treatments of psychoemotional disturbances. Many patients, choosing to avoid the stigma associated with specialty mental heath, engage readily in acupuncture to address their symptoms. In a rather poetic explanation, one "activates the dragons to expel the demons" when using the Seven Dragons intervention (Helms, 2009).

Auricular Acupuncture

Auricular acupuncture, a development of modern French acupuncture, is based on a reflex somatotopic system organized on the surface of the external ear, one of many such microsystems in the body (Taillandier, 1989). Auricular acupuncture can be used effectively for a number of pain, organic, functional, and mental health-related syndromes, and can be done as an exclusive treatment or as a complement to full-body or scalp acupuncture (Helms, 2007a). The external auricle is accessed easily and, because of its unusual embryology, is structured from tissue originating from endodermal, mesodermal, and ectodermal layers (Oleson, 1996). Analogous to the cortical homunculus, wherein a "little man" depicts motor and somatosensory cortices, there is a somatotopic map of the external ear that depicts associated body systems (Wong, 1999). During the early 1950s, Paul Nogier in France undertook auricular charting, and assessed concordance between medical and auricular diagnoses to range between 75% and 92% in blinded assessments (Kroening, 1980; Nogier, 1978, 1980) (Figure 6.1).

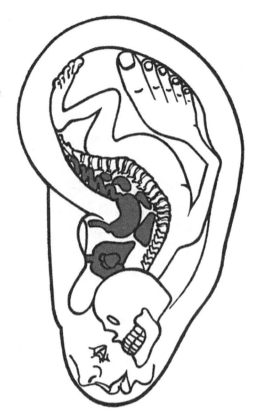

FIGURE 6.1 *Homunculus*

In the case of trauma or pain syndromes, scanning the ear with a battery-operated resistance measuring probe can further identify ear points that correspond to affected areas of the body (Oleson, 1996). Needling these specific zones modulates afferent nociceptive impulses traveling to the brain and, consequently, reduces trauma symptoms and/or the experience of pain (Niemtzow, 2007) (Helms, 2007a).

Points on the ear can be needled with fine acupuncture needles that are left in place for short period of time (e.g., <60 minutes), needled with indwelling studs that are left in place for a longer time (e.g., few days), or needled with very short, superficial needles attached to an adhesive dot (Helms, 2007a). Small commercial magnets, laser devices, and direct electrical stimulating devices may also be used to stimulate ear points (Kenyon, 1983–1985; Naeser, 1994). In addition to following prescribed treatment protocols, acupuncture physicians can scan the ear and needle active points that correspond to patient symptoms. For example, a patient experiencing chronic stress and sleep disturbances might benefit from a prescribed stress protocol plus the needling of points associated with insomnia. This approach could be applied similarly to patients experiencing pain, irritability, depression, or headaches (Figure 6.2).

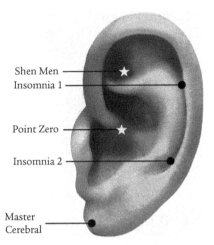

Shen Men
Insomnia 1

Point Zero

Insomnia 2

Master
Cerebral

FIGURE 6.2 *Insomnia Point Pattern*

Military medical acupuncture practitioners have recognized the unique applicability of auricular acupuncture in military populations. Auricular treatments have been used in a variety of deployed and operational environments where pain and sedative hypnotic class medications are less acceptable. Auricular treatments do not reduce performance, impair cognition, or lead to addiction. They can also be offered in austere environments where service members may need to remain in body armor and return to duty after treatment.

Auricular zones allow acupuncture needles to influence the mesodermal tissue of traumatized muscles and also provide easy access to ectodermal and intracranial structures. As a result, acupuncture practitioners have used specific point combinations to target symptoms that present commonly in their practices. One such combination is a collection of five points influencing structures to include the cingulate cortex and thalamic nuclei. The "battlefield acupuncture" combination has been used both in combination with other acupuncture therapies (Niemtzow, & Baxter, 2006) and as a first-line treatment for acute pain (Niemtzow, 2007) (Figure 6.3).

An auricular point combination used to target acute stress and PTSD is the auricular trauma protocol (ATP), which is a six-point collection that influences structures to include the hippocampus, amygdala, hypothalamus, prefrontal cortex, and parasympathetic nervous system.

In military and veteran populations, the ATP can be an early nonpharmacological intervention provided to patients who desire some distance and relief from their torment. Even in urgent and time-constrained practice environments, physicians can use the ATP as a safe and rapid intervention for acute stress symptoms. The ATP can be used as an exclusive treatment or as an adjunct for patients with mild traumatic brain injury (mTBI), acute stress, PTSD, and chronic pain (Figure 6.4).

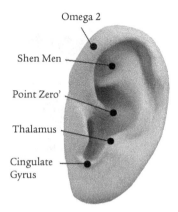

FIGURE 6.3 *Battlefield Acupuncture*

Chinese Scalp Acupuncture

Chinese scalp acupuncture (CSA), an acupuncture development emanating from the Peoples Republic of China, targets the scalp as another body region of somatotopic significance (Shanghai College of Traditional Medicine, 1981). Its practice involves sliding acupuncture needles in the loose connective tissue layer between the aponeurosis and epicranium. Practitioners target specific scalp zones overlying brain structures that influence pain, motor function, balance, vision, and speech. Depending on the problem being treated, CSA effects can be immediate and enduring, immediate and transient, or delayed (Figures 6.5 and 6.6).

CSA has been used to target both acute and chronic pain, and may sometimes be the only intervention required. The technique combines well with allopathic treatments, osteopathic interventions, and other acupuncture approaches. In PTSD, select scalp zones are needled to influence underlying intracranial structures that need rebalancing.

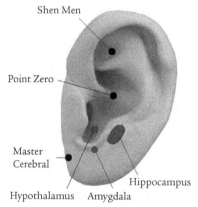

FIGURE 6.4 *Auricular Trauma Protocol*

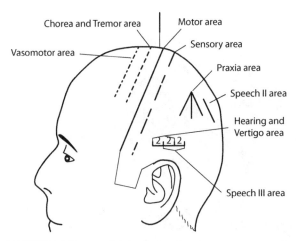

FIGURE 6.5 *Lateral Stimulation Areas*

For example, a patient suffering from traumatic memories and nightmares may receive a CSA treatment pattern over an identified temporal zone targeting hippocampal functions of memory retention and emotional experience integration, as well as amygdala-associated symptoms of irritability, anger, and aggression. Additional needles overlying the prefrontal cortex, orbitofrontal cortex, midline hypothalamus, and limbic structures can target symptoms of diminished focus, impaired executive functioning, and agitation. Needling CSA zones and traditional points can mollify a range of symptoms, including nightmares, thought intrusion, anxiety, fear, helplessness, and overstimulation of the hypothalamic–pituitary–adrenal axis. Additional studies are certainly indicated and, as in most other psychiatric interventions, results are influenced by patient constitution, symptom severity, and practitioner skill (Figures 6.7 and 6.8).

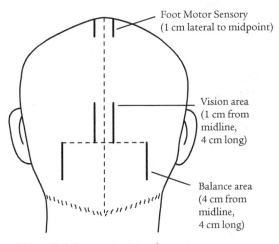

FIGURE 6.6 *Posterior Stimulation Areas*

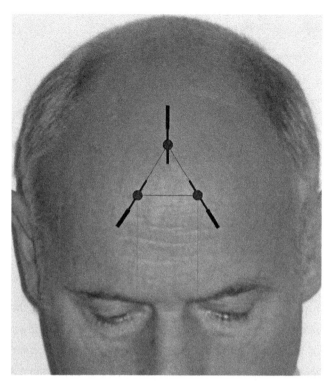

FIGURE 6.7 *Frontal Triangle*

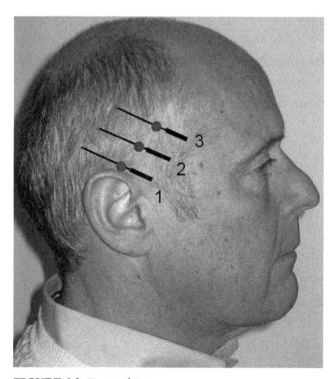

FIGURE 6.8 *Temporal Fan*

ACUPUNCTURE FOR PTSD
AND ASSOCIATED CONDITIONS

Acupuncture is a safe, accessible, nonstigmatizing treatment practice that has endured multiple millennia and, in recent years, has augmented modern medical treatment as well. Medical consumers, empowered by ready access to medical information and peers, have influenced this evolution with demands for new and effective treatments. Patients who experience trauma and anxiety spectrum disorders also experience a high degree of comorbid mood, substance, and pain disorders (Bradley et al., 2005). The following is a brief summary of evidence for acupuncture's impact on PTSD as well as comorbid symptoms commonly associated with PTSD as well as other mood, substance, and pain disorders.

Posttraumatic Stress Disorder

Errington-Evans (2011) examined the recent evidence base of articles supporting use of acupuncture in the treatment of anxiety-related disorders by conducting a literature review of all English-language articles published after 2000 and concluded, despite variability in a number of treatment factors, there were very real, positive outcomes obtained for patients with anxiety who were resistant to conventional interventions.

Hollifield et al. (2007) evaluated the efficacy of acupuncture for PTSD by randomizing 84 people to acupuncture treatment, group cognitive–behavioral therapy (CBT), or a wait-list control. The acupuncture intervention arm defined a standard minimum point prescription for all participants and, to replicate real-world practice, allowed practitioners to tailor treatments by choosing additional points based on patient characteristics, responses, and symptoms. This design is analogous to pharmacological studies that define a standard minimum-dose prescription for all participants and, to replicate real-world practice, allow clinicians to tailor treatments by modifying doses based on patient responses and symptoms. In an interesting contrast, practitioners of acupuncture, compared with practitioners of clinical psychopharmacology, have long understood the need factor individual patient characteristics as a factor in their treatment protocols.

The primary outcome measure for the study was change in PTSD symptoms based on the Posttraumatic Symptom Scale-Self Report (PSS-SR). Secondary outcomes included depression, anxiety, daily functioning, and treatment satisfaction assessment. The self-rated Hopkins Symptom Checklist-25 was used to assess symptoms of anxiety and depression, and the Sheehan Disability Inventory was used to assess impairment in the areas of work, social, and home/family life. Participant satisfaction for those randomized to acupuncture and CBT was assessed at the end of treatment using a 10-item rating scale (0 point, strongly disagree; 10 points, strongly agree) developed for the study using expert consensus methods.

Self-reported PTSD symptoms at baseline, the end of treatment, and at the 3-month follow-up revealed large treatment effects of acupuncture, similar in magnitude to group CBT, compared with wait-list controls. Simple effects analyses for those who completed treatment showed a significant reduction of PSS-SR scores from baseline to the end treatment in both the acupuncture group ($n = 19$) and the CBT group ($n = 21$), but not for the wait-list control group ($n = 21$). By the end of treatment, 68% (13 of 19 people) in the acupuncture group, 43% (9 of 21 people) in the CBT group, and 19% (4 of 21 people) in the wait-list control group had PSS-SR scores below the entry criterion level of 16 points. Parallel contrasts showed the reduction of PTSD symptoms for those who completed treatment with either acupuncture or CBT was maintained at the 3-month follow-up assessment. At 3 months, 68% ($n = 13$) in the acupuncture group remained below the entry criterion score of 16 points and 62% ($n = 13$) in the CBT group were below the entry criterion score. Secondary outcome findings were significant when comparing the acupuncture group versus the wait-list control group for depression, anxiety, and global impairment scores, as well as when comparing the CBT group versus the wait-list control group for depression, anxiety, and global impairment scores. Acupuncture and CBT patients expressed the same level of satisfaction with care on 7 of 10 survey items, including the global satisfaction with care item (a mean acupuncture rating of 9.2 points vs. a mean CBT rating of 9.7 on a 0- to 10-point scale, where 10 points signifies highest satisfaction).

Engel et al. (2014) randomized 55 service members with PTSD to usual PTSD care (UPC) versus UPC plus acupuncture. The acupuncture intervention consisted of 60-minute treatment sessions, twice weekly, for 4 weeks. Acupuncture treatments were selected based on simplicity, safety, and likely efficacy. The first four treatment sessions were standardized for all participants; the second four treatment sessions allowed acupuncturists flexibility to individualize based on standard diagnostic criteria. UPC was guided by existing standards outlined in the *VA/DoD Clinical Practice Guideline for Management of PTSD* (Group, 2012). Outcomes were assessed at baseline and at 4, 8, and 12 weeks using the PTSD Checklist and the Clinician-Administered PTSD Scale. Study results showed that mean improvement in PTSD severity was significantly greater among those receiving acupuncture than those receiving UPC (PTSD Checklist $\Delta = 19.8 \pm 13.3$ points vs. 9.7 ± 12.9 points, $p < .001$; Clinician-Administered PTSD Scale $\Delta = 35.0 \pm 20.26$ points vs. 10.9 ± 20.8 points, $p < .0001$).

In addition, acupuncture was associated with significantly greater improvement in secondary outcome measures of depression, pain, physical health functioning, and mental health functioning. For depression, participants showed a significant decrease in the mean Beck Depression Inventory, second edition (BDI-II), score in the acupuncture-with-UPC group from baseline to 4 weeks (22.3 ± 10.7 points vs. 12.5 ± 9.8 points; t250 =7.7, $p < .0001$), and in maintenance of treatment gains at 8 weeks (13.5 ± 12.0 points; t174 =5.7, $p < .0001$) and 12 weeks (12.0 ± 13.4 points; t160 = 11.3, $p < .0001$). In contrast, among those in the UPC-alone group, BDI-II scores exhibited much smaller changes. For pain, among participants receiving acupuncture with UPC, the mean Numerical Rating Scale score of acupuncture participants dropped significantly from baseline to 4 weeks (4.3 ± 2.6 points vs. 3.4 ± 2.0 points; t252 = 3.3, $p < .001$), and maintained the reduction at 8 weeks (2.5 ± 2.0 points; t216 = 6.0, $p < .0001$) and 12 weeks (2.8 ± 2.2 points; t211 = 4.9, $p < .0001$). In contrast, the Numerical Rating Scale score increased in the UPC-alone group at 4, 8, and 12 weeks. For mental health functioning, the mental health component summary score on the Short Form-36 for those in the acupuncture-with-UPC group showed significant improvement from baseline to 12 weeks (27.6 ± 13.7 points vs. 40.7 ± 17.6 points; t158 = 6.0, $p < .0001$) as it did for UPC participants (28.8 ± 11.2 points vs. 35.7 ± 12.0 points; t245 = 4.8, $p < .0001$). For physical health functioning, the physical health functioning composite score on the Short Form-36 for those in the acupuncture-with-UPC group evidenced modest improvement (47.5 ± 8.7 points vs. 50.1 ± 9.5 points; t180 = 2.1, $p < .05$) compared with the UPC-alone group.

Depression

Depression is a frequent comorbid condition in patients impacted by PTSD (Bradley et al., 2005; Hoge et al., 2004, 2008). Antidepressants are a first-line treatment for depression (VA/DoD Clinical Practice Guideline, 2009); yet, inadequate response (Fava, 2003) and poor medication adherence is a common problem (Effective Health Care Bulletin, 2005) (VA/DoD Clinical Practice Guideline, 2010). Patients are often concerned about overreliance on medications and frequently seek nonpharmacological options when available. Supportive psychotherapy—or counseling—is a commonly accepted and prescribed depression intervention.

MacPherson et al. (2013) conducted an open parallel-arm randomized controlled trial (RCT) comparing effectiveness of acupuncture plus usual care, counseling plus usual care, and usual care alone in primary care. Acupuncture treatments consisted of customized treatments within a standardized theory-driven framework, provided by registered acupuncturists who had at least 3 years postqualification experience.

Counseling consisted of a manual-driven protocol, using a humanistic approach, provided by members of the British Association for Counseling and Psychotherapy who had completed at least 400 supervised hours of postqualification experience. A total of 755 patients assessed to have depression, as measured by a BDI-II score of 20 points or more, were evaluated via the PHQ-9 at baseline, and at 3 months and 12 months. Patients attended a mean of 10 sessions for acupuncture and nine sessions for counseling. Compared with usual care, there was a statistically significant reduction in mean PHQ-9 score at 3 months and 12 months for both acupuncture and counseling. Differences between acupuncture and counseling were not significant.

Sexual Side Effects

Sexual side effects to selective serotonin reuptake inhibiters (SSRIs) and serotonin norepinephrine reuptake inhibiters (SNRIs) are commonly experienced by patients who are treated with either of these two medication classes (Clayton et al., 2006; Ferguson, 2001; Hirschfeld, n.d.). Although comorbid sexual dysfunction is a complex issue with multiple biopsychosocial antecedents, patients who experience these side effects when taking antidepressant medications are less likely to remain treatment adherent (Trivedi et al., 2007).

Khamba et al. (2013) examined the potential benefits of acupuncture in the management of sexual dysfunction secondary to SSRIs and SNRIs in a tertiary mood and anxiety disorder clinic. In this small, investigational, open-label case study, 35 subjects who had no previous history of sexual difficulties and who were experiencing adverse sexual side effects secondary to the use of antidepressant medications received a fixed acupuncture treatment protocol for 12 consecutive weekly sessions. There was no randomized control group. During the 15-minute sessions, nine standardized acupuncture points where used throughout the protocol. Of the nine points, five were "tonified," using a common rotating needle action, at the 5- and 10-minute marks, and the remaining four points where left untouched, in the "neutral" position, throughout the treatment. The standard treatment protocol targeted two traditional Chinese medicine diagnoses associated with sexual dysfunction: heart yin deficiency and kidney qi deficiency (Maciocia, 2005). Point selection was also influenced by two studies that had demonstrated improvement in sexual dysfunction (Engelhardt, 2003; Kho et al., 1999).

At the time of enrollment, all patients were taking either an SSRI or an SNRI medication and reporting sexual dysfunction resulting from its use. Twenty-nine of 35 patients completed the study. The reasons for premature termination included inability to attend weekly sessions and an inability to tolerate further acupuncture. Patients completed a weekly questionnaire package that included the Beck Anxiety

Inventory, the BDI-II, the Sexual Function Visual Analogue Scale, and the Arizona Sexual Experience Questionnaire.

At the conclusion of the study, male participants were found to have significant improvement in all five categories of the Sexual Function Visual Analogue Scale and in three of five categories of the Arizona Sexual Experience Questionnaire. Female participants were found to have significant improvement in desire/libido and lubrication only, with less improvement in orgasm, drive, frequency, or arousal. Secondary outcome measures found males had mean Beck Anxiety Inventory scores that decreased from 7.88 ± 5.80 points to 5.00 ± 5.02 ($p = .010$), whereas mean BDI-II scores decreased from 9.94 ± 7.86 points to 7.61 ± 8.73 points ($p = .040$). Secondary outcome measures found women reported some reductions in depression and anxiety, but neither measure reached statistical significance.

The study authors note that concomitant improvement in sexual function and mental health can be explained in several ways because both of these aspects of health are very related (e.g., Does acupuncture improve sexual function directly or does acupuncture improve depression and anxiety directly, which then contributes to improved sexual function?). Further research is certainly recommended, but there is some evidence to suggest acupuncture may have a potential role in the treatment of medication-induced sexual side effects in some patients.

Insomnia

Insomnia is a comorbid condition of PTSD. Although insomnia can have multiple biopsychosocial antecedents, it frequently presents early during the disease course and may persist throughout treatment as a symptom that can impair recovery.

Cao et al. (2009) performed a systemic review of RCTs evaluating acupuncture as a treatment for various types of insomnia. The review included 46 randomized trials involving 3811 patients. The quality of all studies was assessed to be generally fair with respect to randomization, blinding, and intent-to-treat analysis. Meta-analyses showed a beneficial effect of acupuncture compared with no treatment, as well as a beneficial effect of real acupuncture compared with sham acupuncture on total scores of the Pittsburgh Sleep Quality Index. Acupuncture was found to be superior to medications regarding number of patients with total sleep duration that increased more than 3 hours; but there was no difference between acupuncture and medications in average sleep duration. No definitive conclusions regarding these differences were offered, but future studies might seek to assess the correlation between efficacy of various interventions and the baseline sleep deficit. Most important, perhaps, acupuncture plus medications was shown to improve sleep duration more than medications alone.

There were no serious adverse effects in the included trials and Cao et al. (2009) concluded a beneficial effect of acupuncture on insomnia. They noted the heterogeneity of insomnia type and variety of acupuncture interventions used in the trials, and stated the methodological limitations of the included studies required larger and more rigorously designed RCTs.

Yeung et al. (2011) evaluated the efficacy and safety of electroacupuncture as an additional treatment for insomnia associated with major depressive disorder. The randomized, single-blinded, parallel-group study included 78 patients with DSM, fourth edition-diagnosed major depressive disorder who were being treated by usual care, including taking the same fixed-dose antidepressant for 12 weeks before baseline. Eligible subjects were randomized to electroacupuncture, minimal acupuncture, or noninvasive placebo acupuncture and were treated three times per week for three consecutive weekly sessions.

The Insomnia Severity Index (ISI), Pittsburgh Sleep Quality Index, Hamilton Depression Rating Scale, 1-week sleep diaries, and 3-day actigraphy were administered at baseline and 1 week and 4 weeks after treatment. Comparisons revealed electroacupuncture and minimal acupuncture were more efficacious than placebo acupuncture via the ISI and Pittsburgh Sleep Quality Index at 1 week and 4 weeks posttreatment. There was no difference in any measures between electroacupuncture and minimal acupuncture.

Zollman et al. (2012) assessed the efficacy of acupuncture versus a usual care control group in patients experiencing insomnia associated with chronic traumatic brain injury to determine whether acupuncture had fewer cognitive and affective effects in this population. In this small study of 24 adult survivors of traumatic brain injury, the ISI, actigraphy, Hamilton Depression Rating Scale, Repeatable Battery for the Assessment of Neuropsychological Status, and the Paced Auditory Serial Addition Test were administered at baseline and postintervention. Examiners noted medication use was scant in both study arms, limiting statistical comparison of this parameter, and acupuncture showed a beneficial effect on patient's perception of sleep quality and cognition. Larger and more rigorously designed RCTs are needed for definitive conclusions to be made.

Substance Use Disorders

Substance abuse is a comorbid condition commonly experienced by patients who have PTSD. Samuels et al. (2008) conducted a literature survey and noted a number of clinical studies of auricular acupuncture treatment for substance abuse, but states results were not conclusive. In an RCT of 82 cocaine-dependent methadone-maintained patients, Avants et al. (2000) found that patients assigned to acupuncture treatment were significantly more likely to provide cocaine-negative urine samples than control subjects. Margolin et al. (2002), however, repeated the study protocol ($N = 620$) but found no difference between the groups. They posited the discrepancy in outcome could have resulted from factors that include differences in counseling protocols. Larger and more rigorously designed RCTs are needed for definitive conclusions to be made.

Chronic Pain

Pain is a comorbid condition commonly experienced by patients who have PTSD. Although the etiology of pain can vary significantly, and can have multiple biopsychosocial antecedents, the strongest literature support is for acupuncture to reduce pain and thus impact the amount of potentially addictive medications required to manage that pain.

Vickers et al. (2012) conducted a systematic review to identify RCTs of acupuncture for chronic pain. Individual patient data meta-analyses were conducted using data from 29 of 31 eligible RCTs with a total of 17,922 patients analyzed (in one study, data were corrupted; in another, data could not be obtained). In the primary analysis of included RCTs, acupuncture was superior to both the sham and no-acupuncture control for each of four selected pain conditions (spine, osteoarthritis, headache, and shoulder). Even after excluding an outlying set of RCTs that favored acupuncture strongly, the effect sizes were similar across pain conditions. Patients receiving acupuncture had less pain, with scores that were 0.23 standard deviations (SDs) less (95% confidence interval [CI], 0.13–0.33) for back and neck pain, 16 SDs less (95% CI, 0.07–0.25) for osteoarthritis, and 0.15 SDs less (95% CI, 0.07–0.24) for chronic headache compared with sham control subjects.

ACUPUNCTURE TREATMENT IN VARIOUS SETTINGS

PTSD or depression affects nearly one in five returning veterans, and these phenomena, and their associated comorbid symptoms, can continue long after the transition to civilian life (Tanielian & Jaycox, 2008). Patients engage their medical care system in a variety of locations, including emergency departments, primary care clinics, specialty clinics, or hospitals, and acupuncture is a treatment modality available in all these settings. Patients experiencing musculoskeletal or pain problems, for example, often respond to needles inserted over or surrounding, contracted, inflamed, or traumatized muscles (Koffman & Helms, 2013). These interventions can be performed readily in an emergency department or primary care setting. As patients progress in their care path, the initial local treatments can be reinforced with more complex acupuncture treatments that consider an individual's constitution, biopsychotype, and energy status. In these cases, needles are placed distant to the affected site to impact the autonomic activity of the affected region. Treatments for acute pain are repeated as frequently as necessary until resolution (Helms, 2007a).

Improvised Explosive Device Blast Injury: mTBI–ATP

In theater, while deployed in support of Operation Enduring Freedom, three soldiers were seen in a BAS within days following blunt force (blast) trauma secondary to an improvised explosive device. All three were experiencing pounding, bilateral, migrainelike headaches associated with their mTBI. The soldiers also complained of assorted musculoskeletal pain and soft tissue injuries as a result of having been thrown around their mine-resistant ambush-protected vehicle. With a profound sense of loss and overwhelming grief, all were angry about the death of their battle buddies/friends killed in the attack. On arrival at the BAS, after being cleared medically for "red flags" associated with head injury, such as acute mental status changes, unequal pupils (anisocoria), protracted vomiting, and so on, the soldiers were placed on cots, three abreast. Each had the combination of six auricular needles (15-mm sterile Serine needles) inserted and then left in place for 20 minutes. In addition, the scalp was palpated for tender areas called *ah-she* points (translation: alarm points) while similarly needling these temporal–parietal areas for 20 minutes concurrently. After their treatment, all three soldiers reported their headaches had decreased and they were experiencing significantly reduced pain. Importantly—as irritability and mood changes frequently accompany the presentation of mTBI (Blyth, 2010)—all three soldiers reported a state of calm they had not experienced since their blast injury.

Operational Stress Reaction: Combat/Operational Stress Reaction–ATP, Seven Dragons

A young enlisted soldier, deployed in support of Operation Enduring Freedom, was seen at a BAS in Afghanistan. He was weary from months of sustained battlefield operations and presented to the behavioral health specialist with a chief complaint of "I just can't sleep" and endorsed symptoms of intrusive recollections, hyperarousal, and profound sleep disturbance. He complained of initial and middle insomnia, nightmares, restlessness, and nonrestorative sleep. He had already been prescribed trazodone (a 5HT2A receptor antagonist) for the previous 2 weeks, and then the nonbenzodiazepine sleep agent zolpidem for the preceding few days, but neither agent provided sustained relief. The soldier expressed concerned about taking these medications, considering he was working in a combat zone and needed to be able to respond immediately in the event of a nighttime attack.

The patient was diagnosed with combat/operational stress reaction, a functional equivalent to acute stress disorder, and the operational psychiatrist implemented core military combat/operational stress reaction management principles of BICEPS (brevity, immediacy, centrality, expectancy, and simplicity) for management. In addition to referring the patient to Combat Stress, where the BICEPS care could be delivered, the patient was informed that acupuncture was available, and the patient agreed to a treatment.

The soldier had six auricular needles placed in ATP combination and, after 20 minutes, reported unexpected relaxation. On the 10-point Subjective Unit of Distress scale, the patient's changed from 6 points to 1 point. When seen for follow-up the next day, the patient reported "solid sleep for the first time in months" and agreed to a second acupuncture treatment. During this second intervention, the patient was given the Seven Dragons treatment, targeting symptoms of hyperarousal, anger, and avoidance. The patient reported continued relief from symptoms and was soon returned to duty.

Sexual Trauma: Trauma–Four Gates, Body Points

A middle-age female in her 30s presented with both subacute and chronic psychological symptoms as well as acute physical symptoms. The patient had experienced sexual trauma and her symptoms, including sleep disturbance, irritability, and hypervigilance, were exacerbated by legal proceedings related to her trauma. The patient was also complaining of increased pelvic pain associated with her previously diagnosed dysmenorrhea.

The patient, initially reporting a pain level of "nine or a ten," agreed to a course of acupuncture. She received an initial treatment of Four Gates, selected because of its immediate ability to decrease pain, as well as to quiet and calm the patient's PTSD-associated symptoms. An additional body points session that targeted her pelvic symptoms was proposed to augment the treatment. During her initial 20-minute treatment session, the patient reported significant relief and, when she awoke, reported she was "amazed to be nearly pain free."

mTBI and PTSD: PTSD—Four Gates, Midline Points, ATP

An enlisted soldier, approximately 1 year past her combat experience, was admitted to an in-patient psychiatric ward secondary to PTSD flashback symptoms that had been interfering with social and occupational functioning, and had become too difficult to manage in the outpatient setting. The patient received a biopsychosocial informed assessment and treatment plan consistent with Veterans Affairs/Department of Defense Guidelines (Group, 2012) while on the ward. After a few weeks, the patient's symptoms stabilized sufficiently and she was transferred for to an open-ward hospital bed for ongoing assessment and treatment of diagnoses, including mTBI, headache, PTSD, and insomnia. The patient was engaging and motivated, and able to form solid bonds with a therapy dog that never left her side. The patient continued to experience poor sleep, periodic headaches, and flashbacks of increasing severity. The treatment team became concerned about the patient's persistent symptoms and requested she be transferred back to the in-patient ward. The patient, who was not suicidal, did not desire to return to the in-patient ward, however, and was open to alternative modes of therapy.

The primary treatment team agreed to have a psychiatrist trained in medical acupuncture consult on the patient. After evaluation, the patient was given treatments that included Four Gates, two midline points, and the ATP. The patient fell asleep during initiation of therapy and needles were left in place for 40 minutes. After the first treatment, the patient reported experiencing feelings of "centering, calming, relaxation ... unlike any experienced [since her trauma]." She was seen for three additional weekly sessions during which the base treatment was repeated and her ears were scanned and needled as indicated. The patient remained on the open ward as the frequency and intensity of her flashbacks decreased, her sleep improved, and her headaches lessened. The patient was also noted to be requesting less as-needed medications for anxiety and headaches.

CONCLUSION

The types of acupuncture described in this chapter are all useful in the myriad of civilian treatment settings and military operational environments alike. Although acupuncture may seem "alternative" to the newcomer, acupuncture shares at least one phenomenon with more recognized mainstream or modern therapies: the existence of a trusting and comfortable therapeutic relationship. Key to the collaborative relationship between provider and patient is the realization that service members want—and demand—effective choices when it comes to the treatment of psychoemotional syndromes and associated comorbid symptoms. Although medications may remain a primary treatment course, pharmacotherapy interventions may be eschewed by the patient and sometimes even prohibited in combat situations.

When engaged and empowered, patients who accept acupuncture often report a victory of sorts over their psychological trauma. They have engaged their symptoms on their own terms and, anecdotally, in deployed environments, accept acupuncture treatments, perhaps only for "bragging rights" with their buddies or with family and friends back home. In addition, combat service members often experience the perplexing existential conundrum or moral injury, and the professional who is equipped to integrate acupuncture and psychotherapy has a unique opportunity to explore loss, identify cognitive distortions, and facilitate recovery.

In summary, medical acupuncture is a uniquely and perfectly suited complement to modern western medical care of patients experiencing psychoemotional trauma and associated comorbid physical symptoms. Acupuncture engages the patient as a whole, and provides an alternative treatment approach for those who decline medication or who have not responded to it. Acupuncture fosters and facilitates a trusting relationship between patient and provider, and at times, catalyzes emotional release as part of healing. Expanding opportunities for acupuncture will provide a path for patients who choose to come for the needles and stay for the therapy.

KEY POINTS

- Persons with PTSD experience a higher prevalence of other psychiatric and physical comorbid conditions to include mood, pain, and substance use disorders
- Patients bring to their illness experience a unique perspective, constitution and perpetuating factors that must be recognized by treatment professionals
- Acupuncture is recognized by patients and professionals to be an effective augment to western medical treatments for PTSD and associated comorbid symptoms
- Acupuncture is a safe, accessible, non-stigmatizing treatment practice that has endured multiple millennia and can be provided in a variety of treatment settings
- There is a growing body of evidence supporting acupuncture's impact in treating PTSD as well as comorbid conditions to include mood, pain, and substance use disorders
- Medical acupuncture, the hybrid practice of acupuncture by physicians trained in western medicine, engages the patient as a whole, and complements modern western medical treatments

- Acupuncture approaches to acute problems include interventions that activate the energy of select meridians and/or select acupuncture points
- Acupuncture approaches to chronic and more complex problems include consideration of an individual's biopsychotype to inform treatment selection and energy needs of a governing meridian(s)
- Acupuncture shares one phenomenon with modern medicine—the foundation of a trusting and comfortable therapeutic relationship
- Patients want—and demand—effective choices when it comes to treatment of their psychoemotional syndromes and associated comorbid symptoms

REFERENCES

American Psychiatric Association. (2013). *Diagnostic and Statistical Manual of Mental Disorders 5th Edition.* Washington D.C.: American Psychiatric Publishing.

Avants, S., et al. (2000). A randomized controlled trial of auricular acupuncture for cocaine dependence. *Archives of Internal Medicine*, 160(15):2305–2312.

Barnes, P. e. (2008). Complementary and alternative medicine use among adults and children: United States, 2007. *National Health Stat Report, 12*, 1–23.

Blyth, B. J. (2010). Traumatic alterations in consciousness: Traumatic Brain Injury. *Emergency Medicine Clinics of North America, 28*(3), 571–594.

Bradley, R., et al. (2005). Multidimensional meta-analysis of psychotherapy for PTSD. *American Journal of Psychiatry, 162*, 214–227.

Breslau, N., et al. (1996). Trauma and posttraumatic stress disorder in the community: The 1996 Detroit Area Survey of Trauma. *Archives of General Psychiatry, 55*, 626–632.

Cabyoglu, M. T., et al. (2006). The Mechanism of Acupuncture and Clinical Applications. *International Journal of Neuroscience, 116*(2), 115–125.

Cao, H., et al. (2009). Acupuncture for Treatment of Insomnia: A Systematic Review of Randomized Controlled Trials. *Journal of Alternative and Complementary Medicine, 15*(11), 1171–1186.

Clayton, A., et al. (2006). Major depressive disorder, anti-depressants, and sexual dysfunction. *Clinical Psychiatry, 67*, 33–37.

Dhond, R. e. (2007). Neuroimaging acupuncture effects in the human brain. *Journal of Alternative and Complementary Medicine, 13*, 603–616.

Effective Health Care Bulletin. (2005). *Improving the recognition and management of depression in primary care.* University of York, York: Centre for Reviews and Dissemination.

Engel, C. C., Cordova, E. H., Benedek, D. M., Liu, X., Gore, K. L., Goertz, C., . . . Ursano, R. J. (2014, December). Randomized Effectiveness Trial of a Brief Course of Acupuncture for Posttraumatic Stress Disorder. *Medical Care, 52*(12 Suppl 5), S57–S64.

Engelhardt, P. (2003). Acupuncture in the treatment of psychogenic erectile dysfunction: First results of a prospective randomized placeo-controlled study. *Int J Impot Res, 15*, 343–346.

Errington-Evans, N. (2011). Acupuncture for Anxiety. *CNS Neuroscience and Therapeutics, 18*(4), 277–284.

Fava, M. (2003). Diagnosis and definition of treatment resistent depression. *Biological Psychiatry, 53*, 649–659.

Ferguson, J. (2001). Antidepressant medications: Adverse effects and tolerability. *Primary Care Companion Journal Clinical Psychiatry, 3*, 22–27.

Group, M. o.-T. (2012). *VA/DoD Clinical Practice Guideline for the Management of Post-Traumatic Stress.* Washington, DC: Dept of Veterans Affairs and Dept of Defense.

Haker, E., et al. (2000). Effect of sensory stimulation (acupuncture) on sympathetic and parasympathetic activities in health subjects. *Journal of Autonomic Nervous System, 79*, 52–59.

Helms, J. M. (2007a). *Acupuncture Energetics: A Clinical Approach for Physicians.* New York, NY: Thieme Publishers.

Helms, J. M. (2007b). *Getting to Know You.* Berkeley, CA: Medical Acupuncture Publishers.

Helms, J. M. (2009). Medical Acupuncture for Physicians. *Course Syllabus.* Berkeley: Helms Medical Institute.

Helms, J. M., Elorriaga-Claraco, A., & Ng, A. (2001). *Point Locations and Functions.* Berkeley, CA: Medical Acupuncture Publishers.

Hirschfeld, R. (n.d.). Care of the sexually active depressed patient. *Journal of Clinical Psychiatry, 199*(60), 32–35.

Hoge, C., et al. (2004). Combat Duty in Iraq and Afghanistan, mental health problems, and barriers to care. *New England Journal of Medicine, 351,* 13–22.

Hoge, C., Castro, C., Messer, S., McGurk, D., & Thomas, J. C. (n.d.). Combat Duty in Iraq and Afghanistan, Mental Health Problems, and Barriers to Care. *New England Journal of Medicine, 351*(1), 13–22.

Hoge, C., McGurk, D., Thomas, J., & Cox, A. E. (2008). Mild Traumatic Brain Injury in U.S. Soldiers Returning from Iraq. *New England Journal of Medicine, 358*(5), 453–463.

Hollifield, M., et al. (2007). Acupuncture for Posttraumatic Stress Disorder—A Randomized Controlled Pilot Trial. *Journal of Nervous and Mental Disease, 195*(6), 3–13.

Hollifield, M. (2011). Acupuncture for Posttraumatic Stress Disorder: Conceptual, Clinical, and Biological Data Support Further Research. *CNS Neuroscience and Therapeutics, 17,* 769–779.

Hui, K. K., et al. (2000). Acupuncture modulates the limbic system and subcortical gray structures of the human brain: Evidence from fMRI studies in normal subjects. *Human Brain Mapping, 9*(1), 13–25.

Kaptchuk, T. J. (2002). Acupuncture: Theory, Efficacy, and Practice. *Ann Intern Med, 136*(5), 374–383.

Kenyon, J. (1983–1985). *Modern Techniques of Acupuncture* (Vol. 2). Wellingsborough, Northamptonshire: Thorsons.

Kessler, R., et al. (2008). *The National Comorbidity Survey Replication (NCS-R): Cornerstone in improving mental health and mental health care in the United States.*

Khamba, B., et al. (2013). Efficacy of Acupuncture Treatment of Sexual Dysfunction Secondary to Antidepressants. *Journal of Alternative and Complementary Medicine, 19*(11), 862–9. doi: 10.1089/acm.2012.0751. Epub 2013 Jun 21.

Kho, H., et al. (1999). The use of acupuncture in the treatment of erectile dysfunction. *Int J Impot Res, 11,* 41–46.

Kim, Y.-D., et al. (2013). Acupuncture for Posttraumatic Stress Disorder: A Systematic Review of Randomized Controlled Trials and Prospective Clinical Trials. *Evidence-Based Complementary and Alternative Medicine,* 2013, 1–12.

Koffman, R. L., & Helms, J. M. (2013, May). Acupuncture and PTSD: 'Come for the Needles, Stay for the Therapy'. *Psychiatric Annals, 43*(5), 236–239.

Kong, J., et al. (2002). A pilot study of functional magnetic resonance imaging of the brain during manual and electroacupuncture stimulation of acupuncture point (LI-4 Hegu) in normal subjects reveals differential brain activation between methods. *Journal of Alternative and Complementary Medicine, 8,* 411–419.

Kroening, R. (1980). *Personal Communication—as reported in Acupuncture Energetics (Helms).* Berkeley: Medical Acupuncture Publishers.

Lee, C., et al. (2012). The effectiveness of acupuncture research across components of trauma spectrum response (tsr): a systematic review of reviews. *Systematic Reviews, 1*(46), 1–18.

Maciocia, G. (2005). *Foundations of Chinese Medicine* (2nd ed.). Edinburgh: Churchill Livingstone.

MacPherson, H., et al. (2013). Acupuncture and Counselling for Depression in Primary Care: A Randomized Controlled Trial. *PLOS Medicine,* 1–13. http://dx.doi.org/10.1371/journal.pmed.1001518

Margolin, A., et al. (2002). Acupuncture for the treatment of cocaine addiction: a randomized controlled trial. *JAMA, 287*(1), 55–63.

Miller, M. e. (2012). The prevalence and latent structure of proposed DSM-5 posttraumatic stress disorder symptoms in U.S. national and veteran samples. *Psychological Trauma: Theory, Research, Practice, and Policy, 5*(6), Nov 2013, 501–512.

Naeser, M. (1994). *Laser Acupuncture - An Introductory Textbook.* Boston: Boston Chinese Medicine.

Napadow, V. e. (2005). Effects of electroacupuncture vs. manual acupuncture on the human brain as measured by MRI. *Human Brain Mapping, 24*, 193–205.

Niemtzow Richard C., Belard J.-Louis, and Nogier Raphael. Medical Acupuncture. October 2015, 27(5): 344–348. doi:10.1089/acu.2014.1055.

Niemtzow, R. C., Gambel, J., Helms, J., Pock, A., Burns, S., & Baxter, J. (2006). Integrating Ear and Scalp Acupuncture Techniques into the Care of Blast-Injured United States Military Service Members with Limb Loss. *Journal of Alternative and Complementary Medicine, 12*(7), 596–599.

Nogier, P. (1978). *Introduction Pratique A L'Auriculotherapie.* Moulins-les-Metz, France: Maisonneuve.

Norris, F. H., & Slone, L. B. (2013). *PTSD Research Quarterly.* White River Junction: National Center for PTSD.

Oleson, T. (1996). *Auriculotherapy Manual: Chinese and Western Systems of Ear Acupuncture* (Second ed.). Los Angeles, CA: Health Care Alternatives, Inc.

Oleson, T. e. (1980). An experimental evaluation of auricular diagnosis: the somatotopic mapping of musculokeletal pain at ear acupunture points. *Pain, 8*, 217–229.

Peets, J. e. (1978). CXBK Mice deficient in opiate receptors show poor electroacupuncture analgesia. *Nature, 273*(5664), 675–676.

Pilkington, K., et al. (2007). Acupuncture for anxiety and anxiety disorders—a systematic literature review. *Acupunct Med, 25*(1–2), 1–10.

Samuels, N., et al. (2008). Acupuncture for Psychiatric Illness: A Literature Review. *Behavioral Medicine, 34*, 55–62.

Shanghai College of Traditional Medicine. (1981). *Acupuncture: A Comprehensive Text.* (J. O'Connor, & D. Bensky, Eds.) Seattle: Eastland Press.

Sherman, K. e. (2005). The practice of acupuncture: who are the providers and what do they do? *Ann Fam Med, 3*(2), 151–158.

Shin, L. e. (2005). A functional magnetic resonance imaging study of amygdala and medial prefrontal cortex responses to overtly presented fearful faces in posttraumatic stress disorder. *Archives General Psychiatry, 62*, 273–281.

Taillandier, J. (1989). *Reflexotherapies et microsystemes en acupuncture.* Paris: Encyclopedie des Medecines Naturelles, II-1.

Tanielian, T., & Jaycox, L. H. (2008). *Invisible Wounds of War—Psychological and Cognitive Injuries, Their Consequences, and Services to Assist Recovery.* Arlington, VA, USA: Rand Corporation.

Trivedi, M., et al. (2007). Consensus recommendations for improving adherence, self-management, and outcomes in patients with depression. *CNS Spectr, 12*(1), 1–27.

VA/DoD Clinical Practice Guideline. (2009). *Management of Major Depressive Disorder.* VA/DoD Evidence Based Practice.

VA/DoD Clinical Practice Guideline. (2010). *Management of Post-Traumatic Stress.* VA/DoD Evidence Based Practice.

Vickers, A. J., et al. (2012, October 22). Acupuncture for Chronic Pain—Individual Patient Data Meta-analysis. *Archives of Internal Medicine, 172*(19), 1444–1453.

Vincent, C., et al. (1995). Placebo controls for acupuncture studies. *Journal of the Royal Society of Medicine, 88*, 199–202.

Wahbeh, H., et al. (2014). Complementary and Alternative Medicine for Posttraumatic Stress Disorder Symptoms: A Systematic Review. *Journal of Evidence-Based Complementary and Alternative Medicine, 19*(3), 161–175.

White, A. (2009). Editorial Board of Acupuncture in Medicine—Western medical acupuncture; a definition. *Acupuncture Medicine, 27*(1), 33–35.

Wong, J. Y. (1999). *Manual of Neuro-Anatomical Acupuncture.* Toronto, Ontario: The Toronto Pain and Stress Clinic, Inc.

Yeung, W.-F., et al. (2011). Electroacupuncture for Residual Insomnia Associated with Major Depressive Disorder: A Randomized Controlled Trial. *Sleep, 34*(6), 807–816.

Zhang, W. (2004). Evidence from brain imaging with fMRI supporting functional specificity of acupoints in humans. *Neurosci Lett, 354*(1), 50–53.

Zollman, F. S., et al. (2012). Acupuncture for Treatment of Insomnia in Patients with Traumatic Brain Injury: A Pilot Intervention Study. *Journal of Head Trauma Rehabilitation, 27*(2), 135–142.

SEVEN

Alternative Medicine Pharmacology

ROBERT N. McLAY, DEREK M. MILETICH,
NATHANIEL A. BROWN, AND LESLEY ROSS

THE WORD *PHARMACOLOGY* DERIVES FROM THE GREEK *PHARMAKON,* WHICH MEANS "drug" in modern Greek, but has the older connotation of "poison." To many alternative medicine adherents, the more ancient meaning may represent how they think about most pharmacology. Giving a pill to treat disease is the very stereotype against which alternative medicine is supposedly rebelling. That being said, there are times when a chemical compound is prescribed and yet the practice clearly falls under the rubric of alternative medicine. An obvious example of this would the use of medical marijuana. In between the use of Food and Drug Administration (FDA)–approved medications and marijuana lies a whole spectrum of pharmacological practices that may or may not be considered alternative.

To understand what alternative pharmacology might be, one first has to think about what it is not. For a pharmaceutical manufacturer to market a compound for treatment or prevention of posttraumatic stress disorder (PTSD) the company must submit two preapproved, large-scale, randomized, placebo-controlled trials, both of which demonstrate the drug has efficacy. The completion of such trials does not by itself guarantee approval, because the FDA weighs other factors, such as safety or comparative effectiveness, when deciding to approve a drug for a particular purpose. Because the approval process is both cumbersome and expensive, it is very rare that any entity would seek FDA approval unless it controls the patent on the pharmaceutical. Only two compounds have gone through this process to gain approval for the treatment of PTSD: sertraline (Zoloft) and paroxetine (Paxil), both of which are selective serotonin reuptake inhibitors (SSRIs).

Having FDA approval does not always mean that everyone agrees those medications have the ideal (or even a sufficient) evidence base. The Harvard Psychopharmacology Algorithm Project recommends medications that target sleep and nightmares, trazodone and prazosin, before SSRIs for the treatment of PTSD (Bajor, Ticlea, & Osser 2011). Some have argued that such use of medications with expired patents is itself is a type of rebellion that needs to be encouraged. An example of this is use of the anesthetic ketamine as a treatment for PTSD or depression (Covvey, Crawford, & Lowe 2012).

Off-label use of pharmaceuticals may or may not be alternative medication. Here, however, we opt not review the basics of off-label medications, not because we wish to come down on one side of the debate, but simply because this sort of pharmacology has been reviewed in so many other places (Bernardy & Friedman 2015; Richardson, Sareen, & Stein 2012; Stein, Ipser, & Seedat 2006) and are already used by most physicians.

While considering the topic of alternative medicine pharmacology we attempt to cover subjects that fall outside standard practice. We first discuss how broader concepts of stress and symptom management might be used to guide pharmacological treatment in PTSD. We then describe medications, which although fairly standard (and FDA approved) compounds, can be used in nonstandard ways. Next we cover products such as certain hormones or vitamins that occur either as natural products or as synthetics. Then, we describe natural products that contain a variety of compounds that may have psychoactive properties that influence PTSD. Last, we cover compounds, both synthetic and herbal, that are not FDA approved for any medical purpose and that are banned for use outside of research studies in the United States.

CONCEPTS IN CHOOSING ALTERNATIVE
PHARMACOLOGICAL TREATMENTS FOR PTSD

In concept, pharmacology follows from mechanism to effectiveness—that is, there is an understanding of healthy physiology and why it is perturbed in a disease state. A pharmacological compound is chosen as a treatment because it interrupts the disease process, and the result is a return to healthy function.

The best examples of this in practice probably exist in the form of antibiotics. The antibiotic hinders a particular disease-causing pathogen while leaving other cells unharmed. The pathogen caused the disease and, when removed, the patient recovers. In addition to working in the test tube, there is very strong evidence that such pharmacological interventions have improved health significantly in patients worldwide (Cutler, Deaton, & Lleras-Muney 2006).

An example of something that is a slight step away from this pharmacological ideal is the use of L-dopa for the treatment of Parkinson's disease. In this case, there is not an understanding of exactly why dopamine levels are falling off in the disease state, but it is clear the deficit of this neurotransmitter is linked to the symptoms of the disease. Providing the precursor L-dopa restores levels of dopamine, and symptoms improve—at least for a time (Calne 1970).

Applying this framework of mechanistic treatment to alternative pharmacology for PTSD encounters two difficulties: (1) there is no universally agreed-on biological mechanism to explain PTSD and (2) many systems of alternative medicine rely on explanations of disease that differ from Western biological understanding of the disease state. These problems notwithstanding, some theoretical basis can still be used to try to guide pharmacological intervention.

Looking at purely biochemical changes, a number of abnormalities have been observed in PTSD. The first of these that was used to support pharmacological intervention was the finding that serotonin function is altered in PTSD (Davis, Suris, Lambert, Heimberg, & Petty 1997). The link is not perfect, but it does inform the idea that SSRIs are a logical intervention. Also observed have been alternations of neuroendocrine pathways, perturbation of neurotransmitter levels and function, as well as changes such as altered immune and inflammatory responses (Friedman 1999). For example, cortisol levels have been found to be low in PTSD, which is why either natural or synthetic versions of the hormone have been proposed as a possible way to prevent or treat PTSD (Yehuda, Teicher, Trestman, Levengood, & Siever 1996).

PTSD is a psychological condition, and therefore even in the cannon of Western medicine many models are biopsychological rather than purely biochemical. A broad swath of behavioral research supports the idea that PTSD is a disorder of failure of extinction learning. This is to say that PTSD disease in which traumatic memories are too strongly entrenched, or at least in which the emotional valance of the memory is too powerful (Silove 1998). This logic would lead to the use of drugs that disrupt memory consolidation or allow new associations to be attached to memories. For example, a drug that produces a euphoric effect might be used in combination with the therapeutic recounting of the trauma story, with the goal of changing the physiological stress response. Along the spectrum of similarly proposed mechanisms is the idea that PTSD represents a failure to forget or habituate

(Cottencin et al. 2006). Authors have pointed out that many of the symptoms of PTSD are normal, or even adaptive, responses to dangerous situations, but that disorder results because the patient fails to return to a more relaxed state after the danger is removed (Wessa & Flor 2007). Drugs that enhance habituation have thus been proposed as treatments for PTSD.

Opening PTSD to an even wider variety of pharmacological interventions is the idea that the pathological state is simply the far end of the normal stress response. The body changes in myriad ways in response to stress. Many compounds alter this response, or may in fact alter the very perception that a particular situation is stressful. This is the basis for use of adaptogens (Sarris, McIntyre, & Camfield 2013). Other compounds may alter a particular aspect of a stressful experience. For example, physical pain is an essential signal to avoid tissue damage. However, excessive pain is itself traumatic, and compounds that mitigate pain might lower the stress response and make PTSD symptoms less stressful. As outlined in the following sections, this is a presumed mechanism by which opiates seem to lower the incidence of PTSD (Holbrook, Galarneau, Dye, Quinn, & Dougherty 2010).

Moving beyond the modern Western cannon of medicine, there are almost an infinite number of different ways by which PTSD could be approached from an alternative medicine point of view. Some of these, such as the idea that PTSD is a disease of soul sickness (Wilson & Moran 1998), might not seem immediately amenable to pharmacological options. However, many pharmacologically active compounds, ranging from the hallucinogen peyote to the alcohol in communion wine, are used as part of spiritual ceremonies and also have been proposed as independent treatments for PTSD. Some other alternative medicine concepts that are worth mentioning include the theory of homeopathy, which purports that compounds that cause symptoms similar to that of a disease will cure that same condition if diluted out to levels at which Western physics would say they are not even present. Also, there is the idea of purgatives, present in many traditions, by which a noxious substance induces the body to cleanse itself of disease, either by direct expulsion such as during bleeding or vomiting, or by more mysterious methods of detoxification. Closely allied to this is the formulation by which disease is caused by an imbalance of certain substances or humors in the body, and that by restoring a more natural state by adding generally healthful substances, balance and health may be restored (Ernst, Pittler, Stevinson, & White 2001; Pandzic, McLay, & Morrison 2013).

All the pharmacological reasoning described so far draws on inductive reasoning— using a framework of ideas to predict response. With the scientific method, inductive reasoning is used to develop hypotheses, which then must be verified by deductive observation—that is, observing what the truth is. The reality of medicine has been, however, that therapeutic compounds often have been discovered by chance observation. In fact, we may end up reasoning backward to determine a particular biochemical must be involved in disease pathology because it was observed that a drug that alters that biochemical helps symptoms.

Deductive reasoning is also a very valid means by which previously "alternative" compounds may enter the mainstream of Western medicine. In this framework, the compound to be used is picked because someone was noticed to improve while taking it. What separates anecdotal claims from scientifically supported evidence is following up the general observation with a more rigorously controlled trial. It is worth noting, however, that even with Western medication it is not uncommon for medications to be used largely based on expert consensus and clinical observation rather than randomized, placebo-controlled trials.

Even when observing that particular compounds help PTSD, there are some questions concerning how Western and alternative medicine might view improvement differently. PTSD as discussed here is defined by Western medicine, based primarily on observations of Western populations, and most commonly by using specific language and criteria from the *Diagnostic and Statistical Manual of Mental Disorders* (American Psychiatric Association 2013). Even within the scientific literature, it has been observed that problematic symptoms after trauma vary across time and cultures (Marsella, Friedman, & Spain 1996). The importance that a particular symptom carries within the scope of PTSD, or where the lines of one condition start and another end, are open to debate.

When using pharmacology to help a patient, it is also helpful to think about symptoms that are impairing to the patient rather than the whole disease model. Even as the definition of a disease changes, the needs of a patient do not. We would be remiss in saying that a symptom-based treatment is "not helpful" for PTSD simply because it does not improve a score on the Clinical-Administered PTSD Scale (Blake et al. 1995). Looking at the current definition, some individuals might say that a medicine that helps limit alcohol misuse has improved PTSD, whereas others would consider that a treatment for a different disease. Another example might be an alternative provider who feels a traumatized patient is more open to spirituality after the use of a particular compound. Although space limitations require us to restrict our review to compounds that help the most common symptoms of PTSD, pharmacological thinking and treatment should always include not just a strict adherence to the evidence, but also a careful consideration of the individual being treated.

ALLOPATHIC MEDICATIONS USED
IN NONTRADITIONAL WAYS

With the exception of considering the time of day or if the medication is to be taken with food, Western medicine rarely considers the context in which pharmacology is applied. This contrasts with alternative medicine practice in which an herb or other compound must be ingested as part of a larger ceremony, ritual, or treatment. The absence of such context is one of the principal criticisms of using randomized, placebo-controlled trials for alternative medicine (Fontanarosa & Lundberg 1998). Behavioral models of PTSD, however, have increased the awareness of how medications might be applied in conjunction with psychotherapy, or at a particular point in trauma processing, to produce therapeutic results different than would be seen if the compound were taken on its own (Table 7.1).

TABLE 7.1 Allopathic Medication Mechanisms of Action in Treating PTSD

Compound	D-cycloserine	Beta-Blocker	Ketamine	Opioids
PTSD prevention		X	X	X
Fear extinction	X	X	X	
BDNF			X	
5HT			X	
NE			X	
D			X	
Pain			X	
GABA			X	
Anti-inflammatory				
HPA Axis modulator				
Sleep				
DNA				
NMDA				
AMPA				
Hallucinogen			X	

5HT, serotonin; AMPA, amino-3-hydroxy-5-methy-4-isoxazolepropionic acid; BDNF, brain-derived neurotropic factor; D, dopamine; GABA, γ-aminobutyric acid; HPA, hypothalamic–pituitary–adrenal; NE, nor-epinephrine; NMDA, N-methyl-D-aspartate; PTSD, posttraumatic stress disorder.

Cycloserine

Cycloserine (4-amino-3-isoxazolidinone) is a cyclic analogue of D-alanine, developed and sold under the brand name Seromycin, for the treatment of tuberculosis. In this context, its mechanism of action occurs by inhibiting enzymes crucial to bacterial cell wall synthesis. For the purposes of treating PTSD, cycloserine probably has its benefit via its role as a partial agonist at glycine receptors and by enhancing *N*-Methyl-D-aspartate (NMDA) receptor-mediated neurotransmission. Unlike other compounds that enhance NMDA-medicated transmission, cycloserine appears to do so without inducing neurotoxicity.

The idea that cycloserine might be useful in treating PTSD came out of observations that the compound enhanced extinction of stress-induced behaviors in animals (Anthony & Nevins 1993). Yamamoto et al. (2008) showed that in a rat model of PTSD cycloserine normalized both fear-induced learning responses and levels of NMDA receptor messenger RNA. Other studies (Hofmann et al. 2006; Ressler et al. 2004) demonstrated that cycloserine facilitated fear extinction in human patients as well.

One of the mainstays for the treatment of PTSD is exposure therapy (Foa, Hembree, & Rothbaum 2007). During exposure therapy, patients recount their trauma in the hope they will desensitize or habituate to the memory. Cycloserine is used in conjunction with some form of exposure therapy to enhance habituation. Exact protocols have varied, but, in general, 50 to 100 mg cycloserine is given about an hour before therapy. Several trials have now tested cycloserine with mixed results. Difede et al. (2014) showed earlier and greater improvement in PTSD symptoms when cycloserine was given before virtual reality exposure therapy. Rothbaum et al. (2014) did not find an advantage of cycloserine over placebo when used with this treatment, but did find both of these options worked better than using a benzodiazepine during therapy. de Kleine, Hendriks, Kusters, Broekman, and van Minnen (2012) found no overall effect of cycloserine on augmentation of imaginal prolonged exposure therapy, but did report greater symptom reduction between therapy sessions in a subgroup with severe PTSD symptoms. In a study by Litz et al. (2012) that used a shorter course of imaginal exposure, participants who used cycloserine actually did significantly worse than those who received placebo during therapy.

Because of the mixed results associated with cycloserine when used in conjunction with psychotherapy, this agent would likely be best considered as a second-line treatment for patients who are nonresponders to psychotherapy alone.

Beta-blockers

As the name implies, beta-blockers are a class of synthetic medications that antagonize beta-adrenergic receptors. Propranolol and pronetholol were the first of these compounds, but there are now at least 19 agents in the class, all of which are named with the ending "olol." Eucommia bark also contains a natural beta-blocker, and there are atypical agents such as butaximine, a beta-2-selective agent. Most of the beta-blockers, however, are either nonselective or are designed to block beta-1 receptors specifically, which are found mostly in cardiac tissue. Some beta-blockers such as carvedilol and labetalol also have some alpha-blocking activity (López-Sendó et al. 2004).

The beta-blockers are best known as cardiac and antihypertensive agents, but blocking catacholamines can be useful in a number of clinical contexts. PTSD is generally regarded as a state in which the fight-or-flight response is exaggerated, so it is not surprising that beta-blockers have been proposed as a potential intervention here. Most often the beta-blocker chosen for such interventions has been propranolol, with the choice made at least in part because of the lipophilic nature of this molecule, and thus its greater likelihood of crossing the blood–brain barrier.

As an independent treatment, beta-blockers showed early promise in the treatment of childhood PTSD (Famularo, Kinscherff, & Fenton 1988), but follow-up studies in adults have been lacking. Greater attention is now paid to the idea that beta-blockers might help prevent PTSD if given early, or that they could alter the physiological reactivity paired with a traumatic memory if they are given in conjunction with retelling and reremembering (Tawa & Murphy 2013).

Data on beta-blockers for preventing PTSD is mixed. A 2015 meta-analysis on the topic of prevention concluded that propranolol did not alter the incidence of PTSD (Argolo, Cavalcanti-Ribeiro, Netto, & Quarantini 2015). The results in individual studies has been quite divergent, leading some to believe that, depending on the dose, timing, and nature of the individual treated, different results may be seen. For example, in the study by Nugent et al. (2010) of propranolol for the prevention of PTSD in children, no overall effect of the medication was found; but, on detailed analysis, it was noted this overall neutral effect consisted of a general improvement of PTSD symptoms in boys but a worsening of such symptoms in girls.

Although there are mixed results, beta-blockers will likely be of most benefit to patients who have high sympathetic reactivity, as evidenced by signs and symptoms such as labile or abnormally elevated blood pressure and heart rate or elevated serum catecholamines. By using beta-blockers to normalize the flight-or-flight response (in those whom it is abnormal), patients may see improvement in prevention and rehabituation of PTSD.

Ketamine

Ketamine (2-(O-chlorophenyl)-2-methylamino cyclohexanone) is a compound similar in structure to phencyclidine (or PCP), tiletamine, and cyclohexamine, and was first approved in 1970 for use in anesthesia (White 2014). Although usually considered an antagonist of glutamate at the NMDA receptor, ketamine also has other pharmacological activity, including at opiate receptors and monoamine transporters (Kohrs & Durieux 1998). As an anesthetic, it acts both as an antinociceptive agent and as a disassociative agent. It has advantages over other anesthetics in that it does not usually cause respiratory depression, but the drawback is that it has high abuse potential, and, if not managed properly, can cause hypertension, tachycardia, delirium, increased salivation, lacrimation, and diaphoresis. Ketamine was approved as an intravenous agent, but oral, intranasal, and other administration formulations have been compounded. The effect of ketamine can vary dramatically based on dosing, combination with other agents, and whether it is given as a bolus or an infusion. In general, as dose escalates, ketamine progresses from an antidepressant and antinociceptive agent to a euphoric, hallucinogenic, and dissociative compound to an adjuvant to anesthesia induction, and finally to a full anesthetic agent.

The first reports with ketamine and PTSD were concerning its negative consequences. Worsening disassociative symptoms is a well-known side effect of ketamine. Accident and burn victims who received ketamine as part of their anesthesia and pain management plan were noted to have more severe PTSD symptoms than those who received other agents (Schönenberg, Reichwald, Domes, Badke, & Hautzinger 2005; Schönenberg, Reichwald, Domes, Badke, & Hautzinger 2008). However, these negative effects of ketamine on the development of disassociation and PTSD were contradicted by other studies, particularly in military populations, in which outcomes appeared better in those who received ketamine (McGhee, Maani, Garza, Gaylord, & Black 2008; Pokorny 2012, Zeng et al. 2013).

The idea that ketamine might be useful in the treatment of PTSD largely grew out of studies for depression. Several randomized controlled trials have now demonstrated a very rapid and powerful antidepressant effect of low-dose ketamine (reviewed in Abdallah, Sanacora, Duman, and Krystal [2014b]). It is thought that ketamine induces brain-derived neurotrophic factor, mammalian target of rapamycin complex 1, and eventually synaptogenesis. These are mechanisms also thought to underlie the benefits of SSRIs, but occur much more quickly with ketamine. Ketamine has also been reported to be effective for the treatment of depression in PTSD (Womble 2013) or in situations such as reduced hippocampal volume, which is known to be a marker for both PTSD and treatment-resistant depression (Abdallah et al. 2014a).

Evidence that ketamine helps PTSD symptoms comes from case reports (de Kleine, Hendriks, Kusters, Broekman, & van Minnen 2012) and one randomized, double-blind, crossover trial (Feder et al. 2014). In the randomized trial, a single infusion of 0.5 mg/kg ketamine improved PTSD symptoms significantly 24 hours postinfusion, with benefits lasting at least 7 days on the Impact of Events Scale, but not on the Clinician-Administered PTSD Scale. Improvements were seen equally in all symptom clusters. No adverse events were associated with the ketamine administration. As with treatment of depression, the study by Feder et al. (2014) of ketamine for PTSD showed some diminishment of the benefit over time. Currently, there is little evidence of how to maintain benefits over time, or whether there is tachyphylaxis with repeated treatment. Studies have so far not been published in which ketamine is combined with psychotherapy; but, in theory, both the euphoric and memory-altering effects of ketamine might be useful in combination with forms of exposure therapy (de Kleine, Rothbaum, & van Minnen 2013).

Opioids

Opioids are a broad class of chemical substances that bind to opiate receptors and that have pharmacological properties similar to morphine. Any compound that works in the same way, whether synthetic or natural, is an opioid. Technically only a subset of opioids are *opiates*—that is, natural derivatives of the opium poppy (*Papaver somniferu*)—but the terms *opioid* and *opiate* are sometimes used interchangeably. Examples of the pharmacological agents include morphine, codeine, hydromorphone, hydrocodone, oxycodone, and oxymorphone; and the synthetic agents meperidine, tapentadol, and buprenorphine. Heroin is a semisynthetic opioid banned for pharmacological use in the United States. There are also a number of endogenous peptides, including the endorphins, enkephalins, and endomorphine, that act as opioids and are the body's natural mechanism for activating and modulating opioid receptors.

Opioids are some of the oldest pharmacological agents known to humans, with evidence that poppy extracts were used as far back as 1500 BC as a "remedy to prevent excessive crying of children" (Brownstein 1993, p. 164) Although they do have other uses, such as cough suppressants, opioids are prescribed primarily as pain relievers. They are also known for their addictive properties and potential for abuse.

It has long been noted that pain sensitivity is altered during and after trauma. During periods of high stress, individuals may be relatively insensitive to pain—a phenomenon that is blocked by the opiate antagonist naloxone (Pitman, Van der Kolk, Orr, & Greenberg 1990). Conversely, after trauma, individuals with PTSD are more likely to have pain, and pain processing may be altered. The direction and biological cause of this alteration has appeared differently in different studies (Moeller-Bertram, Keltner, & Strigo 2012), but this has led to speculation that the endogenous opiate system may be involved in the pathology of PTSD. It has been speculated that, in addition to relieving pain and thus minimizing trauma, opiates may interfere with memory consolidation.

In the treatment of PTSD, opiates are an example of medications that may have diametrically opposite effects, depending on the time and individual to whom they are given. In retrospective studies, the acute administration of opiates after burns or physical combat trauma has been associated with a lower incidence of PTSD (Holbrook, Galarneau, Dye, Quinn, & Dougherty 2010; Saxe et al. 2001). Conversely, in patients in the intensive care unit, higher doses of opiates have been associated with greater incidence of delirium and delusions, which in turn are associated with higher rates of PTSD (Jones et al. 2007). Also, chronic use of opiates after physical trauma is not associated with any improvement in PTSD, but does correlate with a number of negative outcomes (Trevino & Brasel 2013). Individuals who are abusing opiates are more likely to experience trauma and to develop PTSD as a result of that trauma (Cottler, Compton, Mager, Spitznagel, & Janca 1992), and individuals who have PTSD are more likely to use higher doses of opiates for pain control (Schwartz et al. 2006) and are more likely to become addicted to opiates (Jacobsen, Southwick, & Kosten 2001).

In summary, opioids are a prime example demonstrating that a pharmaceutical cannot always be thought of as just "good" or "bad" for PTSD, but may do very different things depending on when, how, and to whom the medication is given.

SYNTHESIZED NATURAL SUBSTANCES

It is said that imitation is the sincerest form of flattery. Much of the history of pharmacology has followed a path in which a natural product is found to help a particular condition, and then scientists attempt to isolate the active ingredient out of the multitude of substances in the natural form. When that active ingredient is found, the substance is then either sold in a purified form from the original product or may be synthesized synthetically. Vitamins, hormones, aspirin, and the opiate subset of opioids all fall into this category. Opiates were described in the previous section of allopathic medications because most of them have been patented and marketed as pharmaceuticals. Because of legal issues involving the patenting, marketing, and regulatory control of naturally occurring substances, most of these compounds have fallen into a legal gray area that has made them both tremendously popular and difficult to market formally for the treatment of PTSD or any other disease state.

In 1994, the Dietary Supplement Health and Education Act defined any substance that is a natural component of any food, or that was sold as a supplement before October 1994, as a food supplement rather than a drug. This meant that, legally, these supplements are considered safe until proved otherwise—the opposite of a pharmaceutical drug, which must be proved safe before it can be brought to market. A supplement can also claim general health benefits without submitting specific evidence of it to any regulatory agency. It is still illegal to market a supplement as useful for the treatment of a disease state such as PTSD without submitting evidence from clinical trials, but the ease of direct marketing has removed the practical impetus for manufacturers to gain a formal disease indication. This has not

TABLE 7.2 Naturally Synthesized Substance Mechanisms of Action in Treating PTSD

Compound	DHEA	Magnesium	Melatonin	Omega-3	SAMe
PTSD prevention	X	X			
Fear extinction	X	X		X	
BDNF				X	
5HT		X			X
NE		X			X
D					
Pain					
GABA	X	X			
Anti-inflammatory	X				
HPA axis modulator	X	X			
Sleep			X		
DNA			X	X	
NMDA					
AMPA					
Hallucinogen					

5HT, Serotonin; AMPA, amino-3-hydroxy-5-methy-4-isoxazolepropionic acid; BDNF, brain-derived neurotropic factor; D, dopamine; DHEA, dehydroepiandrosterone; GABA, γ-aminobutyric acid; HPA, hypothalamic–pituitary–adrenal; NE, nor-epinephrine; NMDA, N-methyl-D-aspartate; PTSD, posttraumatic stress disorder; SAMe, S-adenosyl-l-methionine.

stopped research into the clinical applicability of these compounds, and we review that evidence here.

Of note, because of the vagaries of whether a hormonal product is naturally a component of meat or other foods, there are some seemingly arbitrary decisions concerning what is a drug versus a supplement. The circadian rhythm regulatory hormone melatonin is considered a supplement in the United States, whereas in Europe, melatonin is considered a hormone and cannot be sold over the counter. The endogenous glucocorticoid cortisol, as well as most sex steroids such as testosterone, are treated as pharmaceuticals in the United States, although dehydroepiandrosterone (DHEA) is treated as a supplement. In this chapter we limit ourselves to products that are sold as over-the-counter supplements. This choice is not because natural hormones might not be beneficial for PTSD, but rather because the use of prescription hormones for disease states is well covered in traditional texts and reviews (Fink, Pfaff, & Levine 2011; Steckler & Risbrough 2012) (Table 7.2).

Dehydroepiandrosterone

DHEA and the sulfate ester DHEAS are steroid hormones with multiple described actions and effects including neurogenesis and neuroprotection, catecholamine synthesis, antioxidant effects, anti-inflammatory effects, and antiglucocorticoid effects, as well as direct activity at the γ-aminobutyric acid (GABA)-A receptors and NMDA receptors. DHEA has been studied with relation to a number of neuropsychiatric disorders and illnesses (Maninger, Wolkowitz, Reus, Epel, & Mellon 2009). Studies correlating PTSD and DHEA levels have found increased levels of the hormone. However, it is thought this elevation represents a compensatory effect rather than a pathophysiological one. There is evidence that those with relatively higher levels of DHEA respond better to treatment and have an overall greater ability in coping with PTSD symptoms (Yehuda, Brand, Golier, & Yang 2006). It has also been demonstrated that the response to acute stress is improved in individuals with elevated levels of DHEA (Maninger, Wolkowitz, Reus, Epel, & Mellon 2009).

Magnesium

Magnesium (Mg) is an essential mineral for human nutrition and is needed for more than 300 biochemical reactions in the body, including maintaining normal nerve, cardiac, and skeletal muscle function; supporting a healthy immune system; and strengthening bones. Most dietary magnesium comes from vegetables, specifically dark-green leafy vegetables. Other sources include bananas, avocados, nuts, legumes, and soy products.

Mg is associated with the maintenance of fluidity of neuronal membranes and it is known to modulate NMDA and GABA receptors. It also appears to play a role in regulating the hypothalamic–pituitary–adrenal (HPA) axis and it participates in inactivation of protein kinase C neurotransmission. Depletion of Mg affects the NMDA receptor ion channel, and allows calcium and sodium ions to enter the postsynaptic neuron, resulting in the production of free radicals and subsequent neuronal swelling, and cell dysfunction and death. Furthermore, studies show activity of Mg at serotonergic receptors (5HT1A, 5HT2A/2C), norepinephrine (alpha 1, alpha 2), and dopamine (D) receptors (D1, D2) (Serefko et al. 2013).

Administration of Mg has been shown to be effective in decreasing the incidence and severity of posttraumatic depression significantly in mice (posttraumatic brain injury). In human research, treatment with oral Mg showed therapeutic effects similar to tricyclic antidepressants (TCAs) in depressed patients with hypomagnesemia (Serefko et al. 2013). In addition, a deficiency in Mg has been shown to be associated significantly with increased prevalence of depression in adults (Tarleton & Littenberg 2015). Conversely, studies have shown that higher dietary intakes of magnesium are associated with a decrease in prevalence of depression (Miki et al. 2014).

Due to the evidence of neuroprotection against depression and anxiety that Mg provides, and the potential detrimental effects caused by deficiencies of this mineral, it is suggested that all patients with PTSD have a healthy diet that provides adequate amounts of Mg. Although evaluation for hypomagnesemia in the central nervous system is difficult, because plasma/serum levels of Mg do not correlate well with the actual Mg levels in the human brain (Tarleton & Littenberg 2015), an evaluation for adequate Mg intake and a potential trial of Mg supplementation under the guidance of a physician, when there is suspected deficiency, should be considered in these patients.

Melatonin

Melatonin is a hormone produced from tryptophan in the pineal glands of humans and most other vertebrate animals. It is associated with the regulation of circadian rhythms as well as with immune function. It is also found in plants, fungi, and bacteria, where its role is less clear. In part, its function is an antioxidant and a protector of DNA. Most supplements are derived from pituitary extracts, but melatonin can also be extracted or synthesized from other sources.

The pharmacological action of melatonin likely derives from its actions on the melatonin receptor in the brain. In animals, melatonin is produced at night. It encourages activity in nocturnal animals, and sleep in diurnal animals. It is used pharmacologically to improve sleep. Unlike most sleep aids, melatonin does not seem to induce sedation directly, but rather it advances the sleep phase. It may also have anxiety-reducing properties that assist those with sleep difficulties (Acil et al. 2004).

Sleep disruption is an early symptom of PTSD and may predict the development of the full disorder (McLay, Klam, & Volkert 2010). Similarly, disruption of melatonin metabolites has been shown to predict the development of PTSD after trauma (McFarlane, Barton, Briggs, & Kennaway 2010), which has led to speculation that melatonin could improve sleep in PTSD and, if given early, could perhaps mitigate the course of the condition. However, this has yet to be supported by any direct evidence. In other psychiatric conditions in which sleep is disrupted, such as depression, melatonin has been found to improve sleep, but did not have any benefit for other psychiatric symptoms (Dolberg, Hirschmann, & Grunhaus 2014).

Omega-3 Fatty Acids

The consumption of omega-3 fatty acids has evidence suggesting a benefit for a variety of health concerns. Most notable are the benefits for cardiovascular health (National Institute of Health, Office of Dietary Supplements 2005). There is also increasing evidence that there is benefit from the administration of omega-3 fatty acids in the treatment of neuropsychiatric disorders, including depression and schizophrenia (Peet & Stokes 2005). There are data that illustrate that the administration of omega-3 fatty acids increases brain-derived neurotrophic factor and in turn increases neurogenesis in the hippocampus. There is evidence that, by promoting the neurogenesis of the hippocampus, there is an attenuation of the consolidation of fear-related memories (Matsuoka 2011). This result has led to research examining the role of omega-3 fatty acid supplementation in preventing the development of PTSD after trauma (Matsuoka et al. 2011). It should be noted that a small open-label study examining the effects of supplementation of omega-3 fatty acids on PTSD symptoms had to be cut short because of an increase in avoidance symptoms, in addition to patient dropout (Zeev, Michael, Ram, & Hagit 2005). Additional benefits of omega-3 fatty acids for PTSD, beyond the neuropsychiatric implications, may exist in terms of cardiovascular protection, because persons with PTSD are at an increased risk for cardiovascular disease and other cardiovascular risk factors (Coughlin 2011).

S-Adenosyl-L-Methionine

S-adenosyl-l-methionine (SAMe) is a naturally occurring substance found through-out the body and brain, and is synthesized in the same carbon cycle that involves vitamin B12 and folate.

Low central nervous system levels of SAMe are associated with depression. The exact mechanism of action of SAMe is not fully understood, but there are sev-eral hypotheses proposed to explain its antidepressant effects. SAMe is involved in monoamine and melatonin synthesis, and it serves as the methyl group donor for a number of substrates including phospholipids, DNA, RNA, neurotransmit-ters, and proteins. One theory states that by increasing SAMe, synthesis of the neurotransmitter monoamines (serotonin and norepinephrine thought to be defi-cient in depression and anxiety) is increased. Another theory is that SAMe meth-ylates plasma phospholipids and alters the fluidity of the neuronal membrane, which affects the function of proteins that traverse the membrane, including the monoamine receptors and transporters. Last, it is hypothesized that DNA meth-ylation by SAMe may increase DNA transcription, thereby altering cellular func-tion (Papakostas 2008).

SAMe has been prescribed widely in Europe for more than 30 years. Intramuscular and intravenous SAMe have been shown to be equivalent to TCA in efficacy as monotherapy for depression, and there is some evidence to suggest that high-dose oral SAMe (1600 mg/day) may also have similar efficacy (Larzelere, Campbell, & Robertson 2010). In addition, SAMe was found to be better tolerated compared with TCAs, and the onset of the antidepressant effect may be earlier when SAMe is used as monotherapy or adjunctively compared with monotherapy with antidepressant medi-cations (Di Pierro & Settembre 2015). However, there has been concern and debate over the possibility of SAMe increasing other methylated compounds such as homo-cysteine, which is believed to increase cardiovascular risk. Coadministration of be-taine (a cofactor involved in reducing plasma homocysteine levels) with SAMe may help to mitigate this risk, and a recent study from 2015 shows that SAMe–betaine in combination was as effective as TCAs in treating mild depression (Di Pierro & Settembre 2015). In the application of treating PTSD, based on the current treatment model focusing on correcting deficiencies in neurotransmitters including norepineph-rine, serotonin, and dopamine, SAMe may prove to be an ideal supplement or even monotherapy based on its broad mechanism of action in synthesizing all these mono-amines (Papakostas 2008) and its proved efficacy in the treatment of MDD.

Because there are potential cardiovascular concerns (atherosclerosis) associated with using SAMe, and because there are other alternative medications that have similar mechanisms of action toward PTSD (specifically, increases in monoamine neurotransmitters), this agent may be best considered for use in patients who have abnormities in the B12/folate carbon cycle to correct these deficiencies. As a result of the cardiac risks, consultation with a physician is recommended before starting this supplement in patients who have coronary artery disease risk factors or known disease.

Theanine

Theanine is an amino acid analogue of glutamate and glutamine. It is usually found in the L-enantiomer, and thus is called more correctly *L-theanine*. It gives green tea its particular flavor and is found in high concentrations in tea and gyokuro leaves. Theanine is also present in smaller concentrations in a number of plant and fungal species. It can be isolated from these natural sources or synthesized chemically.

The pharmacological action of theanine probably occurs via its action on glutamate receptors, and glutamine and glycine reuptake transporters. Theanine crosses the blood–brain barrier and can act directly at central cites (Yokogoshi, Kobayashi, Mochizuki, & Terashima 1998). It is an agonist at amino-3-hydroxy-5-methy-4-isoxazolepropionic acid (AMPA) and kainite glutamate receptors, but blocks NMDA receptors, which may enhance some glutamate-mediated transmission while simultaneously helping to prevent glutamate-induced neurotoxicity. Indirect mechanisms for theanine include the upregulation of neurotrophic factors, increasing concentrations of inhibitory neurotransmitters and catecholamines.

A broad spectrum of health claims have been made for theanine, mostly as part of mitigating the stress response, and include improving concentration and learning ability, preventing cancer and cardiovascular disease, decreasing blood pressure, improving schizophrenia, promoting weight loss, and enhancing performance of the immune system (Vuong, Bowyer, & Roach 2011). Relevant to PTSD, in animal models theanine prevents stress-induced cognitive changes (Tian et al. 2013) and normalizes gene expression in PTSD (Ceremuga et al. 2014). There is also evidence that theanine improves cognitive performance during stress in humans (Kimura, Ozeki, Juneja, & Ohira 2007). Theanine does not appear to lower anxiety in all contexts, however (Lu et al. 2004), and to our knowledge there are as, of yet, no direct trials in PTSD.

PLANT-BASED TREATMENTS

It would take the most hardened of cynics to believe there is not, somewhere in nature, an herb or other plant that might be helpful for PTSD. But which one, or ones, remains uncertain. Aiding the search for such a treatment are a wealth of folk medicine and historical reference from which to look for options. Some also argue that the long coexistence of humans and plants means they are generally a safer option than more-recently synthesized chemicals. The most poisonous varieties of plant are well known, and evolution has allowed us to adapt to the side effects of less noxious varieties. This is not to say there cannot be side effects or medication interactions (Abebe 2002). For those who believe in a benevolent creator, there is also the thought that He or She would not have made a disease without also offering an option somewhere to counter it. Setting aside spiritual hopes for the moment, however, we review the evidence.

Even more so than with purified natural compounds, the study of herbal treatments faces significant problems with standardization, regulation, and formal testing. There is little incentive for commercial entities to provide randomized clinical trials to study efficacy formally. Even when studies are conducted, there is a question of whether a plant used in a trial is equivalent to what would be provided to a patient. A manufactured pharmaceutical contains a limited number of active ingredients, but a plant is a plethora growing together. The ingredients for successful treatment may or may not be present in consistent quantities depending on the strain, where or how the plant is grown, storage, processing, or individual variation. Also, an investigation by New York state's attorney general found that four of five herbal supplements sold at major retailers did not contain any of the herb advertised on the packaging (O'Connor 2015). Standardization, however, is not impossible. There are accepted methods to ensure pharmaceutical quality (Mukherjee 2002), and many countries now regulate and test herbal medications in ways similar to manufactured pharmaceuticals.

If variety is the curse of herbal medication research, it is also its blessing. There are vast options from which to choose in terms of compounds that might help PTSD, or at least individual symptoms related to PTSD. We could not hope to cover all plant-based options, and therefore refer you to textbooks of herbal medication if you want to read further (Newall, Anderson, & Phillipson 1996; Wichtl 2004). Here we review some plant-based treatments used for or advocated as potential treatments for PTSD (Table 7.3).

Ayahuasca

Ayahuasca is a hallucinogenic beverage with origins in South America. It has been used by shamans in the Amazon Basin as part of traditional folk medicine and religious practices (McKenna, Luna, & Towers 1986). Ayahuasca is consumed as a tea obtained from

TABLE 7.3 Plant-Based Agent Mechanisms of Action in Treating PTSD

Compound	Theanine	Ayahuasca	Kawa	Passion flower	Saffron	St. John's Wort	Valerian root
PTSD prevention	X						
Fear extinction		X					
BDNF	X						
5HT	X	X		X	X	X	X
NE	X	X		X		X	
D	0				X		
Pain						X	
GABA	X		X	X		X	X
Anti-inflammatory					X		
HPA axis modulator					X	X	
Sleep							
DNA							
NMDA	X						
AMPA	X						
Hallucinogen	X						

5HT, serotonin; AMPA, amino-3-hydroxy-5-methy-4-isoxazolepropionic acid; BDNF, brain-derived neurotropic factor; D, dopamine; GABA, γ-aminobutyric acid; HPA, hypothalamic–pituitary–adrenal; NE, nor-epinephrine; NMDA, N-methyl-D-aspartate; PTSD, posttraumatic stress disorder.

the combination of the plants *Banisteriopsis caapi* and, commonly, *Psychotria viridis*, which combines the 5-HT2A agonist and psychedelic agent N,N-dimethyltryptamine with monoamine oxidase-inhibiting B-carboline alkaloids found in *B. caapi* (Riba et al. 2003). The effects of orally ingested ayahuasca include visual and auditory hallucinations, euphoria, and changes in sensorium (Riba Rodríguez-Fornells et al. 2001). In addition, reports indicate feeling "a sense of inner peace and acceptance of self, others, and the world" and "feelings of connectedness" (Erowid 2015). Individual reports indicate benefit in relief from PTSD symptoms. Anecdotally, individuals report experiencing a reorganization of their traumatic memories, allowing them to cope better with previously identified triggers (Bain 2014; Short 2015). A clue to this may lie in the area of the brain activated during ayahuasca intoxication. Imaging studies indicate activation of the paralimbic and prefrontal regions of the brain thought to play a role in emotional arousal and emotional processing (Riba et al. 2006). Research also suggests benefit from ayahuasca in the treatment of substance use disorders as well as depression and anxiety (dos Santos Landeira-Fernandez, Strassman, Motta, & Cruz 2007; Osório et al. 2015; Thomas, Lucas, Capler, Tupper, & Martin 2013).

Kava

Kava is a perennial shrub native to the South Pacific Islands, including Hawaii. Its rootstock contains the pharmacologically active compounds kavalactones. Street names for kava include ava, intoxicating pepper, kawa, and tonga.

Kava is known to have sedative and anxiolytic properties; however, kavalactones have not been studied extensively, and the mechanism of action has yet to be elucidated fully (Kinrys, Coleman, & Rothstein 2009). Kavalactones may act by stimulating binding of GABA receptors indirectly and increasing the number of GABA binding sites. In addition, Kava may exert anticonvulsant effects through its actions on sodium and calcium voltage-dependent channels (Larzelere, Campbell, & Robertson 2010).

Kava is not a controlled substance in the United States; however, as a result of concerns of liver toxicity, many countries (including Canada, France, Germany, Switzerland, and the United Kingdom) and Australia have placed regulatory controls on kava. Because of its actions on GABA, and its potential anticonvulsant properties, it may be beneficial in symptomatic treatment of PTSD, including insomnia, irritability, and hyperarousal (Ravindran & Stein 2009). As a result of its mechanism of action, this agent may be considered an alternative to benzodiazepines or barbiturates in patients in whom use of these medications may be a concern (for reasons such as abuse, dependence, and so on).

Passion Flower

Passiflora incarnata is a plant indigenous to the southeastern United States, Argentina, and Brazil. Passion flower is a woody vine with flowers that has been used since ancient times for its sedative and anxiolytic properties. The mechanism of action is currently unknown, but monoamine oxidase inhibition and activation of GABA receptors may be involved (Kinrys, Coleman, & Rothstein 2009).

Passion flower has been shown to be effective in the treatment of generalized anxiety disorder. In two clinical trials, *P. incarnata* was as effective as oxazepam and mexazolam in the treatment of anxiety. Onset of action was shown to be more rapid in subjects taking oxazepam, but reported cognitive and functional impairment relating to job performance was decreased in subjects taking *P. incarnata* comparatively

(Kinrys, Coleman, & Rothstein 2009; Larzelere, Campbell, & Robertson 2010). Another study comparing *P. incarnata* with placebo for treatment of preoperative anxiety found *P. incarnata* reduced anxiety significantly but did not induce sedation or change psychomotor functioning compared with placebo (Movafegh, Alizadeh, Hajimohamadi, Esfehani, & Nejatfar 2008). Based on these findings, passion flower may be beneficial in the treatment of anxiety symptoms associated with PTSD, such as irritability, hyperarousal, and hypervigilance.

Because *P. incarnata* shows effective anxiolysis without significant sedation or cognitive impairment, it may be an effective alternative for patients in whom these effects are specifically undesirable, such as shift workers, high-attention occupations, and so on.

Saffron

Saffron is an expensive (retail price up to US$11,000/kg) and coveted cooking spice derived from the blue–purple *Crocus sativus* flower. Saffron has been used in traditional medicine as an antidepressant, anticonvulsant, analgesic, and aphrodisiac, in addition to other uses. It is composed of four main bioactive compounds: crocins, crocetin, safranal, and picrocrocin. The first three compounds are potent antioxidants that have been shown to have a synergistic antioxidant effect when used collectively versus independently (Lopresti & Drummond 2014).

The exact mechanism of action of saffron is still currently unknown, but current research suggests antioxidant, anti-inflammatory (cyclooxygenase 1, cyclooxygenase 2, and prostaglandin E2 inhibition), serotonergic (5HT2C antagonism), HPA axis modulation, and neuroprotective effects.

Several recent studies showed saffron with efficacy comparable with the antidepressants fluoxetine and imipramine in treatment of adults with moderate major depressive disorder (MDD). Doses of 30 mg/day of extract from either the stigma or petal portion of the flower were found to be equivalent in reducing depressive symptoms in adults with MDD. This finding is noteworthy because petals are significantly less expensive (Lopresti & Drummond 2014).

Most interestingly, saffron's mechanisms of action align with the current mechanisms and principles of pharmacological treatment of PTSD. In addition, saffron has an established efficacy in treating MDD (a disorder hypothesized to have alterations in many of the same neurotransmitters altered in PTSD). Although the high cost of saffron may make it unfeasible for medical use, investigation into saffron's mechanism of action and creation of synthetic derivatives holds promise for more effective treatments of PTSD.

Although research is still limited, because saffron is a common (although costly) spice and it has a broad range of mechanisms of action affecting both mental health and physical ailments, it will likely be an ideal agent for patients with PTSD who are seeking a simple, food-based supplement for improvement of mood and stress response.

St. John's Wort

St. John's Wort, *Hypericum perforatum*, is a plant native to Europe, West Asia, and North Africa. Its use for treatment of "nerve-related disorders" can be traced back to Greek and Roman times.

Evidence suggests that St. John's Wort has serotonergic, noradrenergic, dopaminergic, and GABA-minergic activity. In addition, the active components hypericin and hyperforin are believed to inhibit cytokine production, resulting in decreased cortisol production and improved regulation of the HPA axis (Kinrys, Coleman, & Rothstein 2009).

Most evidence with St. John's Wort supports use to treat depression; however, there are data suggesting efficacy in treating anxiety disorders. Dosages of 300 to 1800 mg daily have been used. There have been no reported studies evaluating St. John's Wort for treatment for PTSD; however, because of its activity in increasing serotonin and norepinephrine and stabilizing the HPA axis, there is potential utility in treating PTSD. Additional activity on GABA receptors and dopamine may further potentiate relief of hyperarousal/insomnia and negative alterations in cognitions associated with PTSD (Ravindran & Stein 2009).

One potential negative consequence of St. John's Wort is that it is an inducer of the CYP3A4 enzyme, a pathway used commonly in the metabolism of medications. Care must therefore be taken to avoid drug–drug interactions.

Valerian Root

Valeriana is a perennial plant that grows in temperate climates and is used commonly for its sedative–hypnotic and anxiolytic effects. Depending on the species, the specific chemical components vary; however, all varieties contain GABA, arginine, glutamine, and alanine. Valerian root's proposed mechanisms of action include GABA activity, and 5-HT5a receptor activity (Kinrys, Coleman, & Rothstein 2009).

Clinical trials supporting the use of valerian is limited. A recent review of 37 studies investigating the use of valerian root as a sleep aid found no evidence of efficacy, but no safety concerns and few side effects (Taibi, Landis, Petry, & Vitiello, 2007). Of note, in one clinical trial, a blend of St. John's Wort and valerian was superior to diazepam in reducing anxiety symptoms (Kinrys, Coleman, & Rothstein 2009). Given valerian root's potential activity on serotonin, it may play a role in improving anxiety and mood symptoms associated with PTSD, although current science is lacking to support this assertion. As a result of a lack of evidence showing efficacy in treating insomnia, there appears to be limited benefit for using valerian for treating isolated sleep disturbances associated with PTSD; however, given valerian root's safety profile and theoretical benefit in anxiety-related symptoms, further research into the utility of this plant in treatment of other domains of PTSD is warranted.

Because valerian has limited evidence for efficacy, but overall no significant safety concerns or side effects, it may be a good second-line agent in patients who are nonresponders to other anxiolytics, mood agents, or sleep aids in the treatment of PTSD.

SUBSTANCES OF ABUSE

All medications have the potential for harm. In a few instances, however, a compound is perceived to have such negative consequences that legal authorities feel the need to ban it altogether. These bans have included both synthetic and natural products. Different governments, scientists, and organizations have vehemently disagreed about the risks and benefits of various substances. Most notably, in the United States, marijuana is allowed by some states but prohibited in other states and by federal law. Some individuals may, of course, choose to circumvent the law. This choice may be as part of a personal belief system or a search for a desired euphoric effect that blinds the user to the adverse consequences. In some cases, there may be truth to the idea that an individual with PTSD is self-medicating. Scientists and medical providers may also believe that, although the substance is considered harmful, the administration of the substance in a particular medical context could allow a novel way to treat PTSD within acceptable risk parameters. We do not advocate for breaking any law and strongly caution prescribers who might consider offering these options that there are both legal and health risks involved. With that disclaimer, and given there is a popular belief that some banned pharmaceuticals are effective in treating PTSD, we review the evidence (Table 7.4).

TABLE 7.4 Substances of Abuse Mechanisms of Action in Treating PTSD

Compound	MDMA	Psilocybin	LSD	Marijuana
PTSD prevention				
Fear extinction	X	X		X
BDNF				
5HT	X	X	X	
NE	X			
D	X			
Pain				
GABA				
Anti-inflammatory				
HPA axis modulator				
Sleep				
DNA				
NMDA				
AMPA				
Hallucinogen	X	X	X	
CBD				X

5HT, serotoning; AMPA, amino-3-hydroxy-5-methy-4-isoxazolepropionic acid; BDNF, brain-derived neurotropic factor; CBD, cannabidiol; D, dopamine; GABA, γ-aminobutyric acid; HPA, hypothalamic–pituitary–adrenal; LSD, lysergic acid diethylamide; MDMA, methylene-dioxymethamphetamine; NE, nor-epinephrine; NMDA, N-methyl-D-aspartate; PTSD, post-traumatic stress disorder.

Methylenedioxymethamphetamine

Methylenedioxymethamphetamine (MDMA) is a synthetic drug with both stimulant and mild hallucinogenic properties. Street names include Ecstasy, XTC, E, and X.

MDMA is similar structurally to the combined effects of amphetamines and mescaline. As such, it causes the net release of endogenous catecholamines, particularly norepinephrine and dopamine, and blocks their reuptake into presynaptic vesicles. In addition, because of its structural similarity to serotonin, it also causes a net endogenous release of serotonin and inhibits serotonin reuptake (Kalant 2001). These properties overlap with the effects of standard psychotropic medications used in the treatment of PTSD, most notably antidepressants (Ravindran & Stein 2009). The dopaminergic action of MDMA may improve negative alterations in cognitions associated with PTSD (inability to experience positive emotions, diminished interest in activities, negative emotional state); however, it may also worsen other associated symptoms of PTSD including hyperarousal (irritability, hypervigilance, exaggerated startle response) and psychotic symptoms sometimes seen with PTSD.

In 1985, the U.S. Drug Enforcement Administration labeled MDMA a schedule I drug, making manufacture, transport, sale, and medical use for MDMA illegal. Given MDMA's status as an illegal substance, there was no research on its medical utility between 1985 and 2008. Since 2008, however, three randomized controlled trials have been conducted in participants with refractory PTSD (reviewed in White [2014]). Results of these studies suggest that 125 mg MDMA in conjunction with psychotherapy is effective in improving reexperiencing and avoidance symptoms of PTSD. Of note, in these studies, MDMA was given only in the context of the therapy session, not prescribed on a regular basis. Also, if patients were shown to be nonresponders to MDMA-assisted psychotherapy by the end of the third session, additional use of MDMA was unlikely to be beneficial (White 2014).

Psilocybin

Psilocybin is a naturally occurring compound found in dozens of species of mushrooms, including members of the genus *Psilocybe*. Street names include "magic mushrooms" or "shrooms." It is similar structurally to hallucinogens of the tryptamine class, which includes alpha-methyltryptamine ("Spirals"), N,N-dimethyltryptamine, and 5-methoxydimethyltryptamine ("Foxy," "Foxy methoxy"). Psilocybin is metabolized in the body to psilocin, a potent agonist at serotonin receptors (5-HT1A/2A/2C). The effects of psilocybin and the other tryptamines can be similar to lysergic acid diethylamide (LSD) and MDMA, respectively.

Psilocybin is a schedule I substance. Because of the serotonergic effects inherent in this medication, it may be beneficial in treating negative mood symptoms (depression) and anxiety associated with PTSD. In a 2011 study using psilocybin for the treatment of anxiety in patients with advanced-stage cancer, it was shown to have a positive trend in improving mood and anxiety (Grob et al. 2011). The potential synaptic dopamine increases associated with other drugs in the tryptamine class may also contribute to improvement in negative alterations in cognition, and worsening of hyperarousal and psychotic symptoms, as seen in MDMA.

Lysergic Acid Diethylamide

LSD is a potent synthetic hallucinogen. Common street names include "acid" and "dots," in reference to the common practice of adding LSD to blotter paper in colorful shapes and dots, with each shape/dot equivalent to one dose or "hit."

LSD is a derivative of lysergic acid, which is found in the ergot fungus that grows on rye and other grains. It is considered a serotonin agonist and is specifically hypothesized to have particular activity with the 5HT2A receptor in the frontal cortex, which would explain the significant role in hallucinogenesis and psychosis associated with this drug. It has limited activity at other 5HT receptors (including 1A) (Fantegrossi, Murnane, & Reissig 2008).

LSD is a schedule I substance. Because of its limited action on the primary neurotransmitters hypothesized to be dysfunctional in PTSD (norepinephrine and serotonin (5HT1)), its use may be limited for this disorder when compared with the potential of the other hallucinogens mentioned earlier. Although there has been individual advocacy for the use of LSD to treat PTSD, to our knowledge there are no formal clinical studies in this area, and purported mechanisms of action would not particularly support such investigation.

Marijuana

Marijuana, or *Cannabis sativa*, is a plant that has intoxicating effects when smoked or ingested orally. Up until the 20th century, it was used commonly for medicinal purposes in many parts of the world, including the United States. The wide use of marijuana has led to significant research investigating the effects of the constituents of this plant.

Marijuana has many components, but the two major compounds of interest are tetrahydrocannabinol (THC) and cannabidiol (CBD). THC is the major psychoactive component and it has a strong affinity for the endocannabinoid receptor CB1. CBD, which can make up to 40% of a marijuana extract, is not psychoactive and does not have binding affinity for identified receptors of the endocannabinoid system. However, CBD has been shown to have antipsychotic and anxiolytic effects, countering the intoxicant effects of THC (Passie, Emrich, Karst, Brandt, & Halpern 2012). In addition, it has been shown that CBD reduces the degradation of anandamide, an endogenous cannabinoid with affinity for CB1 (Leweke et al. 2012).

Among those with a diagnosis of PTSD, there is an increased prevalence of cannabis use (Bonn-Miller & Rousseau, 2015). Currently, there is only anecdotal evidence that marijuana use has benefits in terms of alleviating symptoms of PTSD. Animal model research has shown the endogenous cannabinoid system plays a role in the extinction of aversive memories (Mariscano et al. 2002). Imaging studies have shown an increased availability of CB1 receptors in the amygdala and hippocampus, as well as other areas of the brain, in patients with PTSD. This same study also demonstrated a reduced level of circulating anandamide (Neumeister et al. 2013). The proposed effects of the endocannabinoid system on extinction of fear-related memories and the abnormalities of the endocannabinoid system described in patients with PTSD suggest an explanation for the increased use of cannabis among those with PTSD, as well as the potential mechanisms by which benefit is conferred. The relationship of THC, CBD, the endocannabinoid system, and symptoms of PTSD is an area of active research.

CONCLUSION

Clinicians and patients seeking treatment of PTSD using a complementary and alternative medicine approach have several pharmacological options available to them, including nontraditional use of allopathic medications, synthesized natural substances, herbally/plant-based compounds, and substances typically associated with recreational drug use/abuse. As a result of the complex nature of PTSD—each patient affected with this condition must be evaluated and treated based on his or her specific biological and psychological pathology associated with PTSD, with pharmacological treatment tailored for each patient's unique signs and symptoms. By using alternative agents with mechanisms of action correlated to the target symptoms associated with PTSD, clinicians and patients can develop an optimal treatment plan that can augment or potentially replace mainstream pharmacological modalities, with the end result being a holistic approach that has improved efficacy, with better access to care, and with more value.

KEY POINTS

- The clinical condition of PTSD has both biological and psychological components that must be addressed for optimal treatment.
- From a biological perspective, treatment of PTSD is very complex, because PTSD can be caused and perpetuated by abnormalities in many different physiological and anatomic processes, including neuroendocrine, neuroanatomy, and inflammation.
- From a psychological perspective, alternative medicine pharmacology can be used to augment psychotherapy, including techniques used to modulate fear extinction.
- Alternative medicine pharmacological treatment of PTSD includes the nontraditional use of allopathic medications, synthesized natural substances, herbally/plant-based compounds, and substances of abuse.

- Based on their mechanisms of action, alternative pharmacological agents may be used as an alternative or to augment traditional medications in the treatment of PTSD.
- Clinicians and patients can use alternative medicine agents to treat the specific signs and symptoms of PTSD, based on each agent's mechanisms of action.
- As a result of the different mechanisms of action, and therefore symptom targets, the efficacy of each alternative medicine agent is determined in part by the goal of treatment—that being primary, secondary, or tertiary prevention of PTSD.
- Alternative medicine pharmacological agents may be useful to patients and their providers because of their potential superiority on several metrics when compared with traditional medications, including affordability, accessibility, and efficacy. In addition, alternative pharmacology may be useful for patients who cannot use traditional psychotropic medications resulting from social factors such as employment regulations.
- Because of similar mechanism of action to many traditional medications, when using alternative medicine in conjunction with these alternative medicine pharmacological agents, or when multiple alternative medicine agents are used together, proper understanding and care must be taken to avoid adverse reactions.

REFERENCES

Abdallah, C. G., Salas, R., Jackowski, A., Baldwin, P., Sato, J. R., & Mathew, S. J. (2014a). Hippocampal volume and the rapid antidepressant effect of ketamine. *Journal of Psychopharmacology*. [Epub ahead of print].

Abdallah, C. G., Sanacora, G., Duman, R. S., & Krystal, J. H. (2014b). Ketamine and rapid-acting antidepressants: a window into a new neurobiology for mood disorder therapeutics. *Medicine*, *66*, 509–523.

Abebe, W. (2002). Herbal medication: potential for adverse interactions with analgesic drugs. *Journal of Clinical Pharmacy and Therapeutics*, *27*(6), 391–401.

Acil, M., Basgul, E., Celiker, V., Karagoz, A. H., Demir, B., & Aypar, U. (2004). Perioperative effects of melatonin and midazolam premedication on sedation, orientation, anxiety scores and psychomotor performance. *European Journal of Anaesthesiology*, *21*(7), 553–557.

American Psychiatric Association. (2013). *Diagnostic and statistical manual of mental disorders (DSM-5®)*. Philadelphia: American Psychiatric Association.

Anthony, E. W., & Nevins, M. E. (1993). Anxiolytic-like effects of *N*-methyl-D-aspartate-associated glycine receptor ligands in the rat potentiated startle test. *European Journal of Pharmacology*, *250*(2), 317–324.

Argolo, F. C., Cavalcanti-Ribeiro, P., Netto, L. R., & Quarantini, L. C. (2015). Prevention of post-traumatic stress disorder with propranolol: a meta-analytic review. *Journal of Psychosomatic Research*. [E-pub ahead of print].

Bain K. (2014, June 24). *Ayahuasca: a promising treatment for post-traumatic stress disorder.* Available at http://reset.me/story/ayahuasca-promising-treatment-post-traumatic-stress-disorder/. Accessed April 15, 2015.

Bajor, L. A., Ticlea, A. N., & Osser, D. N. (2011). The Psychopharmacology Algorithm Project at the Harvard South Shore Program: an update on posttraumatic stress disorder. *Harvard Review of Psychiatry, 19*(5), 240–258.

Bernardy, N. C., & Friedman, M. J. (2015). Psychopharmacological strategies in the management of post-traumatic stress disorder (PTSD): what have we learned? *Current Psychiatry Reports, 17*(4), 1–10.

Blake, D. D., Weathers, F. W., Nagy, L. M., Kaloupek, D. G., Gusman, F. D., Charney, D. S., et al. (1995). The development of a clinician-administered PTSD scale. *Journal of Traumatic Stress, 8*(1), 75–90.

Bonn-Miller, M. O., & Rousseau, G. S. (2015, March 15). *Marijuana use and PTSD among veterans.* PTSD: National Center for PTSD. Available at http://www.ptsd.va.gov/professional/co-occurring/marijuana_use_ptsd_veterans.asp. Accessed April 15, 2015.

Brownstein, M. J. (1993). A brief history of opiates, opioid peptides, and opioid receptors. *Proceedings of the National Academy of Sciences of the United States of America, 90*(12), 5391–5393.

Calne, D. B. (1970). L-Dopa and parkinsonism. *Nature, 226,* 21–24.

Ceremuga, T. E., Martinson, S., Washington, J., Revels, R., Wojcicki, J., Crawford, D., (2014). Effects of L-theanine on posttraumatic stress disorder induced changes in rat brain gene expression. *The Scientific World Journal.2014,* 419032–419033.

Cottencin, O., Vaiva, G., Huron, C., Devos, P., Ducrocq, F., Jouvent, R., et al. (2006). Directed forgetting in PTSD: a comparative study versus normal controls. *Journal of Psychiatric Research, 40*(1), 70–80.

Cottler, L., Compton, W., Mager, D., Spitznagel, E., & Janca, A. (1992). Posttraumatic stress disorder among substance users from the general population. *The American Journal of Psychiatry, 149*(5), 664–670.

Coughlin, S. S. (2011). Post-traumatic stress disorder and cardiovascular disease. *The Open Cardiovascular Medicine Journal, 5,* 164–170.

Covvey, J. R., Crawford, A. N., & Lowe, D. K. (2012). Intravenous ketamine for treatment-resistant major depressive disorder. *Annals of Pharmacotherapy, 46*(1), 117–123.

Cutler, D. M., Deaton, A. S., & Lleras-Muney, A. (2006). The determinants of mortality *Journal of Economic Perspectives, 20,* 97–120.

Davis, L. L., Suris, A., Lambert, M. T., Heimberg, C., & Petty, F. (1997). Post-traumatic stress disorder and serotonin: new directions for research and treatment. *Journal of Psychiatry & Neuroscience: JPN, 22*(5), 318–326.

de Kleine, R. A., Hendriks, G. J., Kusters, W. J., Broekman, T. G., & van Minnen, A. (2012). A randomized placebo-controlled trial of D-cycloserine to enhance exposure therapy for posttraumatic stress disorder. *Biological Psychiatry, 71*(11), 962–968.

de Kleine, R. A., Rothbaum, B. O., & van Minnen, A. (2013). Pharmacological enhancement of exposure-based treatment in PTSD: a qualitative review. *European Journal of Psychotraumatology, 4.*

Difede, J., Cukor, J., Wyka, K., Olden, M., Hoffman, H., Lee, F. S., et al. (2014). D-cycloserine augmentation of exposure therapy for post-traumatic stress disorder: a pilot randomized clinical trial. *Neuropsychopharmacology, 39*(5), 1052–1058.

Di Pierro, F., & Settembre, R. (2015). Preliminary results of a randomized controlled trial carried out with a fixed combination of S-adenosyl-L-methionine and betaine versus amitriptyline in patients with mild depression. *International Journal of General Medicine, 8,* 73–78

Dolberg, O. T., Hirschmann, S., & Grunhaus, L. (2014). Melatonin for the treatment of sleep disturbances in major depressive disorder. *American Journal of Psychiatry, 155,* 1119–1121.

dos Santos, R. G., Landeira-Fernandez, J., Strassman, R. J., Motta, V., & Cruz, A. P. M. (2007). Effects of ayahuasca on psychometric measures of anxiety, panic-like and hopelessness in Santo Daime members. *Journal of Ethnopharmacology, 112*(3), 507–513.

Ernst, E., Pittler, M. H., Stevinson, C., & White, A. (2001). *The desktop guide to complementary and alternative medicine: an evidence-based approach.* Edinburgh: Mosby.

Erowid. (2015, February 11). *Ayahuasca effects*. Available at https://www.erowid.org/chemicals/aya-huasca/ayahuasca_effects.shtml. Accessed April 15, 2015.

Famularo, R., Kinscherff, R., & Fenton, T. (1988). Propranolol treatment for childhood posttraumatic stress disorder, acute type: a pilot study. *American Journal of Diseases of Children, 142*(11), 1244–1247.

Fantegrossi, W. E., Murnane, K. S., & Reissig, C. J. (2008). The behavioral pharmacology of hallucinogens. *Biochemical Pharmacology, 75*(1), 17–33.

Feder, A., Parides, M. K., Murrough, J. W., Perez, A. M., Morgan, J. E., Saxena, S., et al. (2014). Efficacy of intravenous ketamine for treatment of chronic posttraumatic stress disorder: a randomized clinical trial. *Journal of the American Medical Association Psychiatry, 71*(6), 681–688.

Fink, G., Pfaff, D. W., & Levine, J. E. (Eds.). (2011). *Handbook of neuroendocrinology*. Cambridge: Academic Press.

Foa, E., Hembree, E., & Rothbaum, B. O. (2007). *Prolonged exposure therapy for PTSD: emotional processing of traumatic experiences therapist guide*. Oxford: Oxford University Press.

Fontanarosa, P. B., & Lundberg, G. D. (1998). Alternative medicine meets science. *Journal of the American Medical Association, 280*(18), 1618–1619.

Friedman, M. J. (1999). What might the psychobiology of posttraumatic stress disorder teach us about future approaches to pharmacotherapy? *Journal of Clinical Psychiatry, 61*, 44–51.

Grob, C. S., Danforth, A. L., Chopra, G. S., Hagerty, M., McKay, C. R., Halberstadt, A. L., et al. (2011). Pilot study of psilocybin treatment for anxiety in patients with advanced-stage cancer. *Archives of General Psychiatry, 68*(1), 71–78.

Hofmann, S. G., Meuret, A. E., Smits, J. A., Simon, N. M., Pollack, M. H., Eisenmenger, K., et al. (2006). Augmentation of exposure therapy with D-cycloserine for social anxiety disorder. *Archives of General Psychiatry, 63*(3), 298–304.

Holbrook, T. L., Galarneau, M. R., Dye, J. L., Quinn, K., & Dougherty, A. L. (2010). Morphine use after combat injury in Iraq and post-traumatic stress disorder. *New England Journal of Medicine, 362*(2), 110–117.

Jacobsen, L. K., Southwick, S. M., & Kosten, T. R. (2001). Substance use disorders in patients with posttraumatic stress disorder: a review of the literature. *American Journal of Psychiatry, 158*(8), 1184–1190.

Jones, C., Bäckman, C., Capuzzo, M., Flaatten, H., Rylander, C., & Griffiths, R. D. (2007). Precipitants of post-traumatic stress disorder following intensive care: a hypothesis generating study of diversity in care. *Intensive Care Medicine, 33*(6), 978–985.

Kalant, H. (2001). The pharmacology and toxicology of "Ecstasy"(MDMA) and related drugs. *Canadian Medical Association Journal, 165*(7), 917–928.

Kimura, K., Ozeki, M., Juneja, L. R., & Ohira, H. (2007). L-Theanine reduces psychological and physiological stress responses. *Biological Psychology, 74*(1), 39–45.

Kinrys, G., Coleman, E., & Rothstein, E. (2009). Natural remedies for anxiety disorders: potential use and clinical applications. *Depression and Anxiety, 26*(3), 259–265.

Kohrs, R., & Durieux, M. E. (1998). Ketamine: teaching an old drug new tricks. *Anesthesia & Analgesia, 87*(5), 1186–1193.

Larzelere, M. M., Campbell, J. S., & Robertson, M. (2010). Complementary and alternative medicine usage for behavioral health indications. *Primary Care: Clinics in Office Practice, 37*(2), 213–236.

Leweke, F. M., Piomelli, D., Pahlisch, F., Muhl, D., Gerth, C. W., Hoyer, C., et al. (2012). Cannabidiol enhances anandamide signaling and alleviates psychotic symptoms of schizophrenia. *Translational Psychiatry, 2*(3), e94.

Litz, B. T., Salters-Pedneault, K., Steenkamp, M. M., Hermos, J. A., Bryant, R. A., Otto, M. W., et al. (2012). A randomized placebo-controlled trial of D-cycloserine and exposure therapy for post-traumatic stress disorder. *Journal of Psychiatric Research, 46*(9), 1184–1190.

López-Sendó, J., Swedberg, K., McMurray, J., Tamargo, J., Maggioni, A. P., Dargie, H., et al. (2004). Expert consensus document on β-adrenergic receptor blockers: the Task Force on Beta-Blockers of the European Society of Cardiology. *European Heart Journal, 25*(15), 1341–1362.

Lopresti, A. L., & Drummond, P. D. (2014). Saffron (*Crocus sativus*) for depression: a systematic review of clinical studies and examination of underlying antidepressant mechanisms of action. *Human Psychopharmacology: Clinical and Experimental, 29*(6), 517–527.

Lu, K., Gray, M. A., Oliver, C., Liley, D. T., Harrison, B. J., Bartholomeusz, C. F., et al. (2004). The acute effects of L-theanine in comparison with alprazolam on anticipatory anxiety in humans. *Human Psychopharmacology: Clinical and Experimental, 19*(7), 457–466.

Maninger, N., Wolkowitz, O. M., Reus, V. I., Epel, E. S., & Mellon, S. H. (2009). Neurobiological and neuropsychiatric effects of dehydroepiandrosterone (DHEA) and DHEA sulfate (DHEAS). *Frontiers in Neuroendocrinology, 30*(1), 65–91.

Marsella, A. J., Friedman, M. J., & Spain, E. H. (1996). *Ethnocultural aspects of posttraumatic stress disorder: issues, research, and clinical applications*. Philadelphia: American Psychological Association.

Marsicano, G., Wotjak, C. T., Azad, S. C., Bisogno, T., Rammes, G., Cascio, M. G., et al. (2002). The endogenous cannabinoid system controls extinction of aversive memories. *Nature, 418*(6897), 530–534.

Matsuoka, Y. (2011). Clearance of fear memory from the hippocampus through neurogenesis by omega-3 fatty acids: a novel preventive strategy for posttraumatic stress disorder. *Biopsychosocial Medicine, 5*(3), 1751–1759.

Matsuoka, Y., Nishi, D., Nakaya, N., Sone, T., Hamazaki, K., Hamazaki, T., & et al. (2011). Attenuating posttraumatic distress with omega-3 polyunsaturated fatty acids among disaster medical assistance team members after the Great East Japan Earthquake: the APOP randomized controlled trial. *BMC Psychiatry, 11*(1), 132.

McFarlane, A. C., Barton, C. A., Briggs, N., & Kennaway, D. J. (2010). The relationship between urinary melatonin metabolite excretion and posttraumatic symptoms following traumatic injury. *Journal of Affective Disorders, 127*(1), 365–369.

McGhee, L. L., Maani, C. V., Garza, T. H., Gaylord, K. M., & Black, I. H. (2008). The correlation between ketamine and posttraumatic stress disorder in burned service members. *Journal of Trauma-Injury, Infection, and Critical Care, 64*(2), S195–S199.

McKenna, D. J., Luna, L. E., & Towers, G. N. (1986). *Biodynamic constituents in ayahuasca admixture plants: an uninvestigated folk pharmacopoeia*. Portland: Dioscorides Press.

McLay, R. N., Klam, W. P., & Volkert, S. L. (2010). Insomnia is the most commonly reported symptom and predicts other symptoms of post-traumatic stress disorder in US service members returning from military deployments. *Military Medicine, 175*(10), 759–762.

Miki, T., Kochi, T., Eguchi, M., Kuwahara, K., Tsuruoka, H., Kurotani, K., et al. (2014). Dietary intake of minerals in relation to depressive symptoms in Japanese employees: the Furukawa Nutrition and Health Study. *Nutrition, 31*, 686–690.

Moeller-Bertram, T., Keltner, J., & Strigo, I. A. (2012). Pain and post traumatic stress disorder–Review of clinical and experimental evidence. *Neuropharmacology, 62*(2), 586–597.

Movafegh, A., Alizadeh, R., Hajimohamadi, F., Esfehani, F., & Nejatfar, M. (2008). Preoperative oral *Passiflora incarnata* reduces anxiety in ambulatory surgery patients: a double-blind, placebo-controlled study. *Anesthesia & Analgesia, 106*(6), 1728–1732.

Mukherjee, P. K. (2002). *Quality control of herbal drugs: an approach to evaluation of botanicals*. New Delhi: Business Horizons

National Institute of Health, Office of Dietary Supplements. (2005, October 28). *Omega-3 fatty acids and health*. Available at http://ods.od.nih.gov/factsheets/Omega3FattyAcidsandHealth-HealthProfessional/. Accessed April 15, 2015.

Neumeister, A., Normandin, M. D., Pietrzak, R. H., Piomelli, D., Zheng, M. Q., Gujarro-Anton, A., et al. (2013). Elevated brain cannabinoid CB1 receptor availability in post-traumatic stress disorder: a positron emission tomography study. *Molecular Psychiatry, 18*(9), 1034–1040.

Newall, C. A., Anderson, L. A., & Phillipson, J. D. (1996). *Herbal medicines: a guide for health-care professionals*. London: Pharmaceutical Press.

Nugent, N. R., Christopher, N. C., Crow, J. P., Browne, L., Ostrowski, S., & Delahanty, D. L. (2010). The efficacy of early propranolol administration at reducing PTSD symptoms in pediatric injury patients: a pilot study. *Journal of Traumatic Stress, 23*(2), 282–287.

O'Connor, A. (2015). New York attorney general targets supplements at major retailers. *New York Times*. Available at http://well. blogs. nytimes. com/2015/02/03/new-york-attorney-general-targets-supplements-at-major-retailers. Accessed Jan 15 2016.

Osório, F. D. L., Sanches, R. F., Macedo, L. R., dos Santos, R. G., Maia-de-Oliveira, J. P., Wichert-Ana, L., et al. (2015). Antidepressant effects of a single dose of ayahuasca in patients with recurrent depression: a preliminary report. *Revista Brasileira de Psiquiatria*, *37*(1), 13–20.

Pandzic, I., McLay, R., & Morrison, T. (2013). *Complementary and alternative medicine for treatment of PTSD*. Naval Center for Combat and Operational Stress Control white papers. Available at http://www.med.navy.mil/sites/nmcsd/nccosc/healthProfessionalsV2/reports/Documents/white-paper-complimentary-and-alternative-medicine-for-treatment-of-ptsd.pdf. Accessed 6 April 2016.

Papakostas, G. I. (2008). Evidence for S-adenosyl-L-methionine (SAM-e) for the treatment of major depressive disorder. *Journal of Clinical Psychiatry*, *70*, 18–22.

Passie, T., Emrich, H. M., Karst, M., Brandt, S. D., & Halpern, J. H. (2012). Mitigation of post-traumatic stress symptoms by cannabis resin: a review of the clinical and neurobiological evidence. *Drug Testing and Analysis*, *4*(7–8), 649–659.

Peet, M., & Stokes, C. (2005). Omega-3 fatty acids in the treatment of psychiatric disorders. *Drugs*, *65*(8), 1051–1059.

Pitman, R. K., Van der Kolk, B. A., Orr, S. P., & Greenberg, M. S. (1990). Naloxone-reversible analgesic response to combat-related stimuli in posttraumatic stress disorder: a pilot study. *Archives of General Psychiatry*, *47*(6), 541–544.

Pokorny, M. E. (2012). Experiences of military CRNAs with service personnel who are emerging from general anesthesia. *AANA Journal*, *80*(4), 260–261.

Ravindran, L. N., & Stein, M. B. (2009). Pharmacotherapy of PTSD: premises, principles, and priorities. *Brain Research*, *1293*, 24–39.

Ressler, K. J., Rothbaum, B. O., Tannenbaum, L., Anderson, P., Graap, K., Zimand, E., et al. (2004). Cognitive enhancers as adjuncts to psychotherapy: use of D-cycloserine in phobic individuals to facilitate extinction of fear. *Archives of General Psychiatry*, *61*(11), 1136–1144.

Riba, J., Rodríguez-Fornells, A., Urbano, G., Morte, A., Antonijoan, R., Montero, M., et al. (2001). Subjective effects and tolerability of the South American psychoactive beverage ayahuasca in healthy volunteers. *Psychopharmacology*, *154*(1), 85–95.

Riba, J., Romero, S., Grasa, E., Mena, E., Carrió, I., & Barbanoj, M. J. (2006). Increased frontal and paralimbic activation following ayahuasca, the pan-Amazonian inebriant. *Psychopharmacology*, *186*(1), 93–98.

Riba, J., Valle, M., Urbano, G., Yritia, M., Morte, A., & Barbanoj, M. J. (2003). Human pharmacology of ayahuasca: subjective and cardiovascular effects, monoamine metabolite excretion, and pharmacokinetics. *Journal of Pharmacology and Experimental Therapeutics*, *306*(1), 73–83.

Richardson, D. J., Sareen, J., & Stein, M. B. (2012). *Psychiatric management of military-related PTSD: focus on psychopharmacology*. Rijeka, Croatia: INTECH Open Access Publisher.

Rothbaum, B. O., Price, M., Jovanovic, T., Norrholm, S. D., Gerardi, M., Dunlop, B., et al. (2014). A randomized, double-blind evaluation of D-cycloserine or alprazolam combined with virtual reality exposure therapy for posttraumatic stress disorder in Iraq and Afghanistan war veterans. *American Journal of Psychiatry*, *171*(6), 640–648.

Sarris, J., McIntyre, E., & Camfield, D. A. (2013). Plant-based medicines for anxiety disorders, part 2: a review of clinical studies with supporting preclinical evidence. *CNS Drugs*, *27*(4), 301–319.

Saxe, G., Stoddard, F., Courtney, D., Cunningham, K., Chawla, N., Sheridan, R., et al. (2001). Relationship between acute morphine and the course of PTSD in children with burns. *Journal of the American Academy of Child & Adolescent Psychiatry*, *40*(8), 915–921.

Schönenberg, M., Reichwald, U., Domes, G., Badke, A., & Hautzinger, M. (2005). Effects of peritraumatic ketamine medication on early and sustained posttraumatic stress symptoms in moderately injured accident victims. *Psychopharmacology*, *182*(3), 420–425.

Schönenberg, M., Reichwald, U., Domes, G., Badke, A., & Hautzinger, M. (2008). Ketamine aggravates symptoms of acute stress disorder in a naturalistic sample of accident victims. *Journal of Psychopharmacology*, *22*(5), 493–497.

Schwartz, A. C., Bradley, R., Penza, K. M., Sexton, M., Jay, D., Haggard, P. J., et al. (2006). Pain medication use among patients with posttraumatic stress disorder. *Psychosomatics*, *47*(2), 136–142.

Serefko, A., Szopa, A., Wlaź, P., Nowak, G., Radziwoń-Zaleska, M., Skalski, M., et al. (2013). Magnesium in depression. *Pharmacological Reports*, *65*(3), 547–554.

Short, A. M. (2015, January 8). *Ayahuasca saved this narcotics cop/combat vet on the verge of suicide*. Available at http://reset.me/story/ayahuasca-saved-narcotics-copcombat-vet-verge-suicide/. Accessed April 15, 2015.

Silove, D. (1998). Is posttraumatic stress disorder an overlearned survival response? An evolutionary-learning hypothesis. *Psychiatry*, *61*(2), 181–190.

Steckler, T., & Risbrough, V. (2012). Pharmacological treatment of PTSD: established and new approaches. *Neuropharmacology*, *62*(2), 617–662.

Stein, D. J., Ipser, J. C., & Seedat, S. (2006). *Pharmacotherapy for post traumatic stress disorder (PTSD)*. London: The Cochrane Library.

Taibi, D. M., Landis, C. A., Petry, H., & Vitiello, M. V. (2007). A systematic review of valerian as a sleep aid: safe but not effective. *Sleep Medicine Reviews*, *11*(3), 209–230.

Tarleton, E. K., & Littenberg, B. (2015). Magnesium intake and depression in adults. *The Journal of the American Board of Family Medicine*, *28*(2), 249–256.

Tawa, J., & Murphy, S. (2013). Psychopharmacological treatment for military posttraumatic stress disorder: an integrative review. *Journal of the American Association of Nurse Practitioners*, *25*(8), 419–423.

Thomas, G., Lucas, P., Capler, N. R., Tupper, K. W., & Martin, G. (2013). Ayahuasca-assisted therapy for addiction: results from a preliminary observational study in Canada. *Current Drug Abuse Review*, *6*(1), 30–42.

Tian, X., Sun, L., Gou, L., Ling, X., Feng, Y., Wang, L., et al. (2013). Protective effect of L-theanine on chronic restraint stress-induced cognitive impairments in mice. *Brain Research*, *1503*, 24–32.

Trevino, C. M., & Brasel, K. (2013). Does opiate use in traumatically injured individuals worsen pain and psychological outcomes? *The Journal of Pain*, *14*(4), 424–430.

Vuong, Q. V., Bowyer, M. C., & Roach, P. D. (2011). L-Theanine: properties, synthesis and isolation from tea. *Journal of the Science of Food and Agriculture*, *91*(11), 1931–1939.

Wessa, M., & Flor, H. (2007). Failure of extinction of fear responses in posttraumatic stress disorder: evidence from second-order conditioning. *American Journal of Psychiatry*, *164*(11), 1684–1692.

White, C. M. (2014). 3, 4-Methylenedioxymethamphetamine's (MDMA's) impact on posttraumatic stress disorder. *Annals of Pharmacotherapy*, *48*(7), 908–915.

Wichtl, M. (2004). *Herbal drugs and phytopharmaceuticals: a handbook for practice on a scientific basis*, 3rd edition. London: Medpharm GmbH Scientific Publishers.

Wilson, J. P., & Moran, T. A. (1998). Psychological trauma: posttraumatic stress disorder and spirituality. *Journal of Psychology and Theology*, *26*, 168–178.

Womble, Arthur L. (2013). Effects of ketamine on major depressive disorder in a patient with posttraumatic stress disorder. *AANA J*, *81*(2), 118–119.

Yamamoto, S., Morinobu, S., Fuchikami, M., Kurata, A., Kozuru, T., & Yamawaki, S. (2008). Effects of single prolonged stress and D-cycloserine on contextual fear extinction and hippocampal NMDA receptor expression in a rat model of PTSD. *Neuropsychopharmacology*, *33*(9), 2108–2116.

Yehuda, R., Brand, S. R., Golier, J. A., & Yang, R. K. (2006). Clinical correlates of DHEA associated with post-traumatic stress disorder. *Acta Psychiatrica Scandinavica*, *114*(3), 187–193.

Yehuda, R., Teicher, M. H., Trestman, R. L., Levengood, R. A., & Siever, L. J. (1996). Cortisol regulation in posttraumatic stress disorder and major depression: a chronobiological analysis. *Biological Psychiatry, 40*(2), 79–88.

Yokogoshi, H., Kobayashi, M., Mochizuki, M., & Terashima, T. (1998). Effect of theanine, R-glutamylethylamide, on brain monoamines and striatal dopamine release in conscious rats. *Neurochemical Research, 23*(5), 667–673.

Zeev, K., Michael, M., Ram, K., & Hagit, C. (2005). Possible deleterious effects of adjunctive omega-3 fatty acids in post-traumatic stress disorder patients. *Neuropsychiatric Disease and Treatment, 1*(2), 187.

Zeng, M. C., Niciu, M. J., Luckenbaugh, D. A., Ionescu, D. F., Mathews, D. C., Richards, E. M., et al. (2013). Acute stress symptoms do not worsen in posttraumatic stress disorder and abuse with a single subanesthetic dose of ketamine. *Biological Psychiatry, 73*(12), e37–e38.

PART
3

COMPLEMENTARY TREATMENTS

EIGHT

Canines as Assistive Therapy for Treatment of PTSD

ELSPETH CAMERON RITCHIE,
PERRY R. CHUMLEY, MEG DALEY OLMERT,
RICK A. YOUNT, MATTHEW ST. LAURENT,
AND CHRISTINA RUMAYOR

CANINE-ASSISTED THERAPIES ARE BEING USED INCREASINGLY BOTH BY VETERANS and the civilian community for mental and emotional support. During the past decade, a growing body of scientific research has provided evidence that human–animal interactions can improve social competence and reduce physiological, psychological, and behavioral effects of stress and social isolation. One meta-analysis that evaluated 49 published studies of animal-assisted therapy (AAT), used mainly to target mental health concerns, concluded AAT is effective for medical well-being, for behavioral outcomes in adults, and for improving the therapy participation of children with autism and related disorders. The study also found that AAT was as effective as other interventions studied in comparison (Nimer & Lundahl, 2007).

Although these studies were conducted on a civilian population and did not focus specifically on AAT's effects on posttraumatic stress disorder (PTSD), a 2015 systematic review of the literature did. This survey identified 10 studies (nine of which were published in the last 5 years) that examined the effects of animal-assisted interventions on survivors of child abuse and military veterans. The authors report that the most prevalent outcomes were reduced depression, PTSD symptoms, and anxiety and conclude that AAI shows promise as a complementary intervention for trauma. (O'Haire, Guerin, & Kirkham, 2015).

Taken together, this considerable body of evidence strongly implies that military psychosocial and physiological health could also be improved by AAT, and that research can and should be conducted to evaluate AAT as a viable adjunctive treatment for PTSD. Additional research will also help to answer numerous questions surrounding AAT, such as how it should be defined, which methods are most effective, and which biological mechanisms are engaged to support AAT's therapeutic effects.

In this chapter we outline the history and evolution of canine-assisted therapy in military mental health, discuss the evidence of a neurobiological basis for the therapeutic effects of canine-assisted therapy, and focus on one canine-assisted therapy model that appears to be highly effective at reducing the symptoms of PTSD.

HISTORY OF ANIMALS AND THE MILITARY

In 2012, the Congressional Budget Office reported that the Veterans Health Administration treated 400,000 veterans who served in Iraq and Afghanistan. Despite the great cost and effort to provide our Wounded Warriors with the best empirically supported PTSD interventions, treatment resistance and dropout rates can be as high as 90% (Mott et al., 2014), and other research shows that 50% of those who do complete evidence-based psychotherapy can still meet the criteria for PTSD after treatment (Monson et al., 2006; Schnurr et al., 2007).

The limited efficacy of conventional therapies to provide long-term relief from the symptoms of combat trauma, combined with the increased danger of pharmaceutical use and abuse, and the devastating social and economic cost to military families and the United States, have increased support from military leadership for the use of alternative medical interventions, including AAT.

This latest recognition of the healing potential of AAT has deep roots in U.S. military medical history. The U.S. military promoted the use of dogs as a therapeutic intervention with psychiatric patients in 1919 at Saint Elizabeth's Hospital in Washington, DC (Velde, Cipriani, & Fisher, 2005). Another early documented human–animal bond program involved the Department of Defense at Pawling Army Air Force Convalescent Center, Pawling, New York, during the 1940s. The Center's farm animals were integrated into the treatment milieu for emotionally traumatized veterans and provided a purposeful interaction during Soldiers' convalescence (Bekoff, 2007).

Today, various animal-assisted intervention programs are operating at a number of military medical centers. These programs range from targeted therapeutic interventions (AATs) to less formal environmental and social enrichment activities (Animal-Assisted Activities). The majority of these focus on dogs, but there also some equine (horse) programs. Such programs are supported by the local medical commands and operate with a core of Red Cross and other volunteers. The common purpose of these programs is to bring smiles to the patients, family members, and hospital staff, and thus promote an increased sense of well-being in a more positive healing environment.

In the military operational environment, pairs of certified therapy dogs have been specially trained and deployed to Iraq and Afghanistan with several combat and operational stress control units. The 212th Medical Detachment and the 254th Medical Detachment both used therapy dogs for approved studies related to how the animals' involvement may affect certain attitudes such as mood state, job satisfaction, stress levels, and resilience level. The dogs were reported to be a highly effective means of breaking down perceived barriers and facilitating social interaction between Soldiers and occupational health medical professionals (Fike, Najera, & Dougherty, 2012; Gregg, 2012; Ritchie & Amaker, 2012).

Because of the interest and benefits of having animal-assisted interventions in military healthcare settings, the "DOD Human-Animal Bond Program Principles and Guidelines" published by Headquarters Department of The Army, Washington, DC, 3 August 2015 was written and continues to serve as a reference for establishing programs for various military and even civilian communities.

THE MILITARY SOLIDER POPULATION: AN IDEAL SUBCULTURE

The benefits of human–animal interaction are achieved by the young and the old, regardless of age, gender, or ethnicity (Shubert, 2012). Over time, certain age populations have been studied with regards to AAT benefits. The older adolescent or young adult population (specifically, age 18–25 years) is the largest percentage of the military demographic.

This same population is believed to have the potential to be an ideal candidate to benefit from AAT interventions for the following reasons. Growing up, many service members had pets in their home with whom they engaged on a daily basis. They left their pets at home when they entered into active military service. Those same service members could now be stationed thousands of miles away from home.

For some young service members, it may be their first time ever leaving home. They may experience loneliness, loss, sadness, or countless other financial, occupational, or interpersonal stressors. They can be dealing with issues related to identity development, separation from home, and autonomy, and may also find themselves in a variety of new roles (supervisor, subordinate, parent, spouse, and so on), which can add to the sense of being overwhelmed. Service members occasionally come from chaotic families and homes with a history of abuse or violence. These issues may trigger them to seek out initial treatment with Behavioral Health, where they may find the opportunity to engage with a therapy dog.

Having a therapy dog in session with service members makes the clinic atmosphere feel immediately more homelike. This environment may make them feel comfortable, may hasten patient–provider rapport building, and may enhance patients' disclosure to the therapist. Military males, in general, may feel more awkward or uncertain when talking to a therapist initially. Having a therapy dog present can facilitate relaxation and raise comfort levels to improve therapeutic outcomes (Ritchie and Amaker, 2012).

An AAT interaction could give service members their first opportunity to experience unconditional love. It can also provide an opportunity for physical affection (animal and patient) without worrying about boundary violations in the therapeutic relationship. The human–animal relationship can be beneficial in numerous ways, but the population that self-selects for military service may especially gain benefits from work with animal therapy. This is, however, another area where research is needed to verify this hypothesis

THEORETICAL BASIS FOR THE MENTAL HEALTH BENEFITS OF CANINE THERAPY

Many healthcare professions have recognized the therapeutic potential of human–animal interactions. In 1980, Friedmann et al. demonstrated that dog ownership could even improve the 1-year survival rate of owners who had experienced a heart attack. These impressive findings provided the first clue that the sense of well-being that dogs have instilled in humans for thousands of years has a solid—and measurable—physiological basis. This group then went on to show that the mere presence of a friendly, unfamiliar dog was able to attenuate blood pressure elevation in children while reading aloud, a well known cardiovascular stressor (Friedman, 1983). Since these groundbreaking studies, several other investigations have confirmed that social interaction with a dog can result in a significant reduction in sympathetic arousal during stress. This research also suggests the range of mental and physical health benefits that might be improved by incorporating therapy dogs into clinical treatment settings (Friedmann & Thomas, 1995; Kinsley, Barker, & Barker, 2012).

Odendaal and Meintjes (2003) found that the blood pressure of both humans and dogs decreases during friendly interspecies encounters. Looking even deeper, they discovered that friendly interaction with a dog produces significant modulation of neurohormones related to stress reduction and social reward. They found decreases in cortisol as well as increases in β endorphin, prolactin, and dopamine. The most impressive and intriguing neurohormonal change they measured was in plasma levels of oxytocin, which doubled in both dog and human after an interaction session.

It is now well established that oxytocin release not only triggers labor contractions and breast milk release, but also it instigates and rewards maternal behavior and all kinds of social interaction and cooperation in mammals. Oxytocin coordinates this social agenda via its interactions in all the key brain centers that control behavior and emotion (Heinrichs, von Dawas, & Domes, 2009). Oxytocin has been shown to inhibit the hypothalamic–pituitary–adrenal stress axis and also to modulate the locus coeruleus and other arousal centers of the central nervous system to attenuate stress-induced neuroendocrine activity.

Oxytocin receptor-expressing neural circuits in the central amygdala connect to the medial prefrontal cortex to suppress neurons that produce the freezing reaction to fear while promoting risk assessment and an exploratory response to frightening stimuli. Oxytocin has also been shown to modulate the serotonin system and reduce levels of cytokines, adrenocorticotropin, and cortisol. All these brain systems and neurochemical responses have shown to be important functionally in PTSD (Olff, Langeland, Witteveen, & Denys, 2010; McAllister, 2011; Knobloch et al., 2012).

The ability of friendly interactions between humans and dogs to increase oxytocin in humans gained further support in 2008 when Japanese researchers found that eye contact between humans and dogs increased oxytocin levels in human urine (Nagasawa Kikusui, Onaka, & Ohta, 2008). Miller et al. (2009) found that serum oxytocin levels increased more for women when interacting with their dogs than when reading nonfiction material. Swedish found significant correlations between oxytocin levels of owners and their dogs. For instance, they found higher oxytocin levels (and lower cortisol levels) in both dogs and their owners who reported kissing their dogs more (Handlin et al., 2012). Another study showed a significant increase in serum oxytocin in both dog and owner after 15 minutes of friendly interaction, along with a decrease in the heart rate of their owner s. These authors conclude that this antistress effect, "may be a consequence of oxytocin released in the brain caused by sensory) interaction" (Handlin et al., 2011, p. 313). Neumann (2009) agrees that interactions with dogs most likely active oxytocin's brain pathway, "contributing to the positive mental and physical health effects of dog ownership" (p. 492).

The capacity of dog-assisted therapy to be one of the most potent, natural enhancers of the human oxytocin brain network lies in the fact that oxytocin is released naturally in all mammals through nonnoxious sensory stimuli. A gentle touch, a warm hug, a smile, a soothing voice, even a good meal can elevate levels of oxytocin and a sense of well-being (Karelina et al., 2011). Even when trauma victims have lost the ability to connect with another human being, they may be able to reach out to a dog and experience the kinds of social and sensory stimuli that can trigger the release of oxytocin and its calming and social effects.

Dogs may be "humans' best therapist" because their oxytocin brain network is so similar to ours. Kis et al. (2014) found that the structure of the dog's oxytocin receptor gene is quite similar to its human counterpart. It contains similar coding variations (polymorphisms) that relate to the capacity for social behavior. They identified three oxytocin receptor polymorphisms in Border Collies and German Shepherds that correspond to the dogs' urge to be close to their owners and unfamiliar people, and to the dogs' friendliness toward strangers. Their findings led them to conclude that "the social behavior of dogs towards humans is influenced by the oxytocin system" (Kis et al., 2014, pp. 1–9).

This oxytocin-related social symmetry gained behavioral support from another study that manipulated the dogs' oxytocin system by giving some dogs an oxytocin inhalant. Those dogs (vs. dogs who did not receive a whiff of oxytocin) showed greater social orientation toward their owners, and greater affiliation and approach behaviors with familiar dogs. The oxytocin-inspired dog-to-dog contact increased the release of oxytocin in the dogs, demonstrating the positive social feedback capacity of oxytocin (Romero, Nagasawa, Mogi, Hasegawa, & Kikusui, 2014).

Building on earlier research, Nagasawa et al. (2015) confirmed that mutual gaze between dogs and owners produces a significant increase of oxytocin in both. In addition, when they gave oxytocin inhalants to dogs, it increased the amount of time female dogs gazed at their owners and increased the release of oxytocin in their owners. These findings support the hypothesis that human–dog interactions trigger a positive oxytocin feedback similar to the one that supports mother–infant bonding, and that this is neurobiological basis of the domestication of dogs (Olmert, 2009).

These neurobiological and genetic findings support 30 years of research that has shown that human–animal interactions can improve a wide range of physiological and psychological outcomes. Beetz, Uvnas-Moberg, Julius, and Kortshchal (2012) surveyed 69 peer-reviewed studies that documented the prosocial, antistress, and physiological effects of a wide range of human–animal interactions—from the presence of a dog, friendly contact with dogs, and AATs—and concluded that, "oxytocin and human-animal interaction effects largely overlap" (p. 1). Unfortunately, although few of these studies looked specifically at PTSD, there is a dawning understanding that enhancing the oxytocin system naturally through focused and friendly interaction with dogs can have particular relevance in the treatment of Wounded Warriors suffering from mental and physical disabilities.

In 1993, Pittman, Orr, and Lasko showed that war veterans with PTSD given one dose of oxytocin demonstrated a decreased physiological response to provoked combat memories. A recent study by Hunt and Chizkov (2014) showed the presence of dogs can also decrease anxiety even during a potential PTSD "trigger" stressor. This trauma essay challenge with and without a dog present found that the presence of a dog made the recollection and written reporting of a trauma less unpleasant. The other significant finding from the trauma–essay study was that that introverted participants benefited the most from the presence of a dog. Although this study did not look for biological effects, its findings of a reduction of background anxiety in the presence of a dog are similar to the oxytocin effects measured in the PTSD study of Pittman, Orr, and Lasko (1993). Studies of fear conditioning with rats found that oxytocin produces a unique effect of decreasing background anxiety without affecting learning or memory of a specific traumatic event (Missig, Ayers, Schulkin, & Rosen, 2010).

Oxytocin in humans has also been shown to enhance the processing of positive social information compared with negative information, increase a sense of trust in others, reverse the effect of aversive conditioning of social stimuli, enhance the buffering effect of social support on stress responsiveness, and reduce the stress response in people with a history of early trauma (Striepens, Kendrick, Maier, & Hurlemann, 2011). With respect to pain and sleep disturbances, significant corollary symptoms in PTSD, oxytocin has been shown to modulate pain in humans and has been shown to impact sleep patterns in animal studies (Yang, 1994; Singer et al., 2008; Lancel, Kromer, & Neumann, 2003).

Olff, Langeland, Witteveen, and Denys (2010) suggest PTSD symptom treatment would be improved by increasing endogenous levels of oxytocin through "optimalization of social support." The previously mentioned studies illustrate how dogs can provide such an optimalization of social support and why positive interactions with dogs may offer a safe, effective, and relatively inexpensive way to increase endogenous levels of oxytocin and other important antistress agents naturally in humans.

Although there appears to be both a theoretical rationale and a neurobiological basis for the mental health benefits of human–canine interaction, the question of whether specific interactions (e.g., those involved in the training of a service dog) might have therapeutic benefits for trainers with PTSD is an important, yet unanswered question. The Warrior Canine Connection (WCC) program (described in the next section) is perhaps a first step toward answering this question.

THE WARRIOR CANINE CONNECTION SERVICE DOG TRAINING PROGRAM

Warrior Canine Connection (WCC) engages service members in treatment for PTSD in a healing mission to train valuable service dogs for other Wounded Warriors with disabilities. This volunteer program is based on the warrior ethos and has been shown to appeal to even the most treatment-resistant patients.

WCC's dog-training protocol was founded on clinical theories and practices, and is designed to reduce the symptoms of PTSD. WCC's altruistic mission and positive, nurturing training methodologies engage the psychological, social, and tactile–social engagement that have been shown to be rewarding emotionally and neurobiologically.

This innovative canine therapy model was created by Rick Yount, Licensed Social Worker and Professional Service Dog Trainer, and was piloted at the Menlo Park VA's Men's and Women's Trauma Recovery Program from 2008 to 2009. Clinician observations of patient symptom improvement and patient reports indicated this program was promising as a popular and effective adjunct intervention in the treatment of PTSD (Yount, Lee, & Olmert, 2012) (Box 8.1).

BOX 8.1
ANECDOTAL IMPROVEMENTS REPORTED IN PATIENTS
PARTICIPATING IN THE SERVICE DOG TRAINING
PROGRAM AT THE MEN'S TRAUMA RECOVERY PROGRAM,
PALO ALTO VA FROM 2008 TO2009

- Increase in patience, impulse control, emotional regulation
- Improved ability to display affect, decrease in emotional numbness
- Improved sleep
- Decreased depression, increase in positive sense of purpose
- Decrease in startle responses
- Decrease in pain medications
- Increased sense of belongingness/acceptance
- Increase in assertiveness skills
- Improved parenting skills and family dynamics
- Fewer war stories and more in-the-moment thinking
- Lowered stress levels, increased sense of calm

SERVICE DOG TRAINING AS HIGHLY FLEXIBLE COMPLEMENTARY TREATMENT FOR PTSD AND TRAUMATIC BRAIN INJURY

Although the observations in Box 8.1 are consistent with previous studies of both the prosocial and physiological benefits of human–animal interaction, they are not sufficient to suggest that canine–human interaction should replace traditional approaches to the management of PTSD. They have, however, been compelling enough to encourage the Department of Defense and Veterans Affairs caregivers to incorporate this service dog training model into a wide variety of standard interventions for combat trauma.

Since 2011, WCC has provided its Service Dog Training program (SDTP) as part of the Walter Reed National Military Medical Center's occupational therapy program. Based on its success, the SDTP was expanded to support Fort Belvoir's occupational therapy program in 2014. At both facilities, WCC dogs and trainers provide PTSD therapeutic support under the supervision of occupational therapists.

Occupational therapists use these programs as "work therapy" internships, with the goals of engaging and facilitating patients in interventions that build skill sets for functional independence. Occupational therapy uses purposeful and meaningful participation in a task or occupation as a method to reduce mental health symptoms that impair functional independence. Active patient participation fosters experiential learning, a direct and intimate approach that facilitates interest and habituation leading to skill development for successful functional independence.

Although WCC's therapeutic service dog training model operates as mission-based "internships," it has clear treatment objectives. Clinical observation and patient experiences indicates that the highly social service dog training methods used in this program help patients overcome PTSD and traumatic brain injury (TBI) symptoms by improving confidence, cognition, self-esteem, social competence, communication skills, and affect. The repetitive intimate interactions and bonding between human and animal provides successful experiences leading to a highly trained service dog in support of fellow veterans with physical disabilities, and a sense of accomplishment to struggling patients (Olmert, Nordstrom, Peters, St. Laurent, & Yount, 2015).

Since 2011, WCC's service dog training program has also been integrated with the National Intrepid Center of Excellence's PTSD/TBI patient health care as well as their family support program. In 2013, WCC was invited to provide its service dog training program as part of Palo Alto's Veterans Affairs polytrauma, substance abuse, and homeless veteran's care programs. WCC is also offered to veterans with severe TBI in treatment at NeuroRestorative's Germantown, Maryland, residential facility (Tedeschi, Sisa, Olmert, Parish-Plass, & Yount, 2015).

It takes 2 years to mature, train completely, and certify a mobility service dog. Up to 50 service members and veterans with PTSD/TBI can participate in the training of that dog during this time, depending on the length of their treatment plans. This strategy allows the WWSDT program to maximize the therapeutic effect of a limited number of service dogs.

Between 2011 and 2015 more than 3000 service members and veterans have benefited therapeutically by participating in the training of 25 dogs that now serve Wounded Warriors. Twelve of these dogs have become fully accredited mobility service dogs and have been partnered, at no cost, with veterans in need. Thirteen trained dogs also serve as therapy dogs at military medical facilities and as military family support dogs.

THE FUTURE OF SERVICE DOG TRAINING AS EVIDENCE-BASED THERAPY FOR PTSD

The success of WCC's service dog training program has inspired unprecedented stakeholder support from military, congressional, scientific, and academic leaders. In 2013, Researchers from Uniformed Services University of Health Sciences were awarded federal funding to conduct a rigorous study to measure the psychological, physiological, and neurobiological effects of 2 weeks of participation in the SDTP program. Volunteers with PTSD in treatment at Walter Reed's outpatient behavioral health program will participate in this randomized controlled study.

This groundbreaking pilot study will be followed up by a larger, more in-depth research collaboration between Walter Reed, occupational therapists, NICoE, WCC, and the University of Maryland. These studies will be the first randomized controlled investigations to compare both subjective (self-report) and objective (clinically administered evaluations) measures with physiological and biological markers of stress and resiliency produced by a PTSD intervention.

The findings from the pilot study will be published in 2017. We anticipate the results will support and illuminate the observations and experiences of our patients, clinicians, and family members for the 7 years the program has been in service. We hope the data help to maximize the efficacy of the program and establish it as an "evidence-based" intervention for the reduction of symptoms of combat PTSD.

CONCLUSION

AATs are gaining acceptance as an alternative treatment for a wide range of behavioral health problems. A historical lack of interest and funding for rigorous investigation into the countless anecdotal reports of AAT benefit has hampered our ability to understand more fully the healing capacity of the human–animal bond. Despite this hurdle, considerable evidence of the positive physical and mental health benefits of human–canine interaction has been gathered. It is our contention this research supports the use of canine-assisted therapy as an adjunctive treatment for patients with PTSD.

Given the military's long history in turning to canine-assisted therapies for mental health care, it is fitting it is now taking the lead in conducting a rigorous investigation into the efficacy and biological underpinnings of this promising service dog training program currently being offered for PTSD treatment support at Walter Reed. During the next 5 years, these randomized controlled trials will help shed light on which populations may best benefit from this service dog training therapy model, which symptom clusters are best addressed by this model, how the model can be modified for maximum effect, which Warriors will be best served by being partnered with a service dog, and what the therapeutic standard of service dog training for PTSD support should be. This current research will also provide a baseline against which we can measure the comparative efficacy of this canine-assisted therapy model compared with conventional PTSD treatments currently being offered.

These findings will also provide firm scientific footing on which to base appropriate standards and use of canine-assisted therapies in military medicine, and also will have widespread civilian application. Indeed, the entire field of AAT will be moved forward as a result of military leadership in this critical area of research.

KEY POINTS

- Hundreds of thousands (actual number?) of war veterans suffer from PTSD.
- Treatment resistance and limited efficacy of standard behavioral health interventions have increased support from military leadership for the use of alternative medical interventions.
- A growing body of research provides evidence AAT has the potential to reduce a wide range of stress, social and behavioral symptoms of PTSD.
- The military has long employed dogs for emotional and tactical support. A high percentage of military personnel have experienced a close, supportive relationship with a dog, and may benefit from AAT.
- The WCC service dog training program is designed to overcome treatment resistance and reduce the symptoms of PTSD.
- Clinical and patient observations support that this mission-based AAT model has been highly effective at reducing symptoms of PTSD.

- DoD funded randomized controlled studies will be conducted over the next 5 years to investigate the psychological, physiological, and neurobiological effects of this innovative AAT.

DISCLAIMER

The views of military personnel expressed in the article are those of the authors and do not represent the official views/position of the Department of Defense, U.S. Army, or the U.S. Army Medical Command.

REFERENCES

Beetz, A., Uvnas-Moberg, K., Julius, H., & Kortshchal, K. (2012). Psychological and psycho-physiological effects of human–animal interactions: the possible role of oxytocin. *Frontiers in Psychology*, *3*, 1–15.

Bekoff, M. (2007). Animal assistance to humans: animal-assisted interventions. In: Bekoff, M., ed. *Encyclopedia of human–animal relationships*. Vol. 1. Westport, CT: Greenwood Press, pp. 1–2.

Congressional Budget Office. (2012, February). *Veterans Health Administration's treatment with PTSD and traumatic brain injury among recent combat veterans*. CBO publication no. 4097, p. 10. Washington, DC: U.S. Government Printing Office.

Fike, L., Najera, C., & Dougherty D. (2012). Occupational therapists as dog handlers: the collective experience with animal-assisted therapy in Iraq in canine assisted therapy in military medicine. *The AMEDD Journal, April–June*, 51–54.

Friedmann E., Katcher, A. H., Lynch, J. J., Thomas, S. A. (1980). Animal companions and one-year survival of patients after discharge from a coronary care unit, *Public Health Reports, 95*, 307–312.

Friedmann, E., Katcher, A. H., Thomas, S. A., Lynch, J. J., Messent, P. R. (1983). Social interaction and blood pressure: the influence of companion animals. *Journal of Nervous and Mental Disease, 171*, 461–465.

Friedmann, E., & Thomas, S. A. (1995). Pet ownership, social support, and one-year survival after acute myocardial infarction in the Cardiac Arrhythmia Suppression Trial. *American Journal of Cardiology, 17*, 1213–1217.

Gregg, B. T. (2012). Crossing the berm: an occupational therapist's perspective on animal-assisted therapy in a deployed environment in canine assisted therapy in military medicine. *The AMEDD Journal, April–June*, 55–60.

Handlin, L., Hydbring-Sandberg, E., Nilsson, A., Ejdeback, M., Jansson, A., & Uvnas-Moberg, K. (2011). Short-term interaction between dogs and their owners: effects on oxytocin, cortisol, insulin, and heart rate. *Anthrozoos, 24*(3), 301–315.

Handlin, L., Nilsson, A., Ejdeback, M., Hydbring-Sandberg, E., & Uvnas-Moberg, K. (2012). Associations between the psychological characteristics of the human–dog relationship and oxytocin and cortisol levels. *Anthrozoos, 25*(2), 215–228.

Heinrichs, M., von Dawas, B., & Domes, G. (2009). Oxytocin, vasopressin, and human social behavior. *Frontiers in Neuroendocrinology, 30*, 548–557.

Hunt, M. G., & Chizkov, R. R. (2014). Are therapy dogs like Xanax? Does animal-assisted therapy impact processes relevant to cognitive behavioral psychotherapy? *Anthrozoos, 27*(3), 457–469.

Karelina, K., Stuller, K. A., Jarett, B., Zhang, N., Wells, J., Norman, G. J., et al. (2011). Oxytocin mediates social neuroprotection after cerebral ischemia. *Stroke, 42*, 3606–3611.

Kinsley, J. S., Barker, S. B., & Barker R. T. (2012). Research on the Benefits of Canine-Assisted Therapy for Adults in Nonmilitary Settings, *U.S. Army Medical Department Journal, April–June*, 30–37.

Kis, A., Bence, M., Lakatos, G., Pergel, E., Turcsan, B., Pluijmakers, J., et al. (2014). Oxytocin receptor gene polymorphisms are associated with human directed social behavior in dogs (*Canis familiaris*). *PLoS One*, *9*(1), e83993, 1–9.

Knobloch, H. S., Charlet, A., Hoffamn, L. C., Eliava, M., Khrulev, S., & Grinevich, V. (2012). Evoked axonal oxytocin release in central amygdala attenuates fear response. *Neuron*, *73*(3), 553–566.

Lancel, M., Kromer, S., & Neumann, I. D. (2003). Intracerebral oxytocin modulates sleep–wake behavior in male rats. *Regulatory Peptides*, *114*(2–3), 145–152.

McAllister, T. W. (2011). Neurobiological consequences of traumatic brain injury. *Dialogues in Clinical Neuroscience*, *13*(3), 287–300.

Miller, S. C., Kennedy, C., DeVoe, D., Hickey, M., Nelson, T., & Kogan, L. (2009). An examination of changes in oxytocin levels in men and women before and after interaction with a bonded dog. *Anthrozoos*, *22*(1), 31–42.

Missig, G., Ayers, L. W., Schulkin, J., & Rosen, J. B. (2010). Oxytocin reduces background anxiety in fear-potentiated startle paradigm. *Neuropsychopharmacology*, *35*(13), 2607–2616.

Monson, C. M., Schnurr, P. P., Resick, P. A., Friedman, M. J., Young-Xu, Y., & Stevens, S. P. (2006). Cognitive processing therapy for veterans with military-related posttraumatic stress disorder. *Journal of Consulting and Clinical Psychology*, *74*(5), 898–907.

Mott, J. M., Mondragon, S., Hundt, N. E., Beason-Smith, M., Grady, R. H., & Teng, E. J. (2014). Characteristics of U.S. veterans who begin and complete prolonged exposure and cognitive processing therapy for PTSD. *Journal of Traumatic Stress*, *27*, 265–273.

Nagasawa, M., Kikusui, T., Onaka, T., & Ohta, M. (2008). Dog's gaze at its owner increases owner's urinary oxytocin during social interaction. *Hormones & Behavior*, *55*, 434–451.

Nagasawa, M., Mitsui, S., En, S., Ohtani, N., Ohta, M, Sakuma, Y., et al. (2015). Oxytocin–gaze positie loop and the co-evolution of human–dog bonds. *Science*, *348*(6232), 333–336.

Nimer, J., & Lundahl, B. (2007). Animal assisted therapy: a meta-analysis. *Anthrozoos*, *20*(3), 225–238.

Nuemann, I. D. (2009). The advantage of social living: brain neuropeptides mediate the beneficial consequences of sex and motherhood. *Frontiers in Neuroendocrinology*, *30*, 483–496.

Odendaal, J., & Meintjes, R. (2003). Neurophysiological correlates of affiliative behaviour between humans and dogs, *The Veterinary Journal*, *165*, 296–301.

O'Haire, M. E., Guerin, N. A., & Kirham, A. C. (2015). Animal-assisted intervention for trauma: a systematic literature review. *Frontiers in Psychology*, *6*, 1121, pp 1–13.

Olff, M., Langeland, W., Witteveen, A., & Denys, D. (2010). A psychobiological rationale for oxytocin in the treatment of posttraumatic stress disorder. *CNS Spectrumsr*, *15*(8), 436–444.

Olmert, M. D. (2009). *Made for each other: the biology of the human–animal bond*. Cambridge, MA: DaCapo.

Olmert, M. D., Nordstrom, M., Peters, M., St. Laurent, M., & Yount, R. (2015). Canine connection therapy: finding purpose and healing through the training of service dogs. In: *Posttraumatic stress disorder and related diseases in combat veterans*. Switzerland: Springer International Publishing.

Pitman, R. K., Orr, S. P., & Lasko, N. B. (1993). Effects of intranasal vasopressin and oxytocin on physiologic responding during personal combat imagery in Vietnam veterans with post traumatic stress disorder. *Psychiatry Research*, *48*, 107–117.

Ritchie, E. C., & Amaker, R. (2012). The early years in canine assisted therapy in military medicine. *The AMEDD Journal, April–June*.

Romero, T., Nagasawa, M., Mogi, K., Hasegawa, T., & Kikusui, T. (2014). Oxytocin promotes social bonding in dogs. *PNAS*, *111*(25).

Schnurr, P. P., Friedman, M. J., Engle, C. C., Foa, E. B., Shea, M. T., et al. (2007). Cognitive behavioral therapy for posttraumatic stress disorder in women: a randomized controlled trial. *Journal of the American Medical Association*, *297*, 820–830.

Shubert, J. (2012). Dogs and human health/mental health: from the pleasure of their company to the benefits of their assistance in canine assisted therapy in military medicine. *The AMEDD Journal, April–June*.

Singer, T., Snozzi, R., Bird, G., Petrovic, P., Silani, G., Heinrichs, M., et al. (2008). Effects of oxy-tocin and prosocial behavior on brain responses to direct and vicariously experienced pain. *Emotion*, *8*(6), 781–791.

Striepens, N., Kendrick, K. M., Maier, W., & Hurlemann, R. (2011). Prosocial effects of oxytocin and clinical evidence for its therapeutic potential. *Frontiers in Neuroendocrinology*, *32*(4), 426–450.

Tedeschi, P., Sisa, M. L., Olmert, M. D., Parish-Plass, N., & Yount, R. (2015). Treating human trauma with the help of animals: trauma informed intervention for child maltreatment and adult post-traumatic stress. In: Fine, A. ed. *The Handbook on animal-assisted therapy*, pp. 305–319.

Velde, B.P., Cipriani, J., & Fisher, G. (2005). Resident and therapist views of animal-assisted ther-apy: implications for occupational therapy practice. *Australian Occupational Therapy Journal*, *52*, 43–50.

Yang, J. (1994). Intrathecal administration of oxytocin induces analgesia in low back pain involving the endogenous opiate peptide system. *Spine*, *19*(8), 867–871.

Yount, R. A., Lee, M. R., & Olmert, M. D. (2012). Service dog training program for treat-ment of posttraumatic stress in service members. *The Army Medical Department Journal*, *April–June*, 63–69.

NINE

Family-Focused Interventions for PTSD

Lessons from Military Families

STEPHEN J. COZZA

Posttraumatic stress disorder (PTSD) has been shown to have a variety of negative health and mental health effects on those who are afflicted (Kessler et al., 2000), as well as negative effects on relationships with intimate partners and close relatives (Whisman, Sheldon, & Goering, 2000). Families are likely to be impacted by the specific nature of the sustained trauma. For example, PTSD related to sexual trauma may be solely experienced by the victim and likely to be uniquely impacted by and make an impact on intimate partners, and close family and friends in the victim's life (Campbell, Dworkin, & Cabral, 2009). In contrast, PTSD resulting from exposure to natural disasters or terrorism may affect numerous members of a family, particularly when multiple family members have been exposed to the same event, or when homes, possessions, or neighborhoods have been broadly affected (North & Pfefferbaum, 2013). Although specific circumstances may require tailored approaches to family intervention, different types of traumas also share commonalities related to their effect on interpersonal relationships, communication, and family functioning. Little is known about effective interventions for families affected by PTSD, regardless of circumstances.

PTSD resulting from combat exposure has created new opportunities for understanding. The recent wars in Iraq and Afghanistan have resulted in large numbers of combat veterans returning home with rates of PTSD and other combat-related stress disorders as high as 15% to 20% (Hoge, et al., 2004; RAND Center for Military Health Policy Research, 2008), profoundly affecting relationships within families. Consequently, recent efforts have focused on the needs of these military and veteran families, creating a greater understanding of the interpersonal impact of PTSD, which in turn has contributed to models to assist affected families (Cozza, Holmes, & Van Ost, 2013).

This military family perspective is used to inform the structure and content of this chapter, which describes the challenges military and veteran families face as a result of PTSD, with particular attention to families with children. The chapter reviews several pertinent areas, including military and veteran family demographics; understanding PTSD from a family systems perspective and its impact on relationships and family functioning (e.g., marital relationships and partner intimacy, parenting, children); child developmental considerations; and the limited research examining family interventions for PTSD. The chapter concludes with recommendations for six strategies to effectively assist in mitigating risk in families affected by PTSD. Much of what has been learned within this population is also likely to be relevant to the needs of other families affected by PTSD, regardless of the cause.

MILITARY AND VETERAN FAMILIES

Military family members outnumber service members by a ratio approaching 3:2 (Department of Defense, 2013). This should not be surprising; 57% of the active force are married and 44% of active duty members have children, averaging two children per family. According to the *2013 Demographics Profile of the Military Community* (Department of Defense, 2013) there are approximately 2 million children and adolescents of America's active duty, reserve, or National Guard military members. In total, there are approximately 4 million youth who are the sons and daughters of veterans who have served at any time since 9/11. Of the 1.2 million children of active duty members, almost three-quarters are 11 years of age or younger, and 42% of all children are less than the age of 6 years (Department of Defense, 2013). Approximately 43% of selected reserve members (including both Reserve and National Guard components) have children, and nearly 60% of these children are younger than 12 years (Department of Defense, 2013). These mostly young families live throughout the continental United States, its territories (e.g., Puerto Rico, Guam), Hawaii, and Alaska, and at overseas locations; and they reflect the broad socioeconomic, racial, cultural, and ethnic dimensions of the United States. On separation or retirement from the service, veteran families may reside in geographically remote areas, where clinicians do not always identify them for who they are or their connections to military life or challenges.

Combat deployments to Iraq and Afghanistan have profoundly affected military families (Cozza & Lerner, 2013). Since 2001, more than 2 million military service men and women have deployed, and many families have faced repeated deployments— some as many as five or more. Reports describing military children and families have highlighted their general health and wellness, and capacity for resilience (Easterbrooks, Ginsburg, & Lerner, 2013). Some have reported combat deployment-related elevations in rates of interpersonal conflict (Milliken, Auchterlonie, & Hoge, 2007) and child maltreatment (Gibbs, Martin, Kupper, & Johnson, 2007; Rentz et al., 2007; McCarroll, Fan, Newby, & Ursano, 2008), as well as emotional and behavioral problems, increased mental health utilization, and suicidal behaviors in military children (Flake, Davis, Johnson, & Middleton, 2009; Chandra et al., 2010; Lester et al., 2010; Mansfield, Kaufman, Engel, & Gaynes, 2011; Gilreath et al., 2015); and elevated distress (Lester et al., 2010) and mental health utilization (Mansfield et al., 2010) in military spouses. The greater healthcare burden for children of combat ill and injured service members has also been identified (Hisle-Gorman et al., 2015). Taken together, these findings suggest some military families face complex and distressing family lives, with greater challenges related to combat-related injury and illnesses (Cozza, Holmes, & Van Ost, 2013), including PTSD.

DEMOGRAPHICS OF PTSD IN MILITARY SERVICE MEMBERS AND VETERANS

Nearly 20% of combat-exposed service members report threshold symptoms consistent with a psychiatric disorder (PTSD, depression, anxiety disorder, and substance abuse) on returning home (Hoge, Auchterlonie, & Milliken, 2006). The overall prevalence of PTSD among combat-exposed military personnel is estimated to be between 5% and 15% (Tanielian & Jaycox, 2008), indicating that hundreds of thousands of military service members have been affected by traumatic stress during the recent wars. PTSD is associated with a range of negative outcomes to the sufferer, including occupational and social impairment, poor physical health, neuropsychological impairment, substance use, and risk of death (Hidalgo & Davidson, 2000; Kessler, 2000).

FAMILY SYSTEMS AND AN UNDERSTANDING OF THE EFFECT OF PTSD

Few studies have addressed the complex interactions within families resulting from PTSD that may impact individual adult and child health, and intrafamilial relationships. An ecological framework is helpful in examining the impact of PTSD within families. Bronfenbrenner (1979) defined *ecological systems theory* to characterize the interactive effects of smaller and larger systems of relationships and social connections that influence human health and development. The association between child health and wellness, and parental health has been well documented in trauma-exposed civilian populations (Wickrama & Kaspar, 2008; Chemtob et al., 2010), as well as in military families (Chandra et al., 2010; Lester et al., 2010). Because relationships within the family system impact individual and relationship functioning bidirectionally (Cox & Paley, 1997; Bronfenbrenner & Morris, 2006), service providers caring for service members and veterans with PTSD must be aware of its effects within the family, and be prepared to engage family members to address the complex outcomes that can result.

Although combat veterans have a significant risk of developing mental disorders as a result of their wartime exposure, we must avoid a tendency to use an "illness" model in understanding how military spouses and children respond to parental PTSD. Although some military dependents may develop mental disorders, they are likely to constitute a minority of family members. Most affected adults and children will experience distress. Distress is not an illness, but it can still profoundly affect child development, adult health, families, and communities. In addition to the anguish it can cause, distress can undermine occupational, social, and emotional functioning. Distressed parents are less likely to be attentive to their children and may lose some of the parenting capacity that they possessed previously. Distressed children may become withdrawn, participate in fewer extracurricular activities, find it difficult to concentrate in school, or may demonstrate behavioral symptoms that are unusual or that complicate their normal development.

Several theorists have targeted the interactive skills and routines that can protect family members and therefore promote health in spouses and children during times of stress or trauma. Walsh (2006) outlined Family Resilience Theory, which emphasizes the importance of the following processes to overall family health in traumatic circumstances: the ability to develop and preserve shared beliefs, constructive communication, and healthy patterns of organization. Gewirtz, Forgatch, and Wieling (2008) proposed a preventive framework that incorporates positive parenting practices to achieve important family goals after trauma exposure: by providing a social environment that offers structure, security, and emotional warmth, and can address the traumatic event.

Based on their work with families undergoing the stress of combat deployment and reunification, Saltzman et al. (2011) proposed that military family interventions should also promote (1) increased understanding, support, and forgiveness among family members; (2) improved communication and cohesion; (3) coordinated parental leadership; (4) defined but adjustable roles and responsibilities; and (5) development of shared goals and beliefs. Several groups have highlighted both the theoretical (Wadsworth et al., 2013) and clinical (Cozza, Holmes, & Van Ost, 2013) importance of family-centered approaches to combat-related health conditions. Increasingly, U.S. government agencies are recognizing the importance of attending to military and veteran families, as evidenced by the Army Family Covenant, the Air Force Year of the Family, the Department of Defense's "social compact" with service members and families, and newly developing Veterans Affairs family support initiatives resulting from the President's 2012 Executive Order to support the health and well-being of service members, veterans, and their families (The White House, 2012). Despite these developments, military and veteran family-centered programs continue to be lacking (Wadsworth et al., 2013), particularly for families struggling with PTSD.

IMPACT OF PTSD ON MARRIAGES, INTIMATE RELATIONSHIPS, AND FAMILIES

PTSD has toxic effects within the family environment, negatively affecting relationships between service members and spouses or intimate partners, as well as relationships with children. Studies consistently relate PTSD with relationship problems (Kessler, 2000; Whisman, Sheldon, & Goering, 2000). The combination of risk behaviors and psychological symptoms that characterize PTSD have been associated with poor intimate relationships, negative marital satisfaction, impaired family functioning, greater family distress, higher levels of family violence, and disrupted parenting and parent–child relationships (for a comprehensive review, see Galovski and Lyons [2004]). Avoidance or numbing, hyperarousal, and anger (either service member/veteran or partner) have all been associated with family adjustment problems (Hendrix, Erdmann, & Briggs, 1998; Riggs, Byrne, Weathers, & Litz, 1998; Evans, McHugh, Hopwood, & Watt, 2003; Taft, Schumm, Panuzio, & Proctor, 2008). The negative effects of PTSD broadly impact multiple aspects of marital functioning (including divorce) and are consistent regardless of the type of military mission (Kulka et al., 1990; Gimbel & Booth, 1994; Riggs, Byrne, Weathers, & Litz, 1998; Sherman, Zanotti, & Jones, 2005; Karney & Crown, 2007). In studies of service members from past and current wars, children of service members with PTSD exhibited general distress, depression, lower self-esteem, aggression, impaired social relationships, and school-related difficulties (Rosenheck & Nathan, 1985; reviewed in Galovski and Lyons [2004]). All these effects undermine family health and functioning, and appear to be specific to

PTSD, rather than more generally attributable to trauma exposure. For example, veterans suffering with PTSD divorce at a higher rate compared with similarly trauma-exposed veterans without PTSD (Jordan et al., 1992; Cook et al., 2004).

Spouses and partners of service members with chronic PTSD are more likely than spouses of nonaffected service members to show higher rates of distress, psychological symptoms (including depression and suicidal ideation), and poorer adjustment (Calhoun, Beckham, & Bosworth, 2002; Manguno-Mire et al., 2007). Of note, a spouse's mental health problems have been shown to incur greater harm to children's functioning than a service member's, suggesting additive and interactive risk (Herzog, Everson, & Whitworth, 2011). The caustic effect of PTSD on spouse health and couple relationships may also undermine relationship trust. Distrust within a couple is likely to complicate collaborative parenting and decrease available support to children in PTSD-affected families.

More recently, investigators have examined the negative impact of PTSD on other marital or relationship functions. For example, Allen, Rhoades, Stanley and Markman (2010) described the association of PTSD symptoms with poor marital communication, confidence, relationship dedication, parental alliance, and relationship bonding. Fredman et al. (2014) highlighted the association of veteran PTSD symptoms with distress in both partners, suggesting a dynamic interaction of cognitive, behavioral, and emotional processes requiring further therapeutic attention. These investigators (Fredman et al., 2014) introduced the concept of *partner accommodation*, which refers to the modification of a partner's own behavior or enabling of avoidance in the veteran spouse with PTSD, defining a powerful process that can interfere with couple functioning or undermine service member/veteran health. Allen, Rhoades, Stanley, and Markman (2010) described how such behavior might undermine co-parenting when a well-meaning partner might attempt to decrease hostility in the home by attempting to control all interactions between children and the parent suffering with PTSD.

Caregiver burden—or the perceived impact of caring for one with a chronic illness—on social, emotional, physical, or financial health has also been identified as contributing negatively to marital relationship well-being. Because up to one-third of those suffering with PTSD do not fully recover (Kessler et al., 1995), partners of veterans with PTSD are likely to face a number of ongoing stressors related to caring for someone with a chronic disease (Calhoun, Beckham, & Bosworth, 2002). Caregiver burden has been associated with distress in partners of veterans with PTSD and with the severity of PTSD symptoms (Beckham, Lytel, & Feldman, 1996). These findings suggest the importance of respite and social support services for families coping with chronic PTSD.

The impact of PTSD on relationship intimacy has recently become an area of interest and investigation. Monson, Taft, and Fredman (2009) reported findings identifying the relation between PTSD and intimate partner discord, poorer service member and spouse intimate relationship satisfaction, and spouse's perception of marital distress. They concluded that PTSD symptoms are strongly associated with intimate relationship problems, with avoidance and numbing associated with relationship dissatisfaction and hyperarousal associated with aggression and spousal abuse.

IMPACT OF PTSD ON PARENTING

Not unexpectedly, PTSD has been shown to undermine parenting behaviors and parenting satisfaction (Samper, Taft, Kind, & King, 2004; Berz, Taft, Watkins, & Monson, 2008). PTSD-affected parenting can be impaired by greater emotional reactivity, loss of cognitive capacity, greater levels of interpersonal aggression, or increased avoidance and disconnection from loved ones. In such circumstances, healthier parenting practices that had been in place before the onset of illness can be undermined by a variety of individual, social, family, psychiatric, and other health-related factors affecting the parenting couple.

PTSD may be expected to negatively impact parental cooperation and coordination of efforts necessary in raising children. *Co-parenting* is a term developed and initially applied in circumstances of separation or divorce to minimize conflict and to support cooperation across parent households (Doherty, Beaton, & Wenger, 2013). Since its original usage, the term has been applied to intact families, recognizing the unique and varying contributions of fathers and mothers within a family systems model. Doherty, Beaton, and Wenger (2013) describe multiple influences that affect the co-parenting relationship, including contextual factors (e.g., employment, socio-economics, community support), individual mother and father factors (e.g., physical and psychological well-being, family of origin parenting models, expectation of spouse), child factors (gender, age, family size), and the marital relationship. Given changes in parental health and well-being resulting from PTSD, shifts in preexisting parenting practices are likely to occur, often requiring formal renegotiation of the co-parenting relationship. Mental health problems in the spouse are likely to worsen this effect. Clinical literature contains accounts of the challenges couples face with co-parenting when a spouse has PTSD (Allen, Rhoades, Stanley, & Markman, 2010).

Successful PTSD parenting practices are not likely to be straightforward. Gewirtz et al. (2010) found strong negative relationships between PTSD, self-reported couple adjustment, and positive parenting behaviors, highlighting the need for better understanding of these processes. In a study describing the relationship of injured service member father self-reported post-traumatic symptoms, parenting behaviors, and child internalizing and externalizing symptoms, Holmes et al. (2013a) reported moderating effects of two positive parenting strategies (monitoring/supervision and involvement/engagement) with PTSD, but in opposite directions. Parental monitoring/supervision in the presence of more posttraumatic symptoms decreased children's internalizing symptoms, whereas parental involvement/engagement in the presence of more posttraumatic symptoms increased externalizing symptoms (Holmes et al., 2013a). These preliminary findings indicate that successful parenting with PTSD may require something different than applying traditional positive parenting strategies. Given the changes that PTSD may have on co-parenting capacity, successful parenting with PTSD likely requires a renegotiation between the parents. Further study is needed to outline helpful treatment options.

EFFECT OF PTSD ON CHILDREN

In studies of Vietnam combat veterans, children of service members with PTSD exhibit general distress, depression, low self-esteem, aggression, impaired social relationships, and school-related difficulties (Rosenheck & Nathan, 1985). PTSD-associated aggression and family violence may lead to additional traumas within the family, further undermining child health (Galovski & Lyons, 2004).

A parent's PTSD likely affects children depending on their age, developmental level, temperament, and preexisting conditions. Younger children may struggle more than older children to cope and adapt to changes in a parent's behaviors and the parenting relationship, and very young children may have an especially hard time coping with the disorganized parental behavior that can result from PTSD, such as overreaction or disengagement.

Children's reactions should be expected to vary by their age and maturity, and a developmental perspective is critical. For example, infants and toddlers (birth to 2 years) often respond negatively to family cues, such as changes in schedule and routines, the physical and emotional availability of important adults, as well as changes in the emotional climate (anxiety, interpersonal abruptness, irritability) in their families. An infant may evidence problems in sleeping or eating, or may develop irritability or self-regulatory problems, or disturbance of attachment in the face of a distressed or impaired caregiver.

Preschoolers (3–6 years old) often use *magical thinking*, an immature process that can lead them to assume inappropriate responsibility for a parent's anger, reactivity, avoidance, or depression. Preschoolers may become extremely anxious or disorganized by exposure to PTSD symptoms and are likely to demonstrate distress through regressive behaviors, such as loss of previously established developmental milestones (e.g., enuresis or sleep problems), clinginess to adults, or tantrums.

School-age children possess more mature developmental capacity than younger children, but still may harbor similar anxieties. Fear, guilt, and a desire to be helpful can complicate the school-age child's response. These children may be confused about what is expected of them and they may be unsure how to act, especially toward a parent with PTSD. They may also be uncomfortable bringing up questions that could help them better understand and respond.

Teenagers can face unique developmental challenges related to their parents' illness. Teens normatively anticipate greater independence from parents and less reliance on family. Given their near-adult maturation and greater physical capacity, teenagers may be responsible for increased chores, care for younger siblings, or caregiving responsibilities with the ill or injured parent. Such demands, in contrast to their desire to be with same-age friends, may lead to frustration and conflict with parents.

Parents and healthcare providers should expect that PTSD will result in greater distress or worsening of symptoms in children with preexisting medical, developmental, behavioral, or emotional conditions. Given disruptions in geographic transitions, possible separations from established childcare providers and other distractions related to the care of the parent with PTSD, children's healthcare or educational needs can be neglected or inappropriately delayed. Parents and clinicians should use a lower threshold for referral to appropriate clinical resources for these more vulnerable children.

IMPACT OF PTSD ON INTERPERSONAL VIOLENCE

Historically, data indicate an important relationship among combat exposure, PTSD, and violence or aggression, which can further undermine family safety and stability. Several studies have attempted to disaggregate this effect, examining the relative contribution of combat exposure and PTSD to violence. Recent studies with Operation Iraqi Freedom/Operation Enduring Freedom veterans have found the presence and severity of PTSD symptoms best account for veteran aggression (Hoge, Auchterlonie, & Milliken, 2006; Jakupcak et al., 2007; Taft et al., 2007; Sayers, Farrow, Ross, & Oslin, 2009). Another systematic review and meta-analyses of 16 studies published in the United States and the United Kingdom conducted by MacManus et al. (2015) described contributions to all forms of veteran aggression and found that PTSD mediated the effect between combat and postdeployment violence. In a national study of veteran violence, Elbogen et al. (2012) found that alcohol misuse strengthened that effect, with co-occurring PTSD and alcohol misuse adding further risk of violence.

Studies of Vietnam veterans have examined the impact of PTSD on domestic violence. Petrik, Rosenberg, and Watson (1983) found that combat experience in the absence of PTSD was not a strong predictor of violence. Similarly, Jordan et al. (1992) compared the wives of veterans with and without PTSD and found higher levels of violence in both veterans and spouses in the PTSD versus non-PTSD group. Taft et al. (2005) studied potential risk factors for partner violence in 109 male Vietnam veteran violent offenders comparing those with and without PTSD. They found traumatic experiences, comorbid psychopathology, and relationship problems associated with PTSD were risk factors for partner violence in their sample.

Importantly, Elbogen et al. (2014) have studied protective mechanisms that may serve to diminish community violence in PTSD-affected veterans. They conducted a national longitudinal survey between 2009 and 2011, and randomly sampled 1090 Operation Iraqi Freedom/Operation Enduring Freedom veterans in two waves of data collection. They found socioeconomic (money and stable employment), psychosocial (resilience, sense of control over one's life, and social support) and physical (adequate sleep and lack of pain) factors served as protective mechanisms to decrease community violence in veterans (Elbogen et al., 2014). These protective mechanisms may diminish partner aggression, as well.

INTERVENTION STRATEGIES

There is a paucity of studies of family interventions for PTSD resulting from combat or other causes. Two family-centered approaches that target military parenting and family processes, Families OverComing Under Stress (FOCUS)(Lester et al., 2013) and After Deployment Adaptive Parenting Tools (ADAPT) (Gewirtz, Pinna, Hanson, & Brockberg, 2014), have shown promise in supporting child and family health during and after combat deployments. Although neither was designed to address the specific challenges of PTSD in families, both incorporate trauma-informed strategies to target military families with deployment-related distress. FOCUS and ADAPT share common core components, including a strength-based approach and an emphasis on emotion regulation, communication, problem solving, and understanding and addressing children's developmental needs. In addition, ADAPT highlights several positive parenting practices, including parental limit setting, monitoring, and involvement in school and other activities (Gewirtz, Pinna, Hanson, & Brockberg, 2014).

Several couples-based treatments have been proposed to target family-related stress resulting from PTSD. Glynn et al. (1999) reported mixed results from a trial that included traditional exposure therapy for PTSD, with random assignment to exposure combined with couples' conjoint behavioral therapy. Although improvement in PTSD was noted for exposure therapy, those who also received conjoint behavioral therapy received no additional benefit (Glynn, et al., 1999). The most promising work to date, is Cognitive Behavioral Conjoint Therapy for PTSD, a 15-session intervention that focuses on behavioral and communication strategies, the impact of traumatic experiences and associated maladaptive thoughts on the couple, as well as the impact of additional symptoms of PTSD (Monson et al., 2011). Results of a small pilot study of seven couples were mixed, with PTSD-affected veterans reporting nonsignificant improvements in relationship satisfaction, whereas partners reported statistically significant and large effect size improvements in relationship satisfaction. Studies with larger samples of younger veterans are required (Monson et al., 2011).

As mentioned previously, Elbogen et al. (2014) have studied mechanisms that may protect against veteran aggression and could serve as targets for preventive intervention efforts. These researchers found that protective mechanisms played a vital role in understanding and preventing postdeployment violence. They conceptualized an intervention based on psychosocial rehabilitation theory that focuses on resolving symptoms, promoting collaboration with care providers, and developing skills for improved social functioning (including work and home). Their study identified several opportunities to reduce aggression, including reducing homelessness, helping with the transition to civilian work, improving financial management, and enhancing social support (Elbogen et al., 2014). In addition, Elbogen et al. (2014) recommended addressing PTSD-associated hyperarousal, sleep disturbance, anger, and comorbid psychiatric and medical conditions. All of these outcomes would likely benefit families, however further study is required.

CLINICAL APPLICATION AND INTERVENTION GOALS

Combat-related PTSD has powerful and defining effects on military and veteran families. It can generate toxic levels of distress, secondarily undermining parenting, and disorganizing family roles and healthy functioning. This challenge requires multisystem approaches to support child and family health. Such approaches call for defined family strategies derived from evidence-based principles to assist families at risk, which in turn must be connected to communities capable of support.

Family interventions should be contextualized within broader systems of care. Holmes, Rauch, and Cozza (2013b) described recommendations to support children in these high risk military families. For example, it is important to stabilize the family environment by ensuring access to basic needs, such as housing, education, health care, childcare, and jobs throughout postmilitary transition; to identify and promote services that support family organization, communication, coping, and resilience; and to sustain systems of support for those families who might need help for many years. In addition, service members and veterans, spouses, and their children must have ready access to trauma-informed, evidence-based treatments close to where they live. In circumstances when children require clinical intervention, parents can still provide active support through collaborative involvement in their children's treatment. Given the stigma associated with mental disorders, and hesitation in seeking help for family problems, military service members, veterans, and family members might not seek treatment or assistance, highlighting the need for enhanced outreach and engagement strategies.

Within this context of community and therapeutic support, the following six strategies are recommended for families with PTSD that incorporate the evidence base discussed throughout this chapter (Walsh, 2006; Monson et al., 2011; Saltzman et al., 2011; Lester et al., 2013; Elbogen et al., 2014; Gewirtz, Pinna, Hanson, & Brockberg, 2014). These strategies include (1) maintaining a physically safe and structured environment; (2) engaging required community resources; (3) developing and sharing knowledge within and outside the family that builds shared understanding; (4) building a positive and emotionally safe and warm family environment; (5) mastering and modeling important interpersonal skills, including problem solving and conflict resolution; and (6) maintaining a vision of hope and future optimism for the family (see Table 9.1).

Maintaining a Physically Safe and Structured Environment

Families faced with PTSD often contend with transitions from active military to veteran status, including moves to new communities. Parents must ensure children are integrated safely into these new communities, and that adequate structure and support are provided to ensure healthy development. Positive parenting practices include monitoring of children's whereabouts; peer group participation; compliance with home, school, and civic rules; and active and successful engagement in academic programs. In addition, consistent family schedules (including family meals, family recreational time), clear parental expectations, and appropriate consequence-based nonpunitive discipline will ensure a supportive structure for children. In general, parents must provide

TABLE 9.1 Family Strategies for Managing PTSD

Strategy	Description
1. Maintain a physically safe and structured environment	• Ensure children are integrated safely into new communities • Develop adequate structure and support to provide healthy development • Monitor children's whereabouts and peer groups • Expect compliance with home, school, and civic rules • Anticipate academic engagement • Establish consistent family schedules • Use consequence-based/nonpunitive discipline
2. Engage required community resources	• Engage community support when required • Model proactive help-seeking for children • Address barriers to engagement or stigma that can limit access to required resources • Make use of a broad group of professionals and nonprofessionals (relatives, neighbors, friends, healthcare professionals, school personnel, coaches, spiritual leaders, support organizations, and governmental agencies)
3. Develop and share knowledge to build greater understanding	• Develop a family understanding about what PTSD is and what it is not • Attribute interpersonal conflict or dissatisfaction to PTSD when appropriate • Remind children they are not responsible for family problems resulting from PTSD • Use developmentally appropriate language with children • Use effective communication strategies within the family to foster a sense of shared understanding • Encourage discussions and answer questions to promote effective communication • Decide, as a family, how to share illness-related information outside the family
4. Build a positive, and emotionally safe and warm family environment	• Remind each other that, although the family may be changed, it does not need to be defined by the illness • Use positive parenting strategies as appropriate • Practice personally effective stress reduction strategies • Label and express feelings, and identify when and how positive or negative responses are precipitated • Encourage activities that promote calm and relaxation • Model strategies for self-calming for children

(continued)

TABLE 9.1 Continued

Strategy	Description
5. Master and model important interpersonal skills, including problem solving and conflict resolution	• Practice basic problem-solving methods • Demonstrate how successful problem solving brings a sense of confidence and adds to family strength • Note how conflict resolution can minimize family violence • Learn to identify hot spots and triggers to anticipate reactions • Use reflective listening • Develop violence prevention plans, such as taking "timeouts" or seeking outside help when appropriate
6. Maintain a vision of hope and future optimism	• Model acceptance of the changes in the family resulting from PTSD • Note that successful management of challenges can instill greater hope for the future • Use outside resources to build a greater sense of self-efficacy and confidence • Share new and positive experiences within the family that clarify how PTSD does not restrict opportunities to enjoy life together

PTSD, posttraumatic stress disorder.

their children with opportunities for normal growth and development independent from any at-home struggle the family is having as a result of PTSD.

Ensuring that basic needs are met also provides a sense of order and predictability that allows family members to be less distracted, to function more effectively, and to be supportive of each other as the family accommodates to life outside the military. Adults are calmer, and the frequency of impulsive, threatening, or disruptive behavior among family members is reduced when there is access to systems for household maintenance, meals, medical care, money management, and childcare. Children are calmer when adults provide a predictable daily routine and when they model restraint.

Engaging Required Resources

Many of these families will face challenges that require continued professional or personal support and assistance. Parents can address these challenges by engaging support, including required mental health care, occupational support or assistance from community or veteran support programs. Parents can successfully model resource engagement with their children, who must also learn the importance of asking for help from teachers, coaches, relatives, other caring adults, or friends when they are in need of assistance or instrumental support. Parents and children must recognize any barriers to engagement, such as stigmatization or avoidance resulting from PTSD that can undermine their ability to access help successfully. Parents and children should also recognize they live within communities of care that include relatives, neighbors, friends, healthcare professionals, school personnel, counselors, coaches, spiritual leaders, military and veteran support organizations; as well as local, state, and federal governmental agencies; and they can call on each for assistance. Modeling the use of resources teaches one's children about the importance of asking for help and support when required, and provides a lesson that can be used throughout life.

Developing and Sharing Knowledge within and outside the Family That Builds Shared Understanding

Parents, along with healthcare providers, must provide appropriate information to children about their parents' PTSD and any of the consequences they may have experienced as a result of those stressors. A service member's changed behavior should be attributed directly to his or her psychiatric condition, rather than allowing a child to be confused about its origin. Clinicians and parents must provide helpful information about diagnoses, treatment options, and the likely long-term outcomes of the conditions. Adults as well as children may need to be reminded that emotional distance is a common symptom of combat veterans with PTSD and should be attributed to the illness, rather than to a change in emotional commitment on the part of the parent. A key principle is that everyone, parents and children alike, is affected by PTSD. Children, especially, must be reminded that the tension they see at home is not their fault and that it is not their responsibility to "fix" it.

Given the associated distress and the amount of information that must be shared among loved ones and with professionals, these military families face unique challenges that can compromise communication. A primary goal of effective communication, to be achieved over time through frequent discussion, is to foster the family's *shared understanding* of the impact of PTSD on both adults and children. Effective communication must be ongoing (because situations can change) and include individuals both within and outside of the family. The detail and amount of information to be shared must be tailored to each recipient's "need to know" and "capacity to know." Children should not be provided details about combat experiences or battlefield-related trauma. Communication with outside resources (e.g., extended family, neighbors, care systems, schools, clergy) is essential to the family's sense of safety and stability, but it must also respect each family member's need for a measure of privacy.

Children and adults should adopt a brief, clear, easily repeated, and general description of their family's story when speaking with teachers, coaches, and other concerned adults. When speaking with a coach, for example, a child can be taught to say, "My Dad would love to see me play, but he can't be here today because he is a soldier who was in combat and he gets bothered by crowds."

Because recovery from PTSD can proceed over a period of years, explanations to children must account for the service member's changing capacities and should be commensurate with each child's developmental level. Adults should speak in a calm and matter-of-fact manner, use language that is comprehensible to the child, and exclude any unnecessary or frightening information. Older children and teenagers require more detailed and logical explanations of a military parent's condition, its impact on the family, and reasons for any expansions of their own household responsibilities.

Most important, effective communication creates a family atmosphere in which discussion is encouraged. Children should be prompted to express any emotions, either positive or negative, to let parents know when they are confused, and children should be encouraged to ask questions. Maintaining family dialogue allows both children and adults opportunities to develop a sense of closeness and shared understanding of how the recovery process affects each of them.

Building a Positive and Emotionally Safe and Warm Family Environment

Strength-based family approaches and positive parenting strategies are common to previously discussed interventions (Lester et al., 2013; Gewirtz, Pinna, Hanson, & Brockberg, 2014). Positive strategies include helping children and adults stay identified with strengths that were present before the development of PTSD. In the face of their current stress, both adults and children may need to be reminded that, although their family may be "changed", they do not need to be defined by the illness. They continue to possess their previously held strengths and they can use them effectively in the present and the future. In fact, they can build new strengths.

Family distress sometimes undermines what was previously competent parenting. Parents may need to be reminded or trained on the fundamentals of positive parenting, such as expecting positive behaviors from their children, complimenting them when they are in compliance, encouraging cooperative behavior, taking time to listen, helping with problems, and recognizing and responding to their children's emotions. The latter is extremely important because parental sadness or distress may make it difficult for them to recognize or respond to their children's troubled feelings. Given the greater likelihood of emotional dysregulation in combat-affected PTSD families, children and adults should be taught to practice personally effective stress reduction strategies. This includes instruction on how to monitor changes or extremes in emotional states by learning to label and express feelings, and identifying when and how positive or negative responses are precipitated. Although identifying and sharing feelings is a first step toward the control of emotion, families must also develop and encourage individual and family activities that promote calm and relaxation. Both children and adults can be taught to reduce worry and tension by engaging in positive self-talk, allowing themselves breaks when needed, developing more realistic expectations, and setting priorities. Parents can be particularly helpful as teachers by modeling healthy self-calming behaviors for their children. Families can increase a sense of unity and mutual support by sharing enjoyable activities at times when everyone is relaxed. Similarly, all family members can be encouraged to identify and engage in activities that are calming for all. The more opportunities the family has to enjoy positive family time together, the more everyone will identify him- or herself as healthy and the family as unified.

Mastering and Modeling Important Interpersonal Skills, Including Problem Solving and Conflict Resolution

Like all families, families affected by PTSD are likely to face problems that require attention and solving, although these families may have more problems than most. Any problem that seems unsolvable can lead to a sense of individual or family frustration or incompetence and can undermine a child's, adult's, or family's sense of confidence. Festering problems can also result in increasing interpersonal conflict, alienation, and family unrest. Parents should remind children that everyone has problems—adults as well as children—and that what helps people feel strong is being able to solve the problems with which they are faced. Parents can model for their children by calmly showing them how solving problems is a series of steps that can be mastered. Basic problem-solving methods have been used in a number of interventions and generally include (1) defining the problem, (2) listing possible solutions, (3) evaluating the pros and cons of the choices, (4) choosing one of the options, and (5) planning how best to enact (Dausch & Saliman, 2009). Successful problem solving brings a sense of individual and interpersonal confidence, and adds to family strength.

Conflict resolution is a critical type of problem solving, especially when violence is a concern. Although all families have "hot spots" or issues that tend to provoke more intense emotional responses when they arise (homework, chores, finances, and so on), PTSD can contribute to greater reactivity and therefore make families more easily upset by ordinary stressors. In addition, reminders or "triggers" can prompt memories of previous traumas. For example, the occurrence of an unexpected noise

(a child's shout) may agitate a combat veteran who suffered injury from an improvised explosive device. A child might become upset at the unannounced absence of
a parent, because this is a reminder of when that parent was deployed. Each family
member likely brings sensitivity to mutual interactions that can disrupt their time
together. Families must learn to identify hot spots and trauma triggers so they can
anticipate the service member's reactions to such events, as well as their own. For
example, family members can be helped to control their reaction to a service member's provoking behavior by not taking the triggered behavior personally and by
prompting the service member to use previously developed strategies for calming or
controlling the reaction.

When interpersonal conflicts do occur, adults need to model strategies that promote calm resolution and interpersonal understanding to minimize hurt feelings.
Most important, both children and adults must recognize interpersonal conflicts
are not likely to be improved when either or both parties are frustrated, angry, or
distraught. Taking time to compose oneself and use reflective listening to understand the viewpoint of the other is a way children can learn conflict resolution is less
about "winning the fight" and more about coming to an understanding with another
person. Successful conflict resolution creates patterns of interaction more likely to
repeat themselves and result in fewer future conflicts, more repaired relationships,
and stronger family bonds. In highly volatile families, clinicians should help parents
develop violence prevention plans, including seeking help or resources, or making
use of family "timeout" options before violence erupts.

As mentioned earlier in the chapter, co-parenting in families affected by PTSD
may create opportunities for shared and balanced parenting contributions, but also
can be sources of interpersonal conflict. Although little evidence exists to provide
specific recommendations for co-parenting practices in these families, anecdotal reports suggest parents benefit by maximizing individual strengths and limiting weaknesses between parents. As an example, if a military father with PTSD is both reactive to and avoidant of his teenage daughter and son, respectively, he and his wife
might agree that she will take the lead engaging their daughter about the boyfriend
relationship and he will monitor his son's compliance with an established curfew.
Such co-parenting decisions can be successful. In contrast, if a parent feels excluded
from parenting decisions, it may lead to conflict, dysphoria, or disconnection.

Maintaining a Vision of Hope and Future Optimism for the Family

Military and veteran families faced with PTSD may also need to grieve the loss of
their previous health, functioning, military careers, or communities. The changed

personality and interpersonal skills of a service member or veteran suffering from PTSD can create a sense of loss in family members who mourn previous relationships. Grief over these relationship losses can be further complicated by confusion about whether their loved one will recover over time. Parents can model acceptance of this changed reality while using family-based skills to create a positive vision of the future, helping their children accommodate. If parents are able to sustain a safe and emotionally warm family environment, and help their children master skills to address challenges they face both within and outside their home, then they can all look to the future with greater hope. Families that sustain the capacity to actively engage helpful support also develop a greater sense of self-efficacy and confidence about their ability to shape solutions for future challenges. Sharing new and positive experiences together while recognizing and respecting changes brought about by PTSD can foster a sense of future hopefulness and optimism.

CONCLUSIONS AND FUTURE DIRECTIONS

Military and veteran families face many challenges related to combat-related PTSD. A greater understanding of their experiences will better inform family-centered approaches for military families, as well as other families affected by PTSD. Further study is required to distinguish the parenting and family mechanisms likely to promote health and mitigate risk for children in all of these circumstances. Certain parenting strategies are typically considered helpful, such as emotional engagement with children. However, the effect of such "positive parenting" may be different or even problematic when used by a parent who is suffering from PTSD. For example, what if children who are actively engaged by unpredictable or emotionally reactive parents are worsened by therapeutic recommendations for greater parental emotional closeness? As another example, children typically benefit from enhanced communication with parents. But, what if the children become emotionally distressed when parents share too much information about their own traumatic narrative, such as personal details of combat activities? Future research must better define which parenting strategies are likely to be helpful in differing circumstances, recognizing that the application of traditional "positive parenting" approaches may need to be sculpted and applied contextually depending on family circumstances.

Future research must also examine the impact of PTSD on co-parenting. Parents who are affected by PTSD may need to be taught to remove themselves from circumstances of interpersonal conflict in the family and allow their adult partners to take charge if they are better able to positively contribute to family emotional regulation. Future research must help answer these questions and promote more sensitive and contextually designed interventions for families. Research must also examine unique family member role contributions to successful parenting practices, as well as any unique dyadic contributions (i.e., father–son, stepmother–son, stepfather–daughter, mother–daughter) to child and family outcomes. Finally, family cultural contributions must also be examined more closely, as well as unique needs of nontraditional families, such as single-parent or lesbian, gay, bisexual, transgender families.

KEY POINTS

- PTSD has a variety of negative health and mental health effects on those afflicted, as well as negative effects on relationships with intimate partners and close relatives.
- The association between child health and wellness, and parental health has been well documented in trauma-exposed civilian populations.
- Family-centered approaches to PTSD treatment are warranted, given the bidirectional impact of the disorder on individual and relationship functioning.
- Spouses and partners of service members with chronic PTSD are more likely than spouses of nonaffected service members to show higher rates of distress, psychological symptoms, and poorer adjustment.
- Caregiver burden has also been identified as contributing negatively to marital relationship well-being in families affected by PTSD.
- PTSD-affected parenting can be impaired by greater emotional reactivity, loss of cognitive capacity, greater levels of interpersonal aggression, or increased avoidance and disconnection from loved ones.
- Children of service members with PTSD exhibit general distress, depression, low self-esteem, aggression, impaired social relationships, and school-related difficulties.
- Children's reactions should be expected to vary by their age and maturity, and a developmental perspective is critical.
- Associations exist between combat exposure, PTSD, and alcohol, and violence and aggression, and the latter can undermine family safety and stability.
- Given the stigma associated with mental disorders and hesitation in seeking help for family problems, families might not seek treatment or assistance, highlighting the need for enhanced outreach and engagement strategies.
- Effective family-focused strategies for PTSD should include (1) maintaining a physically safe and structured environment; (2) engaging required community resources; (3) developing and sharing knowledge within and outside the family that builds shared understanding; (4) building a positive and emotionally safe and warm family environment; (5) mastering and modeling important

interpersonal skills, including problem solving and conflict resolution; and (6) maintaining a vision of hope and future optimism for the family.

- Further study is required to distinguish the parenting and family mechanisms likely to promote health and mitigate risk for children and families affected by PTSD resulting from any circumstance.

REFERENCES

Allen, E., Rhoades, G., Stanley, S., & Markman, H. (2010). Hitting home: relationships between recent deployment, posttraumatic stress symptoms, and marital functioning for Army couples. Journal of Family Psychology, 24(3), 280–288.

Beckham, J., Lytel, B., & Feldman, M. (1996). Caregiver burden in partners of Vietnam veterans with posttraumatic stress disorder. Journal of Consulting and Clinical Psychology, 64(5), 1068–1071.

Berz, J., Taft, C., Watkins, L., & Monson, C. (2008). Associations between PTSD symptoms and parenting satisfaction in a female veteran sample. Journal of Psychological Trauma, 7(1), 37–45.

Bronfenbrenner, U. (1979). The ecology of human development. Cambridge, MA: Harvard University Press.

Bronfenbrenner, U., & Morris, P. (2006). The bioecological model of human development. In R. E. Lerner, ed. Handbook of Child Psychology (pp. 793–828). New York, NY: Wiley.

Calhoun, P., Beckham, J., & Bosworth, H. (2002). Caregiver burden and psychological distress in partners of veterans with chronic posttraumatic stress disorder. Journal of Traumatic Stress, 15(3), 2015–212.

Campbell, R., Dworkin, E., & Cabral, G. (2009). An ecological model of the impact of sexual assault on women's mental health. Trauma, Violence, & Abuse, 10(3), 225–246.

Chandra, A., Lara-Cinisomo, S., Jaycox, L., Tanielian, T., Burns, R., Ruder, T., et al. (2010). Children on the homefront: the experience of children from military families. Pediatrics, 125(1), 16–25.

Cook, J., Riggs, D., Thompson, R., Coyne, J., & Sheikh, J. (2004). Posttraumatic stress disorder and current relationship functioning among World War II ex-prisoners of war. Journal of Family Psychology, 18(1), 36–45.

Cox, M., & Paley, B. (1997). Families as systems. Annual Review of Psychology. 48(1), 243–267.

Cozza, S., Chun, R., & Polo, J. (2005). Military families and children during Operation Iraqi Freedom. The Psychiatric Quarterly, 76(4), 371–378.

Cozza, S., Holmes, A., & Van Ost, S. (2013). Family-centered care for military and veteran families affected by combat injury. Clinical Child and Family Psychology Review, 16, 311–321.

Cozza, S., & Lerner, R. (2013). Military children and families: introducing the issue. Future Child, 23(2), 3–11.

Dausch, B., & Saliman, S. (2009). Use of family focused therapy in rehabilitation for veterans with traumatic brain injury. Rehabilitation Psychology, 54(3), 279–287.

Department of Defense. (2013, September 1). 2013 Demographics Profile of the Military Community. Retrieved from http://download.militaryonesource.mil/12038/MOS/Reports/2013-Demographics-Report.pdf.

Doherty, W., Beaton, J., & Wenger, L. (2013). Mothers and fathers co-parenting together. In A. Vangelisti, ed. The Routledge Handbook of Family Communication, 2nd ed. (pp. 225–240). New York, NY: Routledge.

Easterbrooks, M., Ginsburg, K., & Lerner, R. (2013). Resilience among military youth. Future Child, 23(2), 99–120.

Elbogen, E., Johnson, S., Newton, V., Timko, C., Vasterling, J., Van Male, L., et al. (2014). Protective mechanisms and prevention of violence and aggression in veterans. Psychological Services, 11(2), 220–228.

Elbogen, E., Johnson, S., Wagner, R., Newton, V., Timko, C., Vasterling, J., et al. (2012). Protective factors and risk modification of violence in Iraq and Afghanistan war veterans. Journal of Clinical Psychiatry, 73(6), e767–773.

Evans, L., McHugh, T., Hopwood, M., & Watt, C. (2003). Chronic posttraumatic stress disorder and family functioning of Vietnam veterans and their partners. Australian and New Zealand Journal of Psychiatry, 37(6), 765–772.

Flake, E., Davis, B., Johnson, P., & Middleton, L. (2009). The psychosocial effects of deployment on military children. Journal of Developmental and Behavioral Pediatrics, 30(4), 271–278.

Fredman, S., Vorstenbosch, V., Wagner, A., Macdonald, A., & Monson, C. (2014). Partner accommodation in posttraumatic stress disorder: initial testing of the Significant Others' Responses to Trauma Scale (SORTS). Journal of Anxiety Disorders, 28(4), 372–381.

Galovski, T., & Lyons, J. (2004). Psychological sequelae of combat violence: a review of the impact of PTSD on the veteran's family and possible interventions. Aggression and Violent Behavior, 9, 477–501.

Gewirtz, A., Forgatch, M., & Wieling, E. (2008). Parenting practices as potential mechanisms for child adjustment following mass trauma. Journal of Marital and Family Therapy, 34(2), 177–192.

Gewirtz, A., Pinna, K., Hanson, S., & Brockberg, D. (2014). Promoting parenting to support reintegrating military families: after deployment, adaptive parenting tools. Psychological Services, 11(1), 31–40.

Gewirtz, A., Polusny, M., DeGarmo, D., Khaylis, A., & Erbes, C. (2010). Posttraumatic stress symptoms among National Guard soldiers deployed to Iraq: associations with parenting behaviors and couple adjustment. Journal of Consulting and Clinical Psychology, 78(5), 599–610.

Gibbs, D., Martin, S., Kupper, L., & Johnson, R. (2007). Child maltreatment in enlisted soldiers' families during combat-related deployments. Journal of the American Medical Association, 298(5), 528–535.

Gilreath, T., Wrabel, S., Sullivan, K., Capp, G., Roziner, I., Benbenishty, R., et al. (2015). Suicidality among military-connected adolescents in California schools. European Child & Adolescent Psychiatry [Epub ahead of print].

Gimbel, C., & Booth, A. (1994). Why does military combat experience adversely affect marital relations? Journal of Marriage and the Family, 56(3), 691–704.

Glynn, S., Eth, S., Randolph, E., Foy, D., Urbaitis, M., Boxer, L., et al. (1999). A test of behavioral family therapy to augment exposure for combat-related posttraumatic stress disorder. Journal of Consulting and Clinical Psychology, 67(2), 243–251.

Hendrix, C., Erdmann, M., & Briggs, K. (1998). Impact of Vietnam veterans' arousal and avoidance on spouses' perceptions of family life. American Journal of Family Therapy, 26(2), 115–128.

Herzog, J., Everson, R., & Whitworth, J. (2011). Do secondary trauma symptoms in spouses of combat-exposed National Guard soldiers mediate impacts of soldiers' trauma exposure on their children? Child and Adolescent Social Work Journal, 28(6), 459–473.

Hidalgo, R., & Davidson, J. (2000). Posttraumatic stress disorder: epidemiology and health-related considerations. Journal of Clinical Psychiatry, 61(Suppl 7), 5–13.

Hisle-Gorman, E., Harrington, D., Nylund, C., Tercyak, K., Anthony, B., & Gorman, G. (2015). Impact of parents' wartime military deployment and injury on young children's safety and mental health. Journal of the American Academy of Child and Adolescent Psychiatry, 54(4), 294–301.

Hoge, C., Auchterlonie, J., & Milliken, C. (2006). Mental health problems, use of mental health service, and attrition from military service after returning from deployment to Iraq or Afghanistan. Journal of the American Medical Association, 295(9), 1023–1032.

Hoge, C., Castro, C., Messer, S., McGurk, D., Cotting, D., & Koffman, R. (2004). Combat duty in Iraq and Afghanistan, mental health problems, and barriers to care. New England Journal of Medicine, 351(1), 13–22.

Holmes, A., Cozza, S., Anderson, A., Sullivan, J., Fullerton, C., & Ursano, R. (2013a). Child functioning in combat-injured military families: the moderating effects of injured service member parenting and PTSD symptoms. Seattle, WA: Society for Research in Child Development.

Holmes, A., Rauch, P., & Cozza, S. (2013b). When a parent is injured or killed in combat. Future Child, 23(2), 143–162.

Jakupcak, M., Conybeare, D., Phelps, L., Hunt, S., Holmes, H., Felker, B., et al. (2007). Anger, hostility, and aggression among Iraq and Afghanistan war veterans reporting PTSD and subthreshold PTSD. Journal of Traumatic Stress, 20(6), 945–954.

Jordan, B., Marmar, C., Fairbank, J., Schlenger, W., Kulka, R., Hough, R., et al. (1992). Problems in families of male Vietnam veterans with posttraumatic stress disorder. Journal of Consulting and Clinical Psychology, 60(6), 916–926.

Karney, B., & Crown, J. (2007). Families under Stress: An Assessment of Data, Theory, and Research on Marriage and Divorce in the Military. Arlington, VA: RAND Corporation.

Kessler, R. (2000). Posttraumatic stress disorder: the burden to the individual and to society. Journal of Clinical Psychiatry, 61(Suppl 5), 4–12.

Kessler, R., Sonnega, A., Bromet, E., Hughes, M., & Nelson, C. (1995). Posttraumatic stress disorder in the National Comorbidity Survey. Archives of General Psychiatry, 52(12), 1048–1060.

Kulka, R., Schlenger, W., Fairbank, J., Hough, R., Jordan, B., Marmar, C., et al. (1990). Trauma and the Vietnam War Generation: Report of Findings from the National Vietnam Veterans Readjustment Study. Philadelphia, PA: Brunner Mazel.

Lester, P., Peterson, K., Reeves, J., Knauss, L., Glover, D., Mogil, C., et al. (2010). The long war and parental combat deployment: effects on military children and at-home spouses. Journal of the American Academy of Child and Adolescent Psychiatry, 49(4), 310–320.

Lester, P., Stein, J., Saltzman, W., Woodward, K., MacDermid, S., Milburn, N., et al. (2013). Psychological health of military children: longitudinal evaluation of a family-centered prevention program to enhance family resilience. Military Medicine, 178(8), 838–845.

MacManus, D., Rona, R., Dickson, H., Somaini, G., Fear, N., & Wessely, S. (2015). Aggressive and violent behavior among military personnel deployed to Iraq and Afghanistan: prevalence and link with deployment and combat exposure. Epidemiologic Reviews, 37, 196–212.

Manguno-Mire, G., Sautter, F., Lyons, J., Myers, L., Perry, D., Sherman, M., et al. (2007). Psychological distress and burden among female partners of combat veterans with PTSD. Journal of Nervous and Mental Disorders, 195(2), 144–151.

Mansfield, A., Kaufman, J., Engel, C., & Gaynes, B. (2011). Deployment and mental health diagnoses among children of US Army personnel. Archives of Pediatrics & Adolescent Medicine, 165(11), 999–1005.

Mansfield, A., Kaufman, J., Marshall, S., Gaynes, B., Morrissey, J., & Engel, C. (2010). Deployment and the use of mental health services among US Army wives. New England Journal of Medicine, 362(2), 101–109.

McCarroll, J., Fan, Z., Newby, J., & Ursano, R. (2008). Trends in US Army child maltreatment reports: 1990–2004. Child Abuse Review, 17, 108–118.

Milliken, C., Auchterlonie, J., & Hoge, C. (2007). Longitudinal assessment of mental health problems among active and reserve component soldiers returning from the Iraq war. Journal of the American Medical Association, 298(18), 2141–2148.

Monson, C., Fredman, S., Adair, K., Stevens, S., Resick, P., Schnurr, P., et al. (2011). Cognitive–behavioral conjoint therapy for PTSD: pilot results from a community sample. Journal of Traumatic Stress, 24(1), 97–101.

Monson, C., Taft, C., & Fredman, S. (2009). Military-related PTSD and intimate relationships: from description to theory-driven research and intervention development. Clinical Psychology Review, 29(8), 707–714.

North, C., & Pfefferbaum, B. (2013). Mental health response to community disasters: a systematic review. Journal of the American Medical Association, 310(5), 507–518.

Petrik, N., Rosenberg, A., & Watson, C. (1983). Combat experience and youth: influences on reported violence against women. Professional Psychology, Research and Practice, 14(6), 895–899.

RAND Center for Military Health Policy Research. (2008). Invisible Wounds: Mental Health and Cognitive Needs of America's Returning Veterans. Arlington, VA: RAND Corporation.

Rentz, E., Marshall, S., Loomis, D., Casteel, C., Martin, S., & Gibbs, D. (2007). Effect of deployment on the occurrence of child maltreatment in military and nonmilitary families. American Journal of Epidemiology, 165(10), 1199–1206.

Riggs, D., Byrne, Weathers, F., & Litz, B. (1998). The quality of the intimate relationships of male Vietnam veterans: problems associated with posttraumatic stress disorder. Journal of Traumatic Stress, 11(1), 87–101.

Rosenheck, R., & Nathan, P. (1985). Secondary traumatization in children of Vietnam veterans. Hospital and Community Psychiatry, 36, 538–539.

Saltzman, W., Lester, P., Beardslee, W., Layne, C., Woodward, K., & Nash, W. (2011). Mechanisms of risk and resilience in military families: theoretical and empirical basis of a family-focused resilience enhancement program. Clinical Child and Family Psychological Review, 14, 213–230.

Samper, R., Taft, C., Kind, D., & King, L. (2004). Posttraumatic stress disorder symptoms and parenting satisfaction among a national sample of male Vietnam veterans. Journal of Traumatic Stress, 17(4), 311–315.

Sayers, S., Farrow, V., Ross, J., & Oslin, D. (2009). Family problems among recently returned military veterans referred for a mental health evaluation. Journal of Clinical Psychiatry, 70(2), 163–170.

Sherman, M., Zanotti, D., & Jones, D. (2005). Key elements in couples therapy with veterans with combat-related posttraumatic stress disorder. Professional Psychology: Research and Practice, 36(6), 626–633.

Taft, C., Pless, A., Stalans, L., Koenen, K., King, L., & King, D. (2005). Risk factors for partner violence among a national sample of combat veterans. Journal of Consulting and Clinical Psychology, 73(1), 151–159.

Taft, C., Schumm, J., Panuzio, J., & Proctor, S. (2008). An examination of family adjustment among Operation Desert Storm veterans. Journal of Consulting and Clinical Psychology, 76(4), 648–656.

Taft, C., Vogt, D., Marshall, A., Panuzio, J., & Niles, B. (2007). Aggression among combat veterans: relationships with combat exposure and symptoms of posttraumatic stress disorder, dysphoria, and anxiety. Journal of Traumatic Stress, 20(2), 135–145.

Tanielian, T., & Jaycox, L., eds. (2008). Invisible wounds of war: psychological and cognitive injuries, their consequences, and services to assist recovery. Arlington, VA: RAND Corporation.

The White House. (2012, August 31). Executive Order: Improving Access to Mental Health Services for Veterans, Service Members, and Military Families. Retrieved from https://www.whitehouse.gov/the-press-office/2012/08/31/executive-order-improving-access-mental-health-services-veterans-service.

Wadsworth, S., Lester, P., Marini, C., Cozza, S., Sornborger, J., Strouse, T., et al. (2013). Approaching family-focused systems of care for military and veteran families. Military Behavioral Health, 1(1), 31–40.

Walsh, F. (2006). Strengthening Family Resilience, 2nd ed. New York, NY: Guilford Press.

Whisman, M., Sheldon, C., & Goering, P. (2000). Psychiatric disorders and dissatisfaction with social relationships: does type of relationship matter? Journal of Abnormal Psychology, 109(4), 803–808.

Wickrama, K., & Kaspar, V. (2008). Family context of mental health risk in tsunami-exposed adolescents: findings from a pilot study in Sri Lanka. Social Science & Medicine, 64(3), 713–723.

TEN

Recreational Therapy for PTSD

HOLLY J. RAMSAWH AND GARY H. WYNN

T HERE ARE CURRENTLY SEVERAL INTERVENTIONS FOR POSTTRAUMATIC STRESS disorder (PTSD) that meet the definition of "evidence-based therapies" as outlined by the Institute of Medicine (2012). These include several forms of exposure-based behavioral interventions and pharmacotherapies that the Institute of Medicine determined are efficacious and first-line treatments for PTSD. Although exposure-based therapies are efficacious, not all patients respond adequately to treatment (Hofmann & Smits, 2008; Kar, 2011; Schottenbauer, Glass, Arnkoff, Tendick, & Gray, 2008). In some cases, behavioral therapies have been associated with high refusal (Bradley, Greene, Russ, Dutra, & Westen, 2005; Schottenbauer et al., 2008) and attrition rates (Hofmann & Smits, 2008; Schottenbauer et al., 2008). Furthermore, evidence-based behavioral interventions are not yet widely available because relatively few practitioners are adequately trained outside of academic institutions, and there are few trained professionals outside of urban centers. Even when evidence-based behavioral or pharmacological treatments are available, veterans sometimes avoid seeking these out because of perceived stigma about receiving traditional forms of mental health care either from traditional mental healthcare providers or in traditional mental healthcare environments (Chapman et al., 2014; Hoge et al., 2004; Mittal et al., 2013). Despite large numbers of returning veterans being diagnosed with PTSD since the start of the recent conflicts in Iraq and Afghanistan (Hoge et al., 2004), there remains a large number of Americans who have limited access to evidence-based interventions for PTSD (Hoge et al., 2004). Although efforts to expand access to these treatments should continue, there should also be an effort to investigate novel interventions for PTSD—particularly those that may require less training and/or may be associated with less stigma than conventional treatments.

The current chapter examines one such group of interventions: recreational therapy. Recreational therapy refers to treatments designed to help restore prior levels of functioning resulting from injury or illness, or to promote health and wellness. Recreational therapies—which can include both sports and leisure activities such as hiking, gardening, crafts, dance, drama, bird watching, fishing, and other activities—typically involve the assistance of a trained therapist or other facilitator, and may be conducted in small groups of patients or one-on-one. In this chapter, the focus is on recreational therapies that are conducted exclusively outdoors. Several subtypes of recreational therapy—namely, equine-related treatments, adventure/wilderness therapy, and fly fishing—are described. The research evidence for their efficacy—for PTSD if available, as well as other outcomes—is reviewed briefly along with possible mechanisms for their efficacy. The chapter concludes with considerations for future work in recreational therapy research—specifically, what the "active ingredients" of such therapies may entail and how future investigations may clarify active components of each subtype of recreational therapy.

EQUINE-RELATED TREATMENTS

Equine-related treatments (ERTs) encompass a broad range of therapies that typically involve horses, but less commonly may also involve other equine species (e.g., donkeys, mules). Although specific techniques vary by subtype—and by instructor within a given subtype—there are some common factors that seem to be present among all variants. All therapies include exposure to horses, along with some combination of foci on understanding horses, grooming, and general horsemanship. Those that include a riding component can be considered therapeutic horseback riding. Given that horses are sensitive to emotions by nature, other ERT therapies use horses as therapeutic tools to facilitate discussion and processing of thoughts and emotional material, and can be referred to as *equine-assisted psychotherapy*. Both types of ERTs have been found in a small but varied body of literature to confer benefits over a range of outcomes, including severe mental illness (Corring, Lundberg, & Rudnick, 2013), autism symptoms (Bass, Duchowny, & Llabre, 2009; Gabriels et al., 2012), and mixed samples of youth exposed to familial violence (Schultz, Remick-Barlow, & Robbins, 2007). Furthermore, there are a multitude of ERT-related websites that tout far-reaching benefits for various mental health conditions. To date, we are not aware of any empirical investigations of ERTs for PTSD specifically. There is one small

(N = 13) study that reported improvement in functional impairment and depressive symptoms in combat veterans, but it has significant limitations, including high attrition (only seven participants completed treatment), unclear statistical analytic methods, and no control group (Lanning & Krenek, 2013).

Several recent reviews of the empirical evidence for the efficacy of ERTs have been conducted (Anestis, Anestis, Zawilinski, Hopkins, & Lilienfeld, 2014; Kendall, Maujean, Pepping, & Wright, 2014), with a review by Anestis et al. (2014) being one of the most thorough. In it, the authors point out that, for any new intervention, there needs to be evidence of incremental efficacy above and beyond existing evidence-based interventions, such that any increase in costs is justified. They contend the cost associated with ERTs is substantial, and therefore such interventions, either as a stand-alone or adjunctive treatment, should be recommended only if there is sufficient evidence to warrant its use (Anestis et al., 2014). Such limitations to recommending ERT may not apply in cases when nonprofit organizations provide these services for free, and currently numerous nonprofit organizations provide financial support for ERT programs.

Anestis et al. (2014) and others point out several methodological problems with the ERT studies reviewed. First, few studies were randomized controlled trials (RCTs) (Anestis et al., 2014; Kendall et al., 2014). Without randomization, it is difficult to know whether there were meaningful differences between those randomized to ERTs and those randomized to the other treatment arm. It is also difficult to know whether patients receiving ERT would have improved anyway, resulting from regression to the mean (i.e., the tendency for extreme scores to become less so at retesting), common factors present within ERT (e.g., the therapeutic alliance), or concurrent treatments being received by study patients (e.g., pharmacotherapy). Furthermore, of the few studies reviewed that did use randomization, the majority used wait-list control groups. Only one study reviewed used an active treatment, school-based counseling, as the comparison condition (Trotter, Chandler, Goodwin-Bond, & Casey, 2008), and even in that study it was unclear that ERT was compared with an intervention with proven efficacy.

In addition, few studies reviewed by Anestis et al. (2014) provided sufficient details about the treatment. Providing adequate details is important, both in order for readers to understand the content of the treatment and to allow for replication by future investigators. Furthermore, without adequate description of the treatment protocol, typically within a manual or empirical paper in the form of explicit details about the ERT, fidelity checks to ensure the treatment described is actually being provided are not possible. In addition, it appears that several studies allowed modification of the treatment protocol for individual patients as the therapist or facilitator thought appropriate. Finally, the length of treatment varied significantly across studies and even *within* a few studies—for example, the treatment length in one study varied from 1 to 116 sessions (Schultz et al., 2007). Thus, the sufficient "dose" of each ERT is unclear because the treatment length varied widely.

Other problems with the body of existing literature on ERTs noted by Anestis et al. (2014) include a lack of independent, unbiased raters (e.g., as in double-blind RCTs) to guard against experimenter expectancies in 12 of 14 reviewed studies, low statistical power resulting from small sample size, lack of corrections for multiple comparisons leading to inflated Type I error, lack of statistical controls or other means to guard against skewing of results resulting from attrition, lack of posttreatment follow-up data collection to determine durability of any effects detected, use of unvalidated measures, and novelty effects related to ERTs. Anestis et al. (2014) noted that the presence of the most serious of these methodological flaws—specifically, the lack of appropriate controls, proper experimental procedures necessary to test treatment outcomes rigorously, and unbiased raters—would "typically disqualify studies in the psychotherapy outcome literature from serious scholarly consideration" (p. 1117). Furthermore, they noted that promotion and marketing of ERTs as a first-line treatment for a range of outcomes, without clear evidence of specific treatment mechanisms provided nor empirical evidence of its effects for examined outcomes, is problematic ethically and should not be recommended over existing treatments that have at least moderately strong evidence of efficacy. They conclude there is little support for ERTs currently being used as either a stand-alone or adjunctive treatment for any mental disorder. They also state that would be problematic ethically to recommend and market ERTs over evidence-based treatments, especially given the significant costs, without first disclosing the developing and inconclusive nature of efficacy research regarding ERTs.

However, despite the current lack of empirical evidence for ERTs thus far, this should not dissuade future, well-designed ERT studies from being conducted. For example, incorporating an RCT design would address one major concern with ERT studies conducted to date. In addition, posttreatment follow-up data could be collected, either at 3 months, 6 months or 1 year after treatment, to examine whether treatment effects, if detected, are maintained over time. Treatment protocols could be manualized, and treatment fidelity data could be collected to ensure patients actually received the treatment specified in the protocol. Treatment adherence data would assess whether the possibility of therapist drift may be occurring after initial training. Accounting for attrition—for example, by conducting between-group comparisons of dropouts with treatment completers and then controlling for any identified demographic or clinical differences in subsequent analyses, using intent-to-treat analyses, and/or using newer approaches for handling selective attrition such as multiple imputation or maximum likelihood estimation—will help to guard against biased data as well as establish generalizability of findings. Although it will be challenging to design such a study, experimental designs that incorporate identical treatment elements in the comparison arm—for example, identical durations of time outside, contact with a mental health professional or instructor, and other elements—would help to ascertain the extent to which novelty effects may be operating. An especially rigorous (although perhaps logistically difficult) comparison arm might include another large, social animal, such as cows, to discern whether treatment effects are specific to equine species (Anestis et al., 2014).

OTHER RECREATIONAL THERAPY SUBTYPES

There are several other types of recreational therapies that have been somewhat widely available, but have only rarely been examined in the literature. These include adventure therapy, which includes programs such as Outward Bound, and therapeutic fly fishing.

Adventure/Wilderness Therapy

Adventure therapy programs, such as Outward Bound, often involve single- or multiday excursions in a natural setting, and participants typically complete physically challenging tasks as part of a group, such as hiking, rock climbing, and whitewater rafting. Although there are studies in the literature suggesting acute improvements in psychological traits, such as increased internal locus of control (Hans, 2000), there are few studies on the efficacy of adventure therapy for PTSD in particular. One recent study, Duvall and Kaplan (2014) found that psychological well-being, social functioning, and life outlook improved pre- to posttreatment in a mixed sample of veterans with a range of Axis I psychopathology, including 46% with PTSD. However, there was no control group, and the authors noted many improvements had begun to wane by the 1-month follow-up. A study by Hyer, Boyd, Scurfield, Smith, and Burke (1996) that also measured PTSD symptoms found that adventure therapy was associated with improvements in self-esteem, emotional control, and social connectedness, but not in severity of specific PTSD symptoms. The findings of their study are in contrast to other claims in the recreational therapy literature that suggest that because improvements in the former (e.g., attention, positive emotions) have been found, improvement in PTSD could also be reasonably expected (Vella, Milligan, & Bennett, 2013). Notably, a form of adventure therapy involving water sports has been used as a control condition in at least one study examining the effects of dolphin-assisted therapy (Antonioli & Reveley, 2005), although here, again, conclusions about the utility of experimental intervention are limited by the lack of evidence supporting the efficacy of the control condition.

Therapeutic Fly Fishing

Therapeutic fly fishing typically involves an excursion of several days during which fly fishing is a prominent component. It shares several features with adventure therapy, but does not typically involve the same level of physical exertion. To our knowledge, there has only been one published study on the topic. In that study, there appeared to be modest decreases in PTSD symptoms, depression, stress, and anxiety-related symptoms from pre- to posttreatment, along with modest increases in attention and positive emotions (Vella et al., 2013). Unfortunately, PTSD symptoms—which were assessed only at two time points, baseline and the 6-week follow-up, instead of three time points as done with all other self-report measures—were not reduced to a point consistent with clinical remission. Furthermore, a number of methodological weaknesses were present. For example, there was no attempt to control for existing pharmacological treatments, and nonpharmacological concurrent treatments were not ascertained. Most concerning was that by the 6-week follow-up, many scores on self-report measures were elevated relative to the prior evaluation, raising the possibility of a return to baseline—a fact not discussed by the authors. Nonetheless, the authors speculated that the fly-fishing excursion may have enabled participants to "reclaim a sense of self unaffected by the combat experience" (p. 258). Although this study represents an effort to evaluate fly-fishing for PTSD, the totality of the evidence is not suggestive of either a benefit or a lack of efficacy; only that much work is needed to evaluate whether or not there is a benefit.

POSSIBLE RESEARCH CHALLENGES: IDENTIFYING ACTIVE INGREDIENTS OF RECREATIONAL THERAPIES FOR PTSD

As noted throughout this chapter, part of the challenge for empirical investigation of recreational therapies is that treatment content is not well defined. Although there have been attempts to develop a theoretical rationale for some of the approaches, in general recreational therapy treatments have not been well explicated. Furthermore, practitioners often modify the treatment as they see appropriate, so that two treatment regimens for different patients within the same recreational therapy subtype (e.g., fly fishing) may have significant differences in execution (Gelkopf, Hasson-Ohayon, Bikman, & Kravetz, 2013). Although recreational therapy is studied further empirically, its mechanisms should be defined as well. The sections that follow present a discussion of several possible mechanisms for improvement in patient symptoms. Further honing of existing treatments with these components in mind would allow for more scientifically sound empirical investigation, and could ultimately lead to more robust and efficacious treatments in the future.

Behavioral Activation

Behavioral activation is a prominent component of cognitive–behavioral therapies (CBTs) for depression (Sudak, Majeed, & Youngman, 2014). The rationale for behavioral activation is that major depression is often associated with withdrawal, seclusion, and isolation, which exacerbates feelings of sadness and loneliness, and leads to the maintenance of depressed mood over time. Therefore, deliberately scheduling pleasurable events can be associated with distraction from negative affect and cognitions, at least some enjoyment of the activity involved, pleasurable anticipation, and the opportunity to engage in thought experiments (as is done frequently during CBT) by testing negative cognitions related to the activity (e.g., "I'm too depressed to enjoy anything at all"). It involves scheduling pleasant activities that are relatively brief, easy to execute, and typically do not rely on the presence of another person to perform. These vary by person; activities are generated during collaborative work with a trained clinician. *Pleasant event scheduling*, as it is sometimes referred to, may include activities such as going for a morning walk, sitting in the sun, attending a musical performance, watching a funny movie, or planning an upcoming trip. Numerous studies have attested to the efficacy of behavioral activation for depression (Dimidjian, Barrera, Martell, Munoz, & Lewinsohn, 2011; Erickson & Hellerstein, 2011; O'Mahen et al., 2013), and a few studies also suggest improvement in veterans with PTSD (Jakupcak et al., 2006; Wagner, Zatzick, Ghesquiere, & Jurkovich, 2007). It is possible that riding or grooming a horse, going on a hike in the wilderness, and fly fishing act as forms of behavioral activation with positive effects for both PTSD and depression, which often co-occurs with PTSD (Cougle, Resnick, & Kilpatrick, 2009; Ramsawh et al., 2014).

Social Support

Another very likely active ingredient in recreational therapy is social support, considered a common factor of group therapies. Recreational therapies are typically conducted with a facilitator or therapist present, and either with small groups of other patients or alone (one-on-one). Much research suggests that social support, which involves being in the presence of others, sharing experiences, hearing suggestions for coping, and just providing a warm, positive regard in a "safe" context has a powerful association with mood, with studies showing decreased stress (Cohen & Wills, 1985), decreased depression and anxiety symptoms (Moak & Agrawal, 2010), improved physical and mental health (Moak & Agrawal, 2010), and even decreased suicidality (Griffith, 2012). These effects of social support on stress and other mental health outcomes may be indirect, through the influence of multiple biological mechanisms. Indeed, social support has been shown to be associated with lowered blood pressure (Bowen et al., 2014; Piferi & Lawler, 2006). In addition, social support has been linked with several neurological indices, including diminished cortisol reactivity, a hormone associated with stress (Heinrichs, Baumgartner, Kirschbaum, & Ehlert, 2003); decreased activity in the amygdala, a region associated with the fear response (Hyde, Gorka, Manuck, & Hariri, 2011); and decreased activity in both the dorsal anterior cingulate cortex and Brodmann's Area 8, regions associated with distress related to social separation (Eisenberger, Taylor, Gable, Hilmert, & Lieberman, 2007). One question for future researchers would be whether the mechanisms involved in the effects of social support are best harnessed through recreational therapies. In other words, are the effects of social support enhanced by recreational therapy? Regardless of mechanism, the positive effects of social support are likely operating in ERTs, adventure therapy, and fly fishing.

Effects of Exercise on Mood

Several different research studies suggest that exercise has beneficial effects on mood, alertness, and physical health. Acute effects include increased endorphin production in the brain, which is associated with a sense of well-being, and decreased pain perception (Oktedalen, Solberg, Haugen, & Opstad, 2001). Over time, exercise or increased levels of physical activity has a range of positive effects on cardiovascular and other health indices (Blair et al., 1995). Although not as likely to be a factor in fly fishing, exercise is likely to be a factor in various types of adventure therapy (e.g., rock climbing, hiking, sailing) and may also be a limited factor in ERTs that involve walking or riding.

Modified Attentional Focus

It has been suggested that some forms of recreational therapy modify attention in a positive way. In particular, it is possible that being in a natural environment encourages a state of mindful awareness of oneself and surroundings, similar to the cognitive state of mindfulness meditation thought to be operating in many newer CBT interventions such as dialectical behavioral therapy and acceptance and commitment therapy (Hayes, Villatte, Levin, & Hildebrandt, 2011). Indeed, early work suggests mindfulness meditation may be helpful in PTSD (Nakamura, Lipschitz, Landward, Kuhn, & West, 2011). This feature may be an active component of all three types of recreational therapy, but perhaps activities such as fly fishing in particular, given the long periods of calm alertness that this context encourages.

Increased Exposure to Sunlight (Physiological and Emotional Effects)

A modest portion of the putative effects of recreational therapy may be attributable to sunlight exposure. Studies have found that sun exposure improves mood and may even decrease suicide proneness (Preti, 1998). Furthermore, early morning sun exposure may influence melanin production, which is associated with sleep and sleepiness (Yoon & Song, 2002). Given that PTSD is closely associated with sleep disturbance (Germain, 2013; Ross, Ball, Sullivan, & Caroff, 1989), it is possible that sunlight exposure leads to improved sleep, and could have an indirect effect on both mood and PTSD symptoms in particular. Sun exposure is present in all three forms of outdoor recreational therapy discussed in this chapter.

Unique Effects of Interactions with Animals

It is possible there are unique effects of interactions with animals. For example, some research suggests that both humans and domesticated animals such as cats and dogs react positively to touch, with both humans and animals releasing oxytocin in response (Handlin et al., 2011). Other research suggests interactions with animals may be associated with decreases in blood pressure (Barker, Knisely, McCain, Schubert, & Pandurangi, 2010; Odendaal, 2000). These factors may be operating in some forms of ERT, particularly when affectionate touch is encouraged or prescribed as part of the treatment.

SUMMARY AND RECOMMENDATIONS FOR CLINICIANS

Most of the literature on the recreational therapies reviewed here suffers from the same methodological flaws as noted earlier for ERTs—notably, the therapies have only occasionally been subjected to empirical investigation, many have small sample size, the nature of the treatment is unclear and/or contains multiple components, treatment adherence is uncertain because implementation varies across therapists and/or patients, and concurrent medication or psychotherapy is not controlled for. Furthermore, when effects are detected for outcomes of interest, they do not show efficacy directly for the primary symptoms of PTSD, nor other mental disorders, and instead tend to show effects for desirable traits such as increased locus of control, sense of accomplishment, or an appreciation for nature. This is not to say that future research should not be conducted. Instead, greater scientific rigor should be applied to the design of future studies of recreational therapy.

In light of the existing research on recreational therapy, what should the clinician recommend to patients with PTSD? Given that there is currently limited research on recreational therapy, and the available studies have methodological limitations, the clinician should avoid recommending these as first-line or stand-alone treatment at the present time. However, there may be a place for recommending ERTs, adventure therapy, or therapeutic fly fishing as second-line or adjunctive treatments, given that there are often nonprofit organizations that offer such treatments free of charge, there have been no demonstrated negative effects, and recreational therapies may be a more acceptable alternative for those who either refuse to engage in first-line treatments or have not responded adequately to them. For those patients who refuse first-line, evidence-based treatments because of concerns about stigma or other reasons, clinicians may consider suggesting recreational therapy while continuing to recommend treatments with a more robust evidence base. This approach is in accordance with Veterans Affairs/Department of Defense guidelines, which recommend evidence-based treatments for PTSD and also recommend taking patient preferences into account during treatment planning (Management of Post-Traumatic Stress Working Group, 2010). Clinicians must be transparent in describing these as a developing form of treatment without evidence of efficacy, but ones that are unlikely to have any direct ill effects. Such information will allow patients to make an informed decision about the various treatment possibilities. Patients who have a positive experience with recreational therapy may be more open to evidence-based treatments afterward, such that recreational therapy serves as a stepping stone to other treatment options (e.g., by leading to reduced stigma associated with mental health-related interventions). Clinicians should take note of patients' interests and preferences when deciding whether to recommend recreational therapies, and should be aware of possible programs in the local area that may offer or support such treatments.

CHALLENGES FOR THE FUTURE

Given the paucity of empirical research currently available on recreational therapy, it is currently challenging for recreational therapy researchers to show there are factors specific to this form of intervention that lead to effects on PTSD and other mental health outcomes over and beyond novelty effects. Disentangling novelty effects from putative active ingredients will be challenging, but once identified, active ingredients can be incorporated more prominently into existing treatment approaches, and less effective (or iatrogenic) components can be decreased or dropped as appropriate. Next, treatment protocols can be developed and incorporated into research study designs, along with checks of treatment fidelity. Study designs will eventually need to incorporate active comparison groups to show comparative efficacy of recreational therapy. The necessary frequency and duration of each intervention will need to be established, as existing studies suggest that one-time acute interventions may only produce acute improvements in symptoms, followed by a return to baseline (Vella et al., 2013), if there is any improvement noted at all. Depending on effect sizes observed, logistical factors such as costs, and other considerations, researchers will need to determine whether recreational therapies are best conceptualized as stand-alone interventions, adjunctive treatments, or both. Analysis of cost-effectiveness is also necessary to demonstrate the strength of any effects shown are robust enough to justify recommending recreational therapy instead of or in conjunction with other evidence-based interventions. Currently, on balance, clinicians may opt to recommend recreational therapies to patients who decline or refuse first-line treatments, given that patients are made aware of the limitations of current research and understand these interventions are not expected to replace first-line treatments. Recreational therapies may also be recommended enthusiastically as an adjunctive therapy for interested patients who are also receiving evidence-based treatments.

KEY POINTS

- There are several evidence-based interventions available for PTSD; however, these treatments are not yet widely available and are characterized by relatively high refusal rates.
- For patients who do enroll in evidence-based behavioral and pharmacological interventions, a significant proportion drop out of treatment, and of those who remain in treatment, not all respond adequately.
- Recreational therapy, which requires less training and often carries less stigma than traditional mental health treatments, may be an option for such patients.
- ERTs involve exposure to horses, along with foci such as understanding horses, grooming, and general horsemanship.
- Adventure/wilderness therapy programs involve single- or multiday group excursions in an natural setting while participants complete physically challenging tasks such as hiking, rock climbing, and whitewater rafting.

- Therapeutic fly fishing typically involves a multiday excursion during which flying fishing is the primary focus.
- Currently, these recreational therapies have been subject only rarely to empirical scrutiny, either for PTSD or for any other health-related outcomes.
- Of the few empirical studies available in the extant literature, significant methodological problems are apparent, including small sample size, lack of control groups, improper experimental procedures, lack of treatment standardization, and lack of unbiased, independent raters.
- Future investigators should be sure to address these methodological deficits to design more rigorous studies of recreational therapy interventions.
- Furthermore, future investigators should identify possible "active ingredients" of treatment to develop more tailored and robust treatments.
- Possible active ingredients of these recreational therapies include behavioral activation, social support, exercise, attention modification, sunlight exposure, and the unique effects of interactions with animals.
- Given that many of these treatments are offered free and there have been no demonstrated ill effects, clinicians may consider recommending recreational therapy to patients who refuse first-line treatments, while continuing to recommend treatments with a more robust evidence base.

REFERENCES

Anestis, M. D., Anestis, J. C., Zawilinski, L. L., Hopkins, T. A., & Lilienfeld, S. O. (2014). Equine-related treatments for mental disorders lack empirical support: a systematic review of empirical investigations. *Journal of Clinical Psychology, 70*(12), 1115–1132.

Antonioli, C., & Reveley, M. A. (2005). Randomised controlled trial of animal facilitated therapy with dolphins in the treatment of depression. *British Medical Journal, 331*(7527), 1231–1234.

Barker, S. B., Knisely, J. S., McCain, N. L., Schubert, C. M., & Pandurangi, A. K. (2010). Exploratory study of stress-buffering response patterns from interaction with a therapy dog. *Anthrozoos, 23*(1), 79–91.

Bass, M. M., Duchowny, C. A., & Llabre, M. M. (2009). The effect of therapeutic horseback riding on social functioning in children with autism. *Journal of Autism and Developmental Disorders, 39*(9), 1261–1267.

Blair, S. N., Kohl, H. W., Barlow, C. E., Paffenbarger, R. S., Gibbons, L. W., & Macera, C. A. (1995). Changes in physical-fitness and all-cause mortality: a prospective study of healthy and unhealthy men. *Journal of the American Medical Association, 273*(14), 1093–1098.

Bowen, K. S., Uchino, B. N., Birmingham, W., Carlisle, M., Smith, T. W., & Light, K. C. (2014). The stress-buffering effects of functional social support on ambulatory blood pressure. *Health Psychology, 33*(11), 1440–1443.

Bradley, R., Greene, J., Russ, E., Dutra, L., & Westen, D. (2005). A multidimensional meta-analysis of psychotherapy for PTSD. *American Journal of Psychiatry, 162*(2), 214–227.

Chapman, P. L., Elnitsky, C., Thurman, R. M., Pitts, B., Figley, C., & Unwin, B. (2014). Posttraumatic stress, depression, stigma, and barriers to care among U.S. Army healthcare providers. *Traumatology, 20*(1), 19–23.

Cohen, S., & Wills, T. A. (1985). Stress, social support, and the buffering hypothesis. *Psychological Bulletin, 98*(2), 310–357.

Corring, D., Lundberg, E., & Rudnick, A. (2013). Therapeutic horseback riding for ACT patients with schizophrenia. *Community Mental Health Journal, 49*(1), 121–126.

Cougle, J. R., Resnick, H., & Kilpatrick, D. G. (2009). PTSD, depression, and their comorbidity in relation to suicidality: cross-sectional and prospective analyses of a national probability sample of women. *Depression and Anxiety, 26*(12), 1151–1157.

Dimidjian, S., Barrera, M., Martell, C., Munoz, R. F., & Lewinsohn, P. M. (2011). The origins and current status of behavioral activation treatments for depression. In S. Nolen Hoeksema, T. D. Cannon, & T. Widiger (Eds.), *Annual review of clinical psychology, 7,* 1–38.

Duvall, J., & Kaplan, R. (2014). Enhancing the well-being of veterans using extended group-based nature recreation experiences. *Journal of Rehabilitation Research and Development, 51*(5), 685–696.

Eisenberger, N. I., Taylor, S. E., Gable, S. L., Hilmert, C. J., & Lieberman, M. D. (2007). Neural pathways link social support to attenuated neuroendocrine stress responses. *Neuroimage, 35*(4), 1601–1612.

Erickson, G., & Hellerstein, D. J. (2011). Behavioral activation therapy for remediating persistent social deficits in medication-responsive chronic depression. *Journal of Psychiatric Practice, 17*(3), 161–169.

Gabriels, R. L., Agnew, J. A., Holt, K. D., Shoffner, A., Zhaoxing, P., Ruzzano, S., et al. (2012). Pilot study measuring the effects of therapeutic horseback riding on school-age children and adolescents with autism spectrum disorders. *Research in Autism Spectrum Disorders, 6*(2), 578–588.

Gelkopf, M., Hasson-Ohayon, I., Bikman, M., & Kravetz, S. (2013). Nature adventure rehabilitation for combat-related posttraumatic chronic stress disorder: a randomized control trial. *Psychiatry Research, 209*(3), 485–493.

Germain, A. (2013). Sleep disturbances as the hallmark of PTSD: where are we now? *American Journal of Psychiatry, 170*(4), 372–382.

Griffith, J. (2012). Suicide and war: the mediating effects of negative mood, posttraumatic stress disorder symptoms, and social support among Army National Guard soldiers. *Suicide and Life-Threatening Behavior, 42*(4), 453–469.

Handlin, L., Hydbring-Sandberg, E., Nilsson, A., Ejdeback, M., Jansson, A., & Uvnas-Moberg, K. (2011). Short-term interaction between dogs and their owners: effects on oxytocin, cortisol, insulin and heart rate: an exploratory study. *Anthrozoos, 24*(3), 301–315.

Hans, T. A. (2000). A meta-analysis of the effects of adventure programming on locus of control. *Journal of Contemporary Psychotherapy, 30*(1), 33–60.

Hayes, S. C., Villatte, M., Levin, M., & Hildebrandt, M. (2011). Open, aware, and active: contextual approaches as an emerging trend in the behavioral and cognitive therapies. *Annual Review of Clinical Psychology, 7,* 141–168.

Heinrichs, M., Baumgartner, T., Kirschbaum, C., & Ehlert, U. (2003). Social support and oxytocin interact to suppress cortisol and subjective responses to psychosocial stress. *Biological Psychiatry, 54*(12), 1389–1398.

Hofmann, S. G., & Smits, J. A. J. (2008). Cognitive–behavioral therapy for adult anxiety disorders: a meta-analysis of randomized placebo-controlled trials. *Journal of Clinical Psychiatry, 69*(4), 621–632.

Hoge, C. W., Castro, C. A., Messer, S. C., McGurk, D., Cotting, D. I., & Koffman, R. L. (2004). Combat duty in Iraq and Afghanistan, mental health problems, and barriers to care. *New England Journal of Medicine, 351*(1), 13–22.

Hyde, L. W., Gorka, A., Manuck, S. B., & Hariri, A. R. (2011). Perceived social support moderates the link between threat-related amygdala reactivity and trait anxiety. *Neuropsychologia, 49*(4), 651–656.

Hyer, L., Boyd, S., Scurfield, R., Smith, D., & Burke, J. (1996). Effects of Outward Bound experience as an adjunct to inpatient PTSD treatment of war veterans. *Journal of Clinical Psychology, 52,* 263–278.

Institute of Medicine. (2012). *Treatment for posttraumatic stress disorder in military and veteran populations: initial assessment.* Washington, DC: National Academies Press.

Jakupcak, M., Roberts, L. J., Martell, C., Mulick, P., Michael, S., Reed, R., et al. (2006). A pilot study of behavioral activation for veterans with posttraumatic stress disorder. *Journal of Traumatic Stress, 19*(3), 387–391.

Kar, N. (2011). Cognitive behavioral therapy for the treatment of post-traumatic stress disorder: a review. *Journal of Neuropsychiatric Disease and Treatment, 7,* 167–181.

Kendall, E., Maujean, A., Pepping, C. A., & Wright, J. J. (2014). Hypotheses about the psychological benefits of horses. *Explore: The Journal of Science and Healing, 10*(2), 81–87.

Lanning, B. A., & Krenek, N. (2013). Examining effects of equine-assisted activities to help combat veterans improve quality of life. *Journal of Rehabilitation Research and Development, 50*(8), XV–XXI.

Management of Post-Traumatic Stress Working Group. (2010). *VA/DOD clinical practice guideline for management of post-traumatic stress.* From http://www.healthquality.va.gov/guidelines/MH/ptsd/.

Mittal, D., Drummond, K. L., Blevins, D., Curran, G., Corrigan, P., & Sullivan, G. (2013). Stigma associated with PTSD: perceptions of treatment seeking combat veterans. *Psychiatric Rehabilitation Journal, 36*(2), 86–92.

Moak, Z. B., & Agrawal, A. (2010). The association between perceived interpersonal social support and physical and mental health: results from the national epidemiological survey on alcohol and related conditions. *Journal of Public Health, 32*(2), 191–201.

Nakamura, Y., Lipschitz, D. L., Landward, R., Kuhn, R., & West, G. (2011). Two sessions of sleep-focused mind–body bridging improve self-reported symptoms of sleep and PTSD in veterans: a pilot randomized controlled trial. *Journal of Psychosomatic Research, 70*(4), 335–345.

Odendaal, J. S. J. (2000). Animal-assisted therapy: magic or medicine? *Journal of Psychosomatic Research, 49*(4), 275–280.

Oktedalen, O., Solberg, E. E., Haugen, A. H., & Opstad, P. K. (2001). The influence of physical and mental training on plasma beta-endorphin level and pain perception after intensive physical exercise. *Stress and Health, 17*(2), 121–127.

O'Mahen, H. A., Woodford, J., McGinley, J., Warren, F. C., Richards, D. A., Lynch, T. R., et al. (2013). Internet-based behavioral activation–treatment for postnatal depression (Netmums): a randomized controlled trial. *Journal of Affective Disorders, 150*(3), 814–822.

Piferi, R. L., & Lawler, K. A. (2006). Social support and ambulatory blood pressure: an examination of both receiving and giving. *International Journal of Psychophysiology, 62*(2), 328–336.

Preti, A. (1998). The influence of climate on suicidal behaviour in Italy. *Psychiatry Research, 78*(1–2), 9–19.

Ramsawh, H. J., Fullerton, C. S., Mash, H. B. H., Ng, T. H., Kessler, R. C., Stein, M. B., et al. (2014). Risk for suicidal behaviors associated with PTSD, depression, and their comorbidity in the U.S. Army. *Journal of Affective Disorders, 161*(1), 116–122.

Ross, R. J., Ball, W. A., Sullivan, K. A., & Caroff, S. N. (1989). Sleep disturbance as the hallmark of posttraumatic stress disorder. *American Journal of Psychiatry, 146*(6), 697–707.

Schottenbauer, M. A., Glass, C. R., Arnkoff, D. B., Tendick, V., & Gray, S. H. (2008). Nonresponse and dropout rates in outcome studies on PTSD: review and methodological considerations. *Psychiatry–Interpersonal and Biological Processes, 71*(2), 134–168.

Schultz, P. N., Remick-Barlow, G., & Robbins, L. (2007). Equine-assisted psychotherapy: a mental health promotion/intervention modality for children who have experienced intra-family violence. *Health & Social Care in the Community, 15*(3), 265–271.

Sudak, D. M., Majeed, M. H., & Youngman, B. (2014). Behavioral activation: a strategy to enhance treatment response. *Journal of Psychiatric Practice, 20*(4), 269–275.

Trotter, K., Chandler, C., Goodwin-Bond, D., & Casey, J. (2008). A comparative study of the efficacy of group equine assisted counseling with at-risk children and adolescents. *Journal of Creativity in Mental Health, 33,* 254–284.

Vella, E. J., Milligan, B., & Bennett, J. L. (2013). Participation in outdoor recreation program predicts improved psychosocial well-being among veterans with post-traumatic stress disorder: a pilot study. *Military Medicine*, *178*(3), 254–260.

Wagner, A. W., Zatzick, D. F., Ghesquiere, A., & Jurkovich, G. J. (2007). Behavioral activation as an early intervention for posttraumatic stress disorder and depression among physically injured trauma survivors. *Cognitive and Behavioral Practice*, *14*(4), 341–349.

Yoon, I. Y., & Song, B. G. (2002). Role of morning melatonin administration and attenuation of sunlight exposure in improving adaptation of night-shift workers. *Chronobiology International*, *19*(5), 903–913.

ELEVEN

The Use of Yoga-Based Interventions for the Treatment of Posttraumatic Stress Disorder

BRIAN PILECKI, MEGAN OLDEN,

MELISSA PESKIN, LUCY FINKELSTEIN-FOX,

AND JOANN DIFEDE

INTRODUCTION TO YOGA PRACTICES

Yoga is a general term for a range of ancient practices originating in India, including meditation, physical movement, controlled breathing, chanting, and singing, to promote physical and mental health (Feuerstein, 1998; Riley, 2004). Hatha yoga is the most popular form in the West and includes physical poses, or asanas, widely used for physical exercise (Radha, 2006). Other forms of yoga include Agni yoga, which emphasizes meditation and breath control to stimulate creative energy; Iyengar yoga, which uses blocks and straps to enhance physical postures; Kundalini yoga, which focuses on the "chakras," or energy points, of the body; Shavasana yoga, which uses a single posture and emphasizes relaxation; and Sudarshan Kriya yoga (SKY), which uses cycles of alternating deep, slow, and fast breathing patterns (da Silva, Ravindran, & Ravindran, 2009). Although there is a wide variety of yoga traditions, the core set of components common to all yoga practices includes alterations in breathing,

TABLE 11.1 Descriptions of Popular Yoga Terms

Name	Abbreviation	Origin	Features/Emphasis
Hatha yoga	Hatha	General term for most popular western form	Physical poses
Agni yoga	Agni	Roerich family, 1920s	Meditation/breath control
Iyengar yoga	Iyengar	Form of hatha yoga	Props/physical postures
Kundalini yoga	Kundalini	Yogi Bhajan, 1960s	Energy points/"chakras"
Shavasana yoga	Shavasana	Ending segment of many yoga practices	Relaxation/breathing
Krishnamarcharya yoga	Krishnamarcharya	Form of hatha yoga	Breathing/self-awareness
Sudarshan Kriya yoga	SKY	Recent adaptation commonly used to treat mood problems	Cyclical controlled breathing
Vivekananda yoga	VYASA	Swami Vivekananda, early yoga missionary to the West	Integrative form
Sensory-enhanced hatha yoga	Sensory enhanced	General principles of the Yoga Warrior Method	Designed for veterans
Kripalu-based yoga	Kripalu	Swami Kripalu, 1960s	Adapts to individual differences
iRest Yoga Nidra Meditation	iRest	Integrative Restoration Institute	Relaxation/meditation
Prayanama	Prayanama	Common to many forms of yoga	Breathing

mindfulness, physical movement and postures, relaxation, and the development of spiritual beliefs. Yoga practices are believed to enhance the connection between body and mind, and are therefore thought to be beneficial for a variety of mental and physical diseases (Cabral, Meyer, & Ames, 2011) (Table 11.1).

A Review of Yoga and Yoga-Related Interventions

Although research is limited, studies have suggested that yoga-based interventions may be effective in the treatment of mood and anxiety symptoms, such as depression (Brown & Gerbarg, 2005a, 2005b; Butler et al., 2008; Janakiramaiah et al., 2000; Woolery, Myers, Sternlieb, & Zeltzer, 2004) and dysthymia (Naga Venkatesha Murthy, Janakiramaiah, Gangadhar, & Subbakrishna, 1998), and as an augmentation to antidepressant treatment (Janakiramaiah et al., 2000; Krishnamurthy & Telles, 2007). Research has also shown yoga to be beneficial in treating anxiety (Hofmann et al., 2015; Malathi & Damodaran, 1999; Norton & Johnson, 1983; Sahasi, Mohan, & Kacker, 1989; Sharma, Azmi, & Settiwar, 1991; Vahia, Doongaji, Jeste, & Kapoor, 1973), obsessive–compulsive disorder (Shannahoff-Khalsa & Beckett, 1996; Shannahoff-Khalsa et al., 1999), symptoms of schizophrenia (Duraiswamy, Thirthalli, Nagendra, & Gangadhar, 2007), alcohol dependence (Vedamurthachar, Janakiramaiah, Jayaram Hedge, & Suburkaishna, 2002), and medical conditions impacted by stress, such as irritable bowel syndrome (Taneja et al., 2004), hypertension (Labarthe & Ayala, 2002; Silverberg, 1990), and asthma (Nagendra & Nagarathna, 1986). These studies are intriguing in their breadth and scope, although many suffer from significant methodological limitations. Additional research with larger samples, valid and reliable measures, and randomized conditions is needed.

YOGA FOR THE TREATMENT OF NATURAL DISASTER-RELATED POSTTRAUMATIC STRESS DISORDER

A common application of yoga has been in treating trauma-related distress in the context of natural disasters. One such study examined the efficacy of a 1-week yoga program to treat survivors of the 2004 tsunami that impacted the Andaman Islands (Telles, Naveen, & Dash, 2007). Forty-seven participants were taught in small groups of 10 participants led by a certified Vivekananda yoga instructor across eight 1-hour daily sessions. Although there was no control group, results indicated that participants practicing yoga reported significantly less fear, anxiety, sadness, and disturbed sleep by the end of the intervention, as evidenced by ratings on a visual analogue scale. In addition, participants showed a decrease in their respiratory rate as measured by a polygraph. A similar study investigated the effectiveness of yoga for survivors of a flood in northern India (Telles, Singh, Joshi, & Balkrishna, 2010). Twenty-two participants were recruited from refugee camps and randomly assigned to either a yoga group or a wait-list control group. The yoga group received 1 hour of daily instruction for 7 days, including loosening exercises, physical postures, breathing techniques, and guided relaxation. Assessments included visual analogue scales to measure various emotions, a polygraph to measure heart rate variability, and a volumetric pressure transducer to measure respiratory rate. Participants in the yoga group reported a significant decrease in sadness whereas control subjects experienced a significant increase in anxiety; neither group had changes in heart rate variability or respiratory rate. Although this second study included a control group, limitations of both studies included small sample size and short duration of intervention.

Another more well-designed study investigated the impact of a yoga breath intervention on posttraumatic stress disorder (PTSD) and depression in 183 refugees of the 2004 Indian Ocean tsunami on the southeast coast of India (Descilo et al., 2010). Cluster randomization was used, assigning whole refugee camps to one of three conditions: yoga breath, yoga breath followed by exposure therapy, or a 6-week wait list. All participants were screened using the PTSD Checklist (PCL-17 [Weathers, Litz, Herman, Huska, & Keane, 1993]), a well-validated measure of PTSD symptoms. The Beck Depression Inventory (Beck, Ward, Mendelson, Mock, & Erbaugh, 1961) and General Health Questionnaire (Goldberg et al., 1997) were also used. The breath intervention (SKY) involved four different breathing techniques taught in 2-hour sessions over 4 consecutive days. All participants were provided with information about trauma, stress reduction, and meaning-making, and participants shared their experiences in weekly group sessions, thereby fostering a sense of social support. Participants receiving exposure therapy in addition to the yoga breathing intervention were given a form of exposure therapy called *traumatic incident reduction* (Gerbode, 1989), a three- to five-session protocol in which each 1- to 3-hour session is spent focusing on the trauma and associated loss. Results indicated the groups receiving the yoga breathing intervention alone or with exposure therapy demonstrated significant reductions in PTSD and depressive symptoms, as well as improvements in general health compared with the wait-list control group. Participants receiving exposure plus yoga did not differ significantly from those receiving yoga alone. The authors hypothesized that yoga may be more culturally acceptable than psychotherapy in India, highlighting a potential consideration when investigating yoga as a potential PTSD intervention in the West.

Finally, another study investigated the use of a 6-week hatha yoga practice in treating stress-related symptoms of 66 survivors of an Icelandic earthquake in 2008 (Thordardottir, Gudmundsdottir, Zoega, Valdimarsdottir, & Gudmundsdottir, 2014). Participants who sought out local yoga classes were assigned to attend six twice weekly 6-hour yoga sessions or to a wait-list control condition based on their residential location. Measures included the Perceived Stress Scale (Cohen, Kamarck, & Mermelstein, 1983), the Posttraumatic Stress Diagnostic Scale (Foa, Cashman, Jaycox, & Perry, 1997), the Beck Depression Inventory Second Edition (Beck, Steer, & Brown, 1996), the Beck Anxiety Inventory (Beck & Steer, 1993), and the Icelandic Quality of Life scale (Helgason et al., 2000). No significant differences were found in stress, anxiety, PTSD symptoms, and depression between the two conditions, and both groups showed improvement in energy, well-being, and sleep. Limitations included lack of random assignment.

Yoga and Military-Related PTSD

Several studies have investigated the use of yoga with military populations. A series of pilot open trials using yoga as an augmentation for antidepressant treatment in a sample of Vietnam veterans with depression and PTSD indicated that yoga was beneficial in reducing depressive symptoms (Carter & Byrne, 2004). Although standardized measures were used to measure reductions in depressive symptoms, including the Center for Epidemiological Studies–Depression Scale (Potts, Daniels, Burnam, & Wells, 1990) and the Structured Interview Version of the Hamilton Depression Rating Scale (Radloff, 1977), no measures assessed PTSD symptoms. The first of these trials found that Iyengar yoga led to reductions in depression symptoms in eight participants who participated in 1-hour group sessions on a weekly basis and completed home practice, and these gains were upheld after 21 weeks. The second study using the same participants adopted a new set of yoga poses intended to be more beneficial for anxiety, although no further improvement in reported anxiety symptoms or depression measures was found. The authors noted that symptoms of insomnia and anger were particularly resistant to the benefits of Iyengar yoga, and they added more breathing exercises (pranayama) in subsequent trials that resulted in improved sleep and reductions in flashbacks and expressions of anger, as well as continued reductions in Center for Epidemiological Studies–Depression Scale scores.

Another study investigated the impact of sensory-enhanced hatha yoga on symptoms of combat stress in deployed military personnel (Stoller, Greuel, Cimini, Fowler, & Koomar, 2012). Sensory-enhanced hatha yoga was developed specifically for combat veterans and includes sensory integration techniques commonly used in occupational therapy (Cimini & Stoller, 2009). Seventy active-duty military personnel deployed in Kirkuk, Iraq, were assigned to one of two groups. Participants in the treatment group were asked to attend at least two of seven 75-minute sensory-enhanced hatha yoga classes offered weekly for 3 weeks based on the General Principles of the Yoga Warrior Method designed for veterans and military personnel (Cimini, Stoller, & Greuel, 2009); this practice includes elements of centering, breathing techniques, postures, meditation, and relaxation. In addition, the treatment group listened to readings from yoga masters, positive affirmations, and Zen meditation music. Participants in the control group received no intervention and were monitored remotely. Measures included the Adult/Adolescent Sensory Profile (Brown & Dunn, 2002), a measure of sensory processing; as well as the State–Trait Anxiety Inventory for Adults (Spielberger, Gorsuch, Vagg, & Jacobs, 1983) and an unvalidated quality-of-life survey that assessed occupational performance, hyperarousal, mood, interpersonal relations, and cognitive functioning. Twenty-five of 35 participants in the treatment group met attendance requirements, although all 35 participants were retained in the final analysis. Results indicated that sensory-enhanced hatha yoga reduced state and trait anxiety but did not reduce sensory processing features associated with PTSD, such as sensory avoidance. In addition, participants in the treatment group demonstrated decreased concentration difficulties, irritability, social isolation, and boredom, as well as increased interest in pleasurable activities and ability to complete daily tasks as measured by the authors' quality-of-life measure. Qualitative feedback of participants in the treatment group indicated that more than half reported sleep improvements despite deployment in a dangerous combat environment. Limitations included a lack of standardized assessments for PTSD and unvalidated quality-of-life measure.

A more recent pilot study investigated the impact of a yoga program on PTSD symptoms in 12 mixed-era veterans who were receiving outpatient care for military-related PTSD (Staples, Hamilton, & Uddo, 2013). The yoga intervention was developed and taught by certified instructors from the Krishnamacharya Healing and Yoga Foundation and was designed to promote focus, calmness, and self-awareness through a breathing-centered practice; no home-based practice was assigned. Participants showed a significant decrease in PTSD hyperarousal symptoms as measured by the PTSD Checklist–Military Version (Weathers et al., 1993), but not in other PTSD symptoms. No changes were found in state or trait anger, as measured by the State–Trait Anger Expression Inventory-2 (Spielberger, 1999) or overall quality of life as measured by the Outcome Questionnaire 45.2 (Lambert, Kahler, Harmon, Burlingame, & Shimokawa, 2011). The intervention was found to be feasible, and participants had good attendance and provided feedback that the intervention was helpful.

Another study by Seppala et al. (2014) examined the impact of SKY on PTSD in male U.S. combat veterans of the Iraq and Afghanistan conflicts. This longitudinal randomized controlled trial (RCT) included 21 veterans, with 11 randomized to the group SKY intervention and 10 to a wait-list control. Participants completed 1 week, 1 month, and 1 year postintervention follow-ups. The SKY breathing-based intervention used in this study required participants to meet for 3 hours per day for 7 days, and followed the protocol outlined by Brown and Gerbarg (2005b). PTSD symptoms were assessed using the PTSD Checklist–Military Version (Weathers et al., 1993), and anxiety and depression were assessed using the Mood and Anxiety Symptoms Questionnaire (Watson et al., 1995). Startle response was assessed using a psycho-physiological paradigm (Grillon, Morgan, Davis, & Southwick, 1998). Participants receiving the SKY intervention showed significant reductions in hyperarousal and reexperiencing symptoms, as well as symptoms of generalized anxiety and arousal. Reductions in startle response were not significant but correlated with reductions in hyperarousal. Treatment gains were maintained at the 1-year follow-up but were not correlated with continued practice of SKY, suggesting the weeklong intervention was sufficient in producing lasting benefits. Although limitations included a small sample size and lack of participant diversity, results indicate potential clinical utility for this yoga intervention.

Yoga for the Treatment of PTSD in Women

Several studies have examined the impact of yoga for women with PTSD. First, a feasibility study investigated the efficacy of a 12-week trauma-sensitive yoga protocol in 17 female survivors of domestic violence (Clark et al., 2014). All participants attended weekly group therapy sessions; in addition, eight of those participants were randomized to complete a 30- to 40-minute yoga session each week. Both groups experienced equal attrition, and participants receiving the yoga intervention reported enthusiasm about yoga practice, although no measures were used to assess outcome. Another small pilot study investigated an intervention called *iRest Yoga Nidra Meditation* for the treatment of 10 women with sexual trauma (Pence, Katz, Huffman, & Cojucar, 2014). Participants showed significant decreases in PTSD symptoms as measured by the PCL, as well as significant decreases on the Posttraumatic Cognitions Inventory (Foa, Ehlers, Clark, Tolin, & Orsillo, 1999). Qualitative results included reports of improved sleep functioning and stress management, and an increase in joy.

A larger study of yoga investigated 64 women with chronic, treatment-resistant PTSD (van der Kolk et al., 2014). Participants were eligible if they met criteria on the Clinician-Administered PTSD Scale (CAPS [Weathers, Ruscio, & Keane, 1999]). Participants were randomly assigned to a 10-week, 1-hour hatha yoga class that included breathing, postures, and meditation or to a health education control condition equivalent in frequency and duration. Measures included the CAPS; the Inventory of Altered Self-Capacities, a measure of functioning (Briere & Runtz, 2002); the Davidson Trauma Scale (Davidson, Tharwani, & Connor, 2002); and the Beck Depression Inventory Second Edition (Beck et al., 1996). Although both the control and yoga groups reported significant decreases on the CAPS, participants in the yoga group reported a significantly greater decrease in symptoms than those in the control group. Both groups reported significant decreases in PTSD symptoms, depression, and overall functioning midtreatment. However, after treatment, participants in the yoga condition were more likely to maintain gains made at midtreatment.

A second study also investigated a yoga intervention in a sample of nine veteran and 29 civilian women recruited through a Veterans Affairs medical center (Mitchell et al., 2014). The yoga intervention consisted of 12 75-minute sessions of Kripalu-based yoga, taught by a certified instructor, that included tenets of trauma-sensitive yoga (Emerson, Sharma, Chaudhry, & Turner, 2009), such as present-moment awareness, making choices, effective action, and moving in rhythm. The classes were structured to have a weekly theme related to dialectical behavior therapy (Linehan, 1993), a cognitive behavioral therapy that promotes mindfulness and other skills to increase emotion regulation. Participants were randomly assigned to the yoga condition or an assessment-only condition. Measures included the PTSD Symptom Scale–Interview (Foa, Riggs, Dancu, & Rothbaum, 1993), a structured interview to assess PTSD symptoms; the Emotion Regulation Questionnaire (Gross & John, 2003); and a measure of experiential avoidance (Bond et al., 2011). Similar to the previous study (van der Kolk et al., 2014), participants in the yoga group and the control group exhibited a reduction in PTSD symptoms after treatment. However, only the yoga group showed significant decreases in expressive suppression, an ineffective emotion regulation strategy measured by the Emotion Regulation Questionnaire; and decreases in experiential avoidance that mediated reductions in PTSD symptoms (Dick, Niles, Street, DiMartino, & Mitchell, 2014). Participants receiving the yoga condition also showed a trend toward a decrease in alcohol and drug use (Reddy, Dick, Gerber, & Mitchell, 2014) on the Alcohol Use Disorder Identification Test (Babor, Higgins-Biddle, Saunders, & Monteiro, 2001) and the Drug Use Disorder Identification Test (Berman, Bergman, & Palmstierna, 2003).

Spiritually Based Interventions for the Treatment of PTSD

Several studies have investigated individual components of yoga practice. The repeating of a "mantra," a spiritually meaningful phrase, has been found to be beneficial in reducing stress and improving quality of life in veterans with and without PTSD (Bormann et al., 2005, 2009). In an RCT, Bormann, Liu, Thorp, and Lang (2012) randomly assigned 66 participants to a mantra intervention or a control group. The mantra intervention included six 90-minute weekly sessions that used mantra repetition to enhance relaxation and emotion regulation. Participants in the control group attended monthly case management meetings to provide general support, which is a limitation because of the unequal comparison with the treatment group. All participants met criteria for PTSD as assessed by the CAPS and PCL-17, and completed a measure of spiritual well-being (Functional Assessment of Chronic Illness Therapy Spiritual Well-Being [Peterman, Fitchett, Brady, Hernandez, & Cella, 2002]). Results indicated that participants receiving the mantra intervention reported significant reductions in PTSD symptoms and increases in spiritual well-being. A later study by the same group randomly assigned 146 veterans with military-related PTSD randomly to receive a mantra intervention and treatment as usual or a control condition consisting solely of treatment as usual. Mantra practice was tracked using a wrist-worn counter and daily log. Participants in the mantra condition showed increases in mindfulness as measured by the Mindful Attention Awareness Scale (Brown & Ryan, 2003), and the amount of mantra practice was found to mediate increases in mindfulness. Moreover, participants in the mantra intervention compared with the control intervention showed significant decreases in PTSD symptoms as measured by the CAPS, which was also mediated by increases in mindfulness.

Another study investigated the impact of a spiritually oriented group intervention called *building spiritual strength* (BSS), an eight-session, manualized spiritual group intervention designed to address spiritual or existential concerns of trauma survivors (Harris et al., 2011). BSS is based on research showing negative religious coping may inhibit adjustment to trauma (e.g. Witvliet, Phipps, Feldman, & Beckham, 2004). Fifty-four participants who reported experiencing a trauma, as verified by the Traumatic Life Events Questionnaire (Kubany et al., 2000), were randomly assigned to either BSS group or a wait-list control group. Only 65% of participants met criteria for PTSD as measured by the PCL-17. Results indicated that participants in the treatment group showed a significant decrease in PTSD symptoms, although 46% of those participants continued to meet criteria for PTSD (Table 11.2).

TABLE 11.2 Summary of Yoga and Trauma Studies

Study	Population	Type of Trauma	N	Control	Yoga Type	Measures	Results
Telles, Naveen, and Dash (2007)	Tsunami survivors	Natural disaster	47	None	Vivekanana	Visual analogue scale	↓ Fear, anxiety, sadness, sleep
Telles et al. (2010)	Flood survivors	Natural disaster	22	Wait-list control	Yoga	Visual analogue scale	↓ Sadness
Descilo et al. (2010)	Tsunami survivors	Natural disaster	183	Wait-list control	SKY	PCL-17. BDI, GHQ	↓ PTSD and depressive symptoms
Thordardottir et al. (2014)	Icelandic earthquake	Natural disaster	66	Wait-list control	Yoga	PSS, PDS, BDI-II, BAI, IQL	No differences
Carter and Byrne (2004)	Vietnam veterans	military	Not stated	None	Iyengar	CES-D, HDRS	↓ Depressive symptoms
Stoller et al. (2012)	Deployed military	Military	70	Control	Sensory enhanced	Adult/adolescent sensory profile, STAI-AD, quality of life	↓ Anxiety
Staples, Hamilton, and Uddo (2013)	Vietnam veterans	Military	12	Control	Krishmamacharya	PCL-M, STAXI-2, OQ-45.2	↓ Hyperarousal symptoms
Seppala et al. (2014)	Iraq/ Afghanistan male veterans	Military	21	Wait-list control	SKY	PCL-M, MASQ, psychophysiological measures	↓ Hyperarousal and reexperiencing symptoms

Study	Sex	Trauma	N	Control	Intervention	Measures	Outcome
Clark et al. (2014)	Female	Domestic violence	17	Group therapy	Yoga	None	Feasibility
Pence et al. (2014)	Female	Sexual	10	None	iRest	PCL, PTCI	↓ PTSD symptoms
van der Kolk et al. (2014)	Female treatment-resistant PTSD	Varied	64	Control	Hatha	CAPS, IASC, DTS, BDI-II	↓ PTSD and depressive symptoms
Mitchell et al. (2014)	Female	Varied	29	Control	Yoga	PSS-I, ERQ	↓ PTSD symptoms and experiential avoidance

BAI, Beck Anxiety Inventory; BDI, Beck Depression Inventory; BDI-II, Beck Depression Inventory Second Edition; CAPS, Clinician-Administered PTSD Scale; CES-D, Center for Epidemiological Studies-Depression Scale; DTS, Davidson Trauma Scale; ERQ, Emotion Regulation Questionnaire; GHQ, General Health Questionnaire; HDRS, Hamilton Depression Rating Scale; IASC, Inventory of Altered Self-Capacities; IQL, Icelandic Quality of Life scale; MASQ, Mood and Anxiety Symptoms Questionnaire; OQ-45.2, Outcome Questionnaire 45.2; PCL-17, PTSD Checklist-17; PCL-M, PTSD Checklist–Military Version; PDS, Posttraumatic stress Diagnostic Scale: PSS, Perceived Stress Scale; PSS-I, PTSD Symptom Scale–Interview; PTCI, Posttraumatic Cognitions Inventory; PTSD, posttraumatic stress disorder; SKY, Sudarshan Kriya yoga; STAI-AD, State–Trait Anxiety Inventory for Adults, STAXI-2, State–Trait Anger Expression Inventory-2.

PTSD, MEDITATION, AND MINDFULNESS

Another core aspect of yoga practice is mindfulness meditation. Mindfulness is defined as paying attention on purpose, in the present-moment, nonjudgmentally (Kabat-Zinn, 1994) and has been found to be effective in reducing anxiety (Baer, 2003; Grossman, Niemann, Schmidt, & Walach, 2004; Hofmann, Sawyer, Witt, & Oh, 2010). Mindfulness-based stress reduction (MBSR [Kabat-Zinn, 1982]) is an 8-week structured course that focuses on developing a daily meditation practice. One study investigated an MBSR intervention with 27 adult survivors of childhood sexual abuse and found participants experienced a decrease in symptoms related to depression, anxiety, and PTSD and, except for depressive symptoms, these improvements were maintained at 24 weeks (Kimbrough, Magyari, Langenberg, Chesney, & Berman, 2010). Another study investigated the acceptability and feasibility of an MBSR intervention with a sample of 92 veterans with PTSD symptoms (Kearney, McDermott, Malte, Martinez, & Simpson, 2012). Sixty-nine participants (74%) attended at least four classes, demonstrating that MBSR is an acceptable and tolerable treatment for PTSD. Results also indicated that participants showed improvements in PTSD symptoms, mindfulness abilities, and overall health and well-being.

Another study demonstrated that an intervention based on transcendental meditation led to decreases in depression, anxiety, emotional numbness, and family problems in a sample of 18 male Vietnam veterans (Brooks & Scarano, 1985). A more recent study showed that a transcendental meditation intervention led to decreased PTSD symptoms in five Operation Iraqi Freedom and Operation Enduring Freedom veterans (Rosenthal, Grosswald, Ross, & Rosenthal, 2011). Finally, a cross-sectional study of 124 urban firefighters showed that higher levels of mindfulness were correlated with fewer PTSD symptoms, depressive symptoms, and alcohol problems (Smith et al., 2011).

POTENTIAL MECHANISMS OF ACTION

Yoga practices include a variety of components and it remains unknown to what degree each ingredient contributes specifically to therapeutic benefits. Understanding these components and the underlying mechanisms of action in yoga interventions will contribute to the development of more effective and individually tailored interventions that may be used to treat different aspects of PTSD, such as avoidance, hypervigilance, or intrusive thoughts. Potential mechanisms include mindfulness, breathing, positive emotions and social cohesion, and meaning-making and cognitive reappraisal.

Mindfulness

As mentioned earlier, yoga practices are forms of mindfulness training. Experienced meditators have shown increased performance on tasks that demand sustained attention or have specific attentional demands (Kozasa et al., 2012; MacLean et al., 2010; van den Hurk, Giommi, Gielen, Speckens, & Barendregt, 2010). The skill of focused attention developed through mindfulness training may confer clinical utility because it allows for more control of mental resources and increased ability to disengage from ruminative thinking (Feldman, Greeson, & Senville, 2010; Frewen, Evans, Maraj, Dozois, & Partridge, 2008). Mindfulness and present-moment awareness may diminish one's focus on negative or maladaptive cognitions and reduce associated distress. Indeed, worry and rumination are cognitive processes purported to increase the severity of PTSD symptoms (Ehring, Szeimies, & Schaffrick, 2009), whereas increased mindfulness has been associated with decreased PTSD symptoms in trauma-exposed adults (Bernstein, Tanay, & Vujanovic, 2011). Research also suggests that individuals with PTSD are more likely to attend to trauma-related stimuli (Buckley, Blanchard, & Neill, 2000), leading to hypervigilance and increased anxiety. Similarly, individuals with PTSD may be deficient in inhibiting irrelevant or unwanted information while attending to other tasks, a process that may explain the etiology of reexperiencing symptoms (Anderson & Levy, 2009; Miyake et al., 2000).

The nonjudgmental attitude central to mindfulness involves not reacting to or placing value (i.e. "good" or "bad") on one's experience. To be nonjudgmental is to avoid using labels or evaluations and to observe the sensory experiences that one is having (Linehan, 1993). Individuals with PTSD have been found to measure high on anxiety sensitivity, the tendency to negatively evaluate anxiety-related symptoms such as bodily sensations (Lang, Kennedy, & Stein, 2002). One small study demonstrated that increasing observational and descriptive skills of internal experiences led to a decrease in PTSD symptoms (Niles, Klunk-Gillis, Silberbogen, & Paysnick, 2009). Adopting a nonjudgmental stance may increase willingness to experience distressing stimuli and thereby reduce avoidance; in this way, a nonjudgmental stance may help individuals engage with exposure therapies (Vujanovic, Niles, Pietrefesa, Schmertz, & Potter, 2011).

Breathing

Another core component of yoga practice is the regulation of breath conducted in various ways, including slow, deep, and SKY breathing. The process of breathing is linked closely to emotional experience. For example, diaphragmatic breathing is a widely used technique to reduce anxiety (for a review, see Hazlett-Stevens and Craske [2009]) that involves taking slow, deep, deliberate breaths that result in physiological changes and improvements in mood. In general, fast breathing stimulates the sympathetic nervous system, which is associated with arousal and preparedness for danger; slowed breathing stimulates the parasympathetic nervous system, the opposing network associated with relaxation (Kim, Schneider, Kravitz, Mermier, & Burge, 2013).

Yogic breathing may reduce PTSD symptoms through altering emotions by changing the pace of respiration (Zope & Zope, 2013). The physiological effects of breathing practice includes changes in heart rate and improved cognition, perhaps through stimulating the vagal nerve and the parasympathetic nervous system (Kim et al., 2013; Streeter, Gerbarg, Saper, Ciraulo, & Brown, 2012). The vagal nerve is theorized to project indirectly to the hypothalamus, amygdala, stria terminalis, and limbic cortex, thereby impacting autonomic, endocrine, and emotional processes (Brown & Gerbarg, 2005a). It is hypothesized that for mammals, breathing techniques that activate parasympathetic functioning may influence a wide range of physical and mental processes. In addition, heart rate fluctuations that occur naturally with breathing are influenced by parasympathetic activations (Brown & Gerbarg, 2005a). Therefore, slow yoga breathing may exaggerate these normal fluctuations, providing feedback to the vagal nerve and regulating affect (Sovik, 2000). Yogic chanting may also serve a similar function by increasing parasympathetic activity and promoting physiological relaxation (Telles, Nagarathna, & Nagendra, 1995). Deep breathing may decrease the consumption of oxygen, reduce heart rate and blood pressure, and increase parasympathetic activity to produce a calming effect (Jerath, Edry, Barnes, & Jerath, 2006).

A faster breathing technique associated with SKY is known to activate the sympathetic, or fight-or-flight nervous system. Although using SKY for individuals with PTSD may appear counterintuitive, it may actually enhance sympathetic reserves and protect against their depletion, similar to how daily physical exercise provides mild stimulation that is protective and yields greater preparedness to face acute stressors (Brown & Gerbarg, 2005a). Rapid breathing, a form of voluntary hyperventilation, may also have inhibitory effects on the frontal and parieto-occipital cortex (Posse et al., 1997), resulting in decreased executive functions associated with anxiety, including planning, worrying, and anticipation. Finally, yogic breathing may impact hormones related to mood and anxiety. One study found that depressed patients who practiced SKY for 3 weeks had significant decreases in cortisol, a stress hormone, which correlated with decreases in measures of depression (Gangadhar, Janakiramaiah, Sudarshan, & Shety, 2000). SKY interventions have also been found to increase prolactin, a hormone associated with reduced fear responses in mammals (Janakiramaiah et al., 2000).

Positive Emotions and Social Cohesion

Another beneficial component of yoga may be practices intended to produce positive emotions, such as singing, chanting, or mantra repetition. Several studies have demonstrated that participants who completed a loving-kindness meditation, a meditative practice intended to increase feelings of love and compassion, experienced an increase in positive mood and a decrease in negative mood (Fredrickson, Cohn, Coffey, Pek, & Finkel, 2008; Hutcherson, Seppala, & Gross, 2008), even among a sample of individuals with negative symptoms of schizophrenia (Garland et al., 2010). In addition, a study using functional magnetic resonance imaging showed activation in the left medial prefrontal cortex and anterior cingulate gyrus, which are areas related to positive emotions, during a similar type of meditation (Engstrom & Soderfeldt, 2010). Further studies could investigate whether increased prefrontal cortex activity is correlated with decreases in amygdala activity—an area associated with emotional arousal and PTSD symptoms.

Because group formats for yoga interventions are the most commonly studied, social cohesion may be an additional therapeutic mechanism that may address the PTSD symptoms of social isolation and feeling distant from others (Marshall et al., 2006; Schnurr, Lunney, Bovin, & Marx, 2009). Loving-kindness meditation has been found to be associated with increases in positive interactions with others (Hutcherson et al., 2008), which some researchers theorize leads to improved functioning, a stronger sense of mastery and resilience, and increased social support (Fredrickson, 2001). Brown and Gerbarg (2005a) also suggest that SKY breathing practices may elevate oxytocin levels, a hormone implicated in feelings of attachment and affiliation. Therefore, yoga may confer social benefits that are associated with reductions in PTSD symptoms and increased positive emotions.

Meaning-Making, Spirituality, and Cognitive Restructuring

As mentioned previously, some research suggests that spiritual practices may be beneficial for the treatment of PTSD by promoting spiritual beliefs or encouraging individuals to make meaning of their trauma (e.g., Bormann et al., 2012). Many of these studies include a component aimed directly at helping individuals create more adaptive beliefs through spiritual teachings or mantra practice. Many traditions of yoga practice are embedded within a spiritual or cultural context that address the meaning of life, the divine, or living a good life. Because experiencing a trauma often negatively impacts individuals' beliefs about themselves or the world, which can maintain PTSD symptomatology (Ehlers & Clark, 2000; Foa & Cahill, 2001), these belief-modifying aspects of yoga practice may be beneficial in helping individuals develop more adaptive beliefs. Trauma survivors may find comfort in spiritual views that address existential concerns such as why the trauma happened to them. This process can be compared with cognitive restructuring, a cognitive–behavioral technique with evidence of effectiveness in treating PTSD (Marks, Lovell, Noshirvani, Livanou, & Thrasher, 1998; Tarrier et al., 1999), as well as depression (Aderka, Gillihan, McLean, & Foa, 2013), nightmares (Thunker & Pietrowsky, 2012), and physical pain (Liedl et al., 2011). However, importing specific beliefs systems from yoga into therapeutic treatments must be done with caution because the field of mental health exists in a generally secular context. Specifically, patients may not be receptive to techniques if they espouse values or beliefs contrary to their own. In addition, without cultural context, nonspecific factors that contribute to the effects of yoga may be left out. (Cimini et al., 2009).

CONCLUSION AND FUTURE DIRECTIONS

The research reviewed here suggests yoga may be beneficial for the treatment of PTSD, anxiety, and associated depression. However, these preliminary results are tentative in nature and additional research is needed to support the effectiveness of yoga treatments. Furthermore, most studies reported general outcome measures only, such as overall PTSD severity or anxiety, although some studies found yoga to be beneficial in targeting specific factors such as improved physical health, overall sleep patterns, and positive emotions. Specific factors that showed mixed support include quality of life and insomnia, whereas anger, heart rate variability, and respiratory rates seemed to be the most resistant to benefit from yoga. Therefore, it is still too early to make specific recommendations about how various yoga treatments may impact distinctive PTSD symptoms differentially, although this would be a desirable goal for future research. Finally, because yoga is comprised of several components, it is unclear to what degree each may contribute to potential treatment benefits. Although the benefits of increased mindfulness and social cohesion have been investigated more thoroughly and gained more support, the role of other potential mechanisms such as spirituality, meaning-making, and cognitive changes remain largely untested. Finally, the studies reviewed in this chapter include numerous yoga interventions that differ in yoga type, length, and frequency. Because of the limited research available, it is difficult to identify which of these interventions may be the most effective. Therefore, future research in yoga for PTSD may benefit from adopting a unified approach similar to that adopted by Jon Kabat-Zinn (1991) in developing MBSR. For example, the sensory-enhanced yoga developed for veterans may serve as a good candidate because of its development specifically for a population vulnerable to PTSD. Such an approach would facilitate the development of well-designed RCTs to compare yoga with placebo treatments and exposure therapies.

KEY POINTS

- *Yoga* is general term for a range of ancient practices that may confer mental health benefits.
- Yoga-based interventions have been shown to be effective in the treatment of anxiety and depressive symptoms.
- A small body of evidence suggests that yoga-based interventions are feasible and acceptable, and may be helpful in the treatment of PTSD, although there are limitations to many studies, such as small sample size and lack of a true control group.
- Positive research findings for the treatment of PTSD with yoga include reductions in PTSD symptoms, anxiety, depression, and experiential avoidance, as well as increases in quality of life.
- Studies on the use of yoga for the treatment of PTSD have focused mainly on specific populations, such as survivors of natural disasters, military personnel and veterans, and females.
- Interventions that are related to PTSD, such as mantram repetition or meditation, have also been shown to be beneficial in the reduction of PTSD symptoms.
- Because yoga involves a multitude of components, studies are needed to determine the exact mechanisms of action, such as mindfulness, breathing, positive emotions, social cohesion, meaning-making, and cognitive appraisal.
- The adaptation of yoga practices from their cultural context must be done with caution because of potential differences in values and the loss of beneficial nonspecific factors.

REFERENCES

Aderka, I. M., Gillihan, S. J., McLean, C. P., & Foa, E. B. (2013). The relationship between post-traumatic and depressive symptoms during prolonged exposure with and without cognitive restructuring for the treatment of posttraumatic stress disorder. *Journal of Consulting and Clinical Psychology, 81*, 375–382.

Anderson, M., & Levy, B. (2009). Suppressing unwanted memories. *Current Directions in Psychological Science, 18*, 189–194.

Babor, T. F., Higgins-Biddle, J. C., Saunders, J. B., & Monteiro, M. G. (2001). *AUDIT: The Alcohol Use Disorders Identification Test: Guidelines for Use in Primary Care* (2nd ed.). Geneva, Switzerland: World Health Organization, Department of Mental Health and Substance Dependence.

Baer, R. (2003). Mindfulness training as a clinical intervention: a conceptual and empirical review. *Clinical Psychology: Science and Practice, 10*, 125–143.

Beck, A. T., & Steer, R. A. (1993). *Manual for Beck Depression Inventory*. San Antonio, TX: Psychological Corporation.

Beck, A. T., Steer, R. A., & Brown, G. K. (1996). *Manual for the Beck Depression Inventory-II*. San Antonio, TX: Psychological Corporation.

Beck, A. T., Ward, C. H., Mendelson, M., Mock, J., & Erbaugh, J. (1961). An inventory for measuring depression. *Archives of General Psychiatry, 4*, 561–571.

Berman, A. H., Bergman, H., & Palmstierna, T. (2003). *DUDIT-E, the Drug Use Disorders Identification Test- E: Version 1.1. Manual.* Stockholm: Karolinska Institutet.

Bernstein, A., Tanay, G., & Vujanovic, A. A. (2011). Concurrent relations between mindful attention and awareness and psychopathology among trauma-exposed adults: preliminary evidence of transdiagnostic resilience. *Journal of Cognitive Psychotherapy, 25*, 99–113.

Bond, F. W., Hayes, S. C., Baer, R. A., Carpenter, K. M., Guenole, N., Orcutt, H. K., et al. (2011). Preliminary psychometric properties of the Acceptance and Action Questionnaire-II: a revised measure of psychological inflexibility and experiential avoidance. *Behavior Therapy, 42*, 676–688.

Bormann, J. E., Liu, L., Thorp, S. R., & Lang, A. J. (2012). Spiritual wellbeing mediates PTSD change in veterans with military-related PTSD. *International Journal of Behavioral Medicine, 19*, 496–502.

Bormann, J. E., Smith, T. L., Becker, S., Gershwin, M., Pada, L., Grudzinski, A. H., et al. (2005). Efficacy of frequent mantram repetition on stress, quality of life, and spiritual well-being in veterans: a pilot study. *Journal of Holistic Nursing, 23*, 395–414.

Bormann, J. E., Thorp, S., Witherell, J., Golshan, S., Fellows, I., Lang, A., et al. (2009). *Efficacy of a Spiritually-Based Mantram Intervention on Quality of Life in Veterans with Military-Related PTSD.* Paper presented at the annual meeting of the Health Services Research and Development National Meeting, Baltimore, MD.

Briere, J., & Runtz, M. (2002). The Inventory of Altered Self-Capacities (IASC): a standardized measure of identity, affect regulation, and relationship disturbance. *Assessment, 9*, 230–239.

Brooks, J. S., & Scarano, T. (1985). Transcendental meditation in the treatment of post-Vietnam adjustment. *Journal of Counseling and Development, 64*, 212–215.

Brown, C., & Dunn, W. (2002). *Adult/Adolescent Sensory Profile: User's Manual.* San Antonio, TX: Psychological Corporation.

Brown, R. P., & Gerbarg, P. L. (2005a). Sudarshan Kriya yogic breathing in the treatment of stress, anxiety, and depression: part I. Neurophysiologic model. *J Altern Complement Med, 11*, 189–201.

Brown, R. P., & Gerbarg, P. L. (2005b). Sudarshan Kriya Yogic breathing in the treatment of stress, anxiety, and depression: part II. Clinical applications and guidelines. *Journal of Alternative and Complementary Medicine, 11*, 711–717.

Brown, K. W., & Ryan, R. M. (2003). The benefits of being present: mindfulness and its role in psychological well-being. *Journal of Personality and Social Psychology, 84*, 822–848.

Buckley, T. C., Blanchard, E. B., & Neill, W. T. (2000). Information processing and PTSD: a review of the empirical literature. *Clinical Psychology Review, 20*, 1041–1065.

Butler, L. D., Waelde, L. C., Hastings, T. A., Chen, X. H., Symons, B., Marshall, J., et al. (2008). Meditation with yoga, group therapy with hypnosis, and psychoeducation for long-term depressed mood: a randomized pilot trial. *Journal of Clinical Psychology, 64*, 806–820.

Cabral, P., Meyer, H. B., & Ames, D. (2011). Effectiveness of yoga therapy as a complementary treatment for major psychiatric disorders: a meta-analysis. *Primary Care Companion for CNS Disorders*, *13*(4).

Carter, J., & Byrne, G. (2004). A two year study of the use of yoga in a series of pilot studies as an adjunct to ordinary psychiatric treatment in a group of Vietnam War veterans suffering from post traumatic stress disorder. From *http://www.therapywithyoga.com*, 1–11.

Cimini, L., & Stoller, C. (2009). *General priniciples of the Yoga Warrior method*. West Boylston, MA.

Cimini, L., Stoller, C., & Greul, J. (2009). *The Yoga Warrior Lesson Plan*. West Boylston, MA.

Clark, C. J., Lewis-Dmello, A., Anders, D., Parsons, A., Nguyen-Feng, V., Henn, L., et al. (2014). Trauma-sensitive yoga as an adjunct mental health treatment in group therapy for survivors of domestic violence: a feasibility study. *Complementary Therapy and Clinical Practice*, *20*, 152–158.

Cohen, S., Kamarck, T., & Mermelstein, R. (1983). A global measure of perceived stress. *Journal of Health and Social Behavior*, *24*, 385–396.

da Silva, T. L., Ravindran, L. N., & Ravindran, A. V. (2009). Yoga in the treatment of mood and anxiety disorders: a review. *Asian Journal of Psychiatry*, *2*, 6–16.

Davidson, J. R., Tharwani, H. M., & Connor, K. M. (2002). Davidson Trauma Scale (DTS): normative scores in the general population and effect sizes in placebo-controlled SSRI trials. *Depression and Anxiety*, *15*, 75–78.

Descilo, T., Vedamurtachar, A., Gerbarg, P. L., Nagaraja, D., Gangadhar, B. N., Damodaran, B., et al. (2010). Effects of a yoga breath intervention alone and in combination with an exposure therapy for post-traumatic stress disorder and depression in survivors of the 2004 South-East Asia tsunami. *Acta Psychiatrica Scandinavica*, *121*, 289–300.

Dick, A. M., Niles, B. L., Street, A. E., DiMartino, D. M., & Mitchell, K. S. (2014). Examining mechanisms of change in a yoga intervention for women: the influence of mindfulness, psychological flexibility, and emotion regulation on PTSD symptoms. *Journal of Clinical Psychology*, *70*, 1170–1182.

Duraiswamy, G., Thirthalli, J., Nagendra, H. R., & Gangadhar, B. N. (2007). Yoga therapy as an add-on treatment in the management of patients with schizophrenia: a randomized controlled trial. *Acta Psychiatrica Scandinavica*, *116*, 226–232.

Ehlers, A., & Clark, D. M. (2000). A cognitive model of posttraumatic stress disorder. *Behaviour Research and Therapy*, *38*, 319–345.

Ehring, T., Szeimies, A. K., & Schaffrick, C. (2009). An experimental analogue study into the role of abstract thinking in trauma-related rumination. *Behaviour Research and Therapy*, *47*, 285–293.

Emerson, D., Sharma, R., Chaudhry, S., & Turner, J. (2009). Trauma-sensitive yoga: principles, practice, and research. *International Journal of Yoga Therapy*, *19*, 123–128.

Engstrom, M., & Soderfeldt, B. (2010). Brain activation during compassion meditation: a case study. *Journal of Alternative and Complementary Medicine*, *16*, 597–599.

Feldman, G., Greeson, J., & Senville, J. (2010). Differential effects of mindful breathing, progressive muscle relaxation, and loving-kindness meditation on decentering and negative reactions to repetitive thoughts. *Behaviour Research and Therapy*, *48*, 1002–1011.

Feuerstein, G. (1998). *The Yoga Tradition: Its History, Literature, Philosophy, and Practice*. Prescott, AZ: Hohm Press.

Foa, E. B., & Cahill, S. P. (2001). Psychological therapies: emotional processing. In N. J. Smelser & P. B. Bates (Eds.), *International Encyclopedia of Social and Behavioral Sciences* (pp. 12363–12369). Oxford, UK: Elsevier.

Foa, E. B., Cashman, L., Jaycox, L., & Perry, K. (1997). The validation of a self-report measure of posttraumatic stress disorder: the Posttraumatic Diagnostic Scale. *Psychological Assessment*, *9*, 445–451.

Foa, E. B., Ehlers, A., Clark, D. M., Tolin, D. F., & Orsillo, S. M. (1999). The Posttraumatic Cognitions Inventory (PTCI): development and validation. *Psychological Assessment*, *11*, 303–314.

Foa, E. B., Riggs, D. S., Dancu, C. V., & Rothbaum, B. O. (1993). Reliability and validity of a brief instrument for assessing post-traumatic stress disorder. *Journal of Traumatic Stress*, *6*, 459–473.

Fredrickson, B. L. (2001). The role of positive emotions in positive psychology: the broaden-and-build theory of positive emotions. *Am Psychol, 56*(3), 218–226.

Fredrickson, B. L., Cohn, M. A., Coffey, K. A., Pek, J., & Finkel, S. M. (2008). Open hearts build lives: positive emotions, induced through loving-kindness meditation, build consequential personal resources. *Journal of Personality and Social Psychology, 95*, 1045–1062.

Frewen, P. A., Evans, E. M., Maraj, N., Dozois, D. J. A., & Partridge, K. (2008). Letting go: mindfulness and negative automatic thinking. *Cognitive Therapy and Research, 32*, 758–774.

Gangadhar, B. N., Janakiramaiah, N., Sudarshan, B., & Shety, K. T. (2000). *Stress-Related Biochemical Effects of Sudarshan Kriya Yoga in Depressed Patients Study #6.* Paper presented at the Conference on Biological Psychiatry, UN NGO Mental Health Committee, New York, NY.

Garland, E. L., Fredrickson, B., Kring, A. M., Johnson, D. P., Meyer, P. S., & Penn, D. L. (2010). Upward spirals of positive emotions counter downward spirals of negativity: insights from the broaden-and-build theory and affective neuroscience on the treatment of emotion dysfunctions and deficits in psychopathology. *Clinical Psychology Review, 30*, 849–864.

Gerbode, F. A. (1989). *Beyond Psychology: An Introduction to Metapsychology.* Menlo Park, CA: IRM.

Goldberg, D. P., Gater, R., Sartorius, N., Ustun, T. B., Piccinelli, M., Gureje, O., et al. (1997). The validity of two versions of the GHQ in the WHO study of mental illness in general health care. *Psychological Medicine, 27*, 191–197.

Grillon, C., Morgan, C. A., 3rd, Davis, M., & Southwick, S. M. (1998). Effect of darkness on acoustic startle in Vietnam veterans with PTSD. *American Journal of Psychiatry, 155*, 812–817.

Gross, J. J., & John, O. P. (2003). Individual differences in two emotion regulation processes: implications for affect, relationships, and well-being. *Journal of Personality and Social Psychology, 85*, 348–362.

Grossman, P., Niemann, L., Schmidt, S., & Walach, H. (2004). Mindfulness-based stress reduction and health benefits: a meta-analysis. *Journal of Psychosomatic Research, 57*, 35–43.

Harris, J. I., Erbes, C. R., Engdahl, B. E., Thuras, P., Murray-Swank, N., Grace, D., et al. (2011). The effectiveness of a trauma focused spiritually integrated intervention for veterans exposed to trauma. *Journal of Clinical Psychology, 67*, 425–438.

Hazlett-Stevens, H., & Craske, M. G. (2009). Breathing retraining and diaphragmatic breathing techniques. In W. T. O'Donohue & J. E. Fisher (Eds.), *General Principals and Empirically Supported Techniques of Cognitive Behavior Therapy* (pp. 167–172). Hoboken, NJ: Wiley.

Helgason, T., Bjoernsson, J. K., Tomasson, K., Gretarsdottir, E., Jonsson, H.Jr., Zoega, T., et al. (2000). [Validation of an Icelandic version of the Geriatric Depression Scale (GDS)]. *Laeknabladid, 86*(6), 422–428.

Hofmann, S. G., Curtiss, J., Khalsa, S. B. S., Hoge, E., Rosenfield, D., Bui, E., et al. (2015). Yoga for generalized anxiety disorder: design of a randomized controlled clinical trial. *Contemporary Clinical Trials, 44*, 70–76.

Hofmann, S. G., Sawyer, A. T., Witt, A. A., & Oh, D. (2010). The effect of mindfulness-based therapy on anxiety and depression: a meta-analytic review. *Journal of Consulting and Clinical Psychology, 78*, 169–183.

Hutcherson, C. A., Seppala, E. M., & Gross, J. J. (2008). Loving-kindness meditation increases social connectedness. *Emotion, 8*, 720–724.

Janakiramaiah, N., Gangadhar, B. N., Naga Venkatesha Murthy, P. J., Harish, M. G., Subbakrishna, D. K., & Vedamurthachar, A. (2000). Antidepressant efficacy of Sudarshan Kriya yoga (SKY) in melancholia: a randomized comparison with electroconvulsive therapy (ECT) and imipramine. *Journal of Affective Disorders, 57*, 255–259.

Jerath, R., Edry, J. W., Barnes, V. A., & Jerath, V. (2006). Physiology of long pranayamic breathing: neural respiratory elements may provide a mechanism that explains how slow deep breathing shifts the autonomic nervous system. *Medical Hypotheses, 67*, 566–571.

Kabat-Zinn, J. (1982). An outpatient program in behavioral medicine for chronic pain patients based on the practice of mindfulness meditation: theoretical considerations and preliminary results. *General Hospital Psychiatry, 4,* 33–47.

Kabat-Zinn, J. (1991). *Full Catastrophe Living: Using the Wisdom of Your Body and Mind to Face Stress, Pain, and Illness.* New York: Delta.

Kabat-Zinn, J. (1994). *Wherever You Go, There You Are: Mindfulness Meditation in Everyday Life.* New York, NY: Hyperion.

Kearney, D. J., McDermott, K., Malte, C., Martinez, M., & Simpson, T. L. (2012). Association of participation in a mindfulness program with measures of PTSD, depression and quality of life in a veteran sample. *Journal of Clinical Psychology, 68,* 101–116.

Kim, S. H., Schneider, S. M., Kravitz, L., Mermier, C., & Burge, M. R. (2013). Mind–body practices for posttraumatic stress disorder. *Journal of Investigative Medicine, 61,* 827–834.

Kimbrough, E., Magyari, T., Langenberg, P., Chesney, M., & Berman, B. (2010). Mindfulness intervention for child abuse survivors. *Journal of Clinical Psychology, 66,* 17–33.

Kozasa, E. H., Sato, J. R., Lacerda, S. S., Barreiros, M. A., Radvany, J., Russell, T. A., et al. (2012). Meditation training increases brain efficiency in an attention task. *Neuroimage, 59,* 745–749.

Krishnamurthy, M. N., & Telles, S. (2007). Assessing depression following two ancient Indian interventions: effects of yoga and ayurveda on older adults in a residential home. *Journal of Gerontolical Nursing, 33,* 17–23.

Kubany, E. S., Haynes, S. N., Leisen, M. B., Owens, J. A., Kaplan, A. S., Watson, S. B., et al. (2000). Development and preliminary validation of a brief broad-spectrum measure of trauma exposure: the Traumatic Life Events Questionnaire. *Psychological Assessment, 12,* 210–224.

Labarthe, D., & Ayala, C. (2002). Nondrug interventions in hypertension prevention and control. *Cardiological Clinics, 20,* 249–263.

Lambert, M. J., Kahler, M., Harmon, C., Burlingame, G. M., & Shimokawa, K. (2011). *Administration and Scoring Manual for the Outcome Questionnaire-45.2.* Salt Lake City, UT: OQMeasures.

Lang, A. J., Kennedy, C. M., & Stein, M. B. (2002). Anxiety sensitivity and PTSD among female victims of intimate partner violence. *Depression and Anxiety, 16,* 77–83.

Liedl, A., Muller, J., Morina, N., Karl, A., Denke, C., & Knaevelsrud, C. (2011). Physical activity within a CBT intervention improves coping with pain in traumatized refugees: results of a randomized controlled design. *Pain Medicine, 12,* 234–245.

Linehan, M. M. (1993). *Cognitive–Behavioral Treatment of Borderline Personality Disorder.* New York, NY: Guilford Press.

MacLean, K. A., Ferrer, E., Aichele, S. R., Bridwell, D. A., Zanesco, A. P., Jacobs, T. L., et al. (2010). Intensive meditation training improves perceptual discrimination and sustained attention. *Psychol Science, 21,* 829–839.

Malathi, A., & Damodaran, A. (1999). Stress due to exams in medical students: -role of yoga. *Indian Journal of Physiology and Pharmacology, 43,* 218–224.

Marks, I., Lovell, K., Noshirvani, H., Livanou, M., & Thrasher, S. (1998). Treatment of posttraumatic stress disorder by exposure and/or cognitive restructuring: a controlled study. *Archives of General Psychiatry, 55,* 317–325.

Marshall, R. D., Turner, J. B., Lewis-Fernandez, R., Koenan, K., Neria, Y., & Dohrenwend, B. P. (2006). Symptom patterns associated with chronic PTSD in male veterans: new findings from the National Vietnam Veterans Readjustment Study. *Journal of Nervous and Mental Disease, 194,* 275–278.

Mitchell, K. S., Dick, A. M., DiMartino, D. M., Smith, B. N., Niles, B., Koenen, K. C., et al. (2014). A pilot study of a randomized controlled trial of yoga as an intervention for PTSD symptoms in women. *Journal of Traumatic Stress, 27,* 121–128.

Miyake, A., Friedman, N. P., Emerson, M. J., Witzki, A. H., Howerter, A., & Wager, T. D. (2000). The unity and diversity of executive functions and their contributions to complex "frontal lobe" tasks: a latent variable analysis. *Cognitive Psychology, 41,* 49–100.

Naga Venkatesha Murthy, P. J., Janakiramaiah, N., Gangadhar, B. N., & Subbakrishna, D. K. (1998). P300 amplitude and antidepressant response to Sudarshan Kriya yoga (SKY). *Journal of Affective Disorders, 50*, 45–48.

Nagendra, H. R., & Nagarathna, R. (1986). An integrated approach of yoga therapy for bronchial asthma: a 3–54-month prospective study. *Journal of Asthma, 23*, 123–137.

Niles, B. L., Klunk-Gillis, J., Silberbogen, A. K., & Paysnick, A. (2009). *A Mindfulness Intervention for Veterans with PTSD: A Telehealth Approach.* Paper presented at the North American Conference on Integrative Medicine, Minneapolis, MN.

Norton, G. R., & Johnson, W. E. (1983). A comparison of two relaxation procedures for reducing cognitive and somatic anxiety. *Journal of Behavior Therapy and Experimental Psychiatry, 14*, 209–214.

Pence, P. G., Katz, L. S., Huffman, C., & Cojucar, G. (2014). Delivering integrative restoration–Yoga Nidra Meditation (iRest®) to women with sexual trauma at a Veteran's medical center: a pilot study. *International Journal of Yoga Therapy, 24*, 53–62.

Peterman, A. H., Fitchett, G., Brady, M. J., Hernandez, L., & Cella, D. (2002). Measuring spiritual well-being in people with cancer: the Functional Assessment of Chronic Illness Therapy–Spiritual Well-being Scale (FACIT-Sp). *Annals of Behavioral Medicine, 24*, 49–58.

Posse, S., Dager, S. R., Richards, T. L., Yuan, C., Ogg, R., Artru, A. A., et al. (1997). In vivo measurement of regional brain metabolic response to hyperventilation using magnetic resonance: proton echo planar spectroscopic imaging (PEPSI). *Magnetic Resonance in Medicine, 37*, 858–865.

Potts, M. K., Daniels, M., Burnam, M. A., & Wells, K. B. (1990). A structured interview version of the Hamilton Depression Rating Scale: evidence of reliability and versatility of administration. *Journal of Psychiatric Research, 24*, 335–350.

Radha, S. S. (2006). *Hatha Yoga: The Hidden Language, Symbols, Secrets, and Metaphors.* Kootenay Bay, BC: Timeless Books.

Radloff, L. S. (1977). The CES-D scale: a self-report depression scale for research in the general population. *Applied Psychological Measurement, 1*, 385–401.

Reddy, S., Dick, A. M., Gerber, M. R., & Mitchell, K. (2014). The effect of a yoga intervention on alcohol and drug abuse risk in veteran and civilian women with posttraumatic stress disorder. *Journal of Alternative and Complementary Medicine, 20*, 750–756.

Riley, D. (2004). Hatha yoga and the treatment of illness. *Alternative Therapies in Health and Medicine, 10*, 20–21.

Rosenthal, J. Z., Grosswald, S., Ross, R., & Rosenthal, N. (2011). Effects of transcendental meditation in veterans of Operation Enduring Freedom and Operation Iraqi Freedom with posttraumatic stress disorder: a pilot study. *Military Medicine, 176*, 626–630.

Sahasi, G., Mohan, D., & Kacker, C. (1989). Effectiveness of yogic techniques in the management of anxiety. *Journal of Personality Clinical Studies, 5*, 51–55.

Schnurr, P. P., Lunney, C. A., Bovin, M. J., & Marx, B. P. (2009). Posttraumatic stress disorder and quality of life: extension of findings to veterans of the wars in Iraq and Afghanistan. *Clinical Psychology Review, 29*, 727–735.

Seppala, E. M., Nitschke, J. B., Tudorascu, D. L., Hayes, A., Goldstein, M. R., Nguyen, D. T., et al. (2014). Breathing-based meditation decreases posttraumatic stress disorder symptoms in U.S. military veterans: a randomized controlled longitudinal study. *Journal of Traumatic Stress, 27*, 397–405.

Shannahoff-Khalsa, D. S., & Beckett, L. R. (1996). Clinical case report: efficacy of yogic techniques in the treatment of obsessive compulsive disorders. *International Journal of Neuroscience, 85*, 1–17.

Shannahoff-Khalsa, D. S., Ray, L. E., Levine, S., Gallen, C. C., Schwartz, B. J., & Sidorowich, J. J. (1999). Randomized controlled trial of yogic meditation techniques for patients with obsessive–compulsive disorder. *CNS Spectrums, 4*, 34–47.

Sharma, L., Azmi, S. A., & Settiwar, R. M. (1991). Evaluation of the effect of pranayama in anxiety state. *Alternative Medicine, 3*, 227–235.

Silverberg, D. S. (1990). Non-pharmacological treatment of hypertension. *Journal of Hypertension. Supplemental, 8*, S21–S26.

Smith, B. W., Ortiz, J. A., Steffen, L. E., Tooley, E. M., Wiggins, K. T., Yeater, E. A., et al. (2011). Mindfulness is associated with fewer PTSD symptoms, depressive symptoms, physical symptoms, and alcohol problems in urban firefighters. *Journal of Consulting and Clinical Psychology, 79*, 613–617.

Sovik, R. (2000). The science of breathing: the yogic view. *Progress in Brain Research, 122*, 491–505.

Spielberger, C. (1999). *STAXI-2 State–Trait Anger Expression Inventory-2: Professional Manual.* Odessa, FL: Psychological Assessment Resources.

Spielberger, C., Gorsuch, R., R., L., Vagg, P., & Jacobs, G. (1983). *Manual for the State–Trait Anxiety Inventory.* Palo Alto, CA: Consulting Psychologists Press.

Staples, J. K., Hamilton, M. F., & Uddo, M. (2013). A yoga program for the symptoms of post-traumatic stress disorder in veterans. *Miitaryl Medicine, 178*, 854–860.

Stoller, C. C., Greuel, J. H., Cimini, L. S., Fowler, M. S., & Koomar, J. A. (2012). Effects of sensory-enhanced yoga on symptoms of combat stress in deployed military personnel. *American Journal of Occupational Therapy, 66*, 59–68.

Streeter, C. C., Gerbarg, P. L., Saper, R. B., Ciraulo, D. A., & Brown, R. P. (2012). Effects of yoga on the autonomic nervous system, gamma-aminobutyric-acid, and allostasis in epilepsy, depression, and post-traumatic stress disorder. *Medical Hypotheses, 78*, 571–579.

Taneja, I., Deepak, K. K., Poojary, G., Acharya, I. N., Pandey, R. M., & Sharma, M. P. (2004). Yogic versus conventional treatment in diarrhea-predominant irritable bowel syndrome: a randomized control study. *Applied Psychophysiology and Biofeedback, 29*, 19–33.

Tarrier, N., Pilgrim, H., Sommerfield, C., Faragher, B., Reynolds, M., Graham, E., et al. (1999). A randomized trial of cognitive therapy and imaginal exposure in the treatment of chronic post-traumatic stress disorder. *Journal of Consulting & Clinical Psychology, 67*, 13–18.

Telles, S., Nagarathna, R., & Nagendra, H. R. (1995). Autonomic changes during "om" meditation. *Indian Journal of Physiology and Pharmacology, 39*, 418–420.

Telles, S., Naveen, K. V., & Dash, M. (2007). Yoga reduces symptoms of distress in tsunami survivors in the Andaman Islands. *Evidence Based Complementary and Alternative Medicine, 4*, 503–509.

Telles, S., Singh, N., Joshi, M., & Balkrishna, A. (2010). Post traumatic stress symptoms and heart rate variability in Bihar flood survivors following yoga: a randomized controlled study. *BMC Psychiatry, 10*, 18.

Thordardottir, K., Gudmundsdottir, R., Zoega, H., Valdimarsdottir, U. A., & Gudmundsdottir, B. (2014). Effects of yoga practice on stress-related symptoms in the aftermath of an earthquake: a community-based controlled trial. *Complementary Therapies in Medicine, 22*, 226–234.

Thunker, J., & Pietrowsky, R. (2012). Effectiveness of a manualized imagery rehearsal therapy for patients suffering from nightmare disorders with and without a comorbidity of depression or PTSD. *Behaviour Research and Therapy, 50*, 558–564.

Vahia, N. S., Doongaji, D. R., Jeste, D. V., & Kapoor, S. N. (1973). Further experience with therapy based on concepts of Patanjali in the treatment of psychiatric disorders. *Indian Journal of Psychiatry, 15*, 32–37.

van den Hurk, P. A., Giommi, F., Gielen, S. C., Speckens, A. E., & Barendregt, H. P. (2010). Greater efficiency in attentional processing related to mindfulness meditation. *Quarterly Journal of Experimental Psychology, 63*, 1168–1180.

van der Kolk, B. A., Stone, L., West, J., Rhodes, A., Emerson, D., Suvak, M., et al. (2014). Yoga as an adjunctive treatment for posttraumatic stress disorder: a randomized controlled trial. *Journal of Clinical Psychiatry, 75*, e559–e565.

Vedamurthachar, A., Janakiramaiah, N., Jayaram Hedge, M., & Suburkaishna, K. S. (2002). *Effects of Sudarshan Kriya on Alcohol Dependent Patients.* Abstract presented at the "Science of Breath" International Symposium on Sudarshan Kriya, Pranayam & Consciousness, AIIMS, New Delhi: All Indian Institute of Medical Sciences.

Vujanovic, A. A., Niles, B., Pietrefesa, A., Schmertz, S. L., & Potter, C. M. (2011). Mindfulness in the treatment of posttraumatic stress disorder among military veterans. *Professional Psychology: Research and Practice, 42,* 24–31.

Watson, D., Weber, K., Assenheimer, J. S., Clark, L. A., Strauss, M. E., & McCormick, R. A. (1995). Testing a tripartite model: I. Evaluating the convergent and discriminant validity of anxiety and depression symptom scales. *Journal of Abnormal Psychology, 104,* 3–14.

Weathers, F. W., Litz, B. T., Herman, D. S., Huska, J. A., & Keane, T. M. (1993). *The PTSD Checklist (PCL). Reliability, Validity, and Diagnostic Utility.* Paper presented at the annual meeting of the International Society for Traumatic Stress Studies. San Antonio, TX.

Weathers, F., Ruscio, A. M., & Keane, T. (1999). Psychometric properties of nine scoring rules for the Clinician-Administered PTSD Scale. *Psycholical Assessment, 11,* 124–133.

Witvliet, C. V., Phipps, K. A., Feldman, M. E., & Beckham, J. C. (2004). Posttraumatic mental and physical health correlates of forgiveness and religious coping in military veterans. *Journal of Traumatic Stress, 17,* 269–273.

Woolery, A., Myers, H., Sternlieb, B., & Zeltzer, L. (2004). A yoga intervention for young adults with elevated symptoms of depression. *Alternative Therapies in Health and Medicine, 10,* 60–63.

Zope, S. A., & Zope, R. A. (2013). Sudarshan Kriya yoga: breathing for health. *International Journal of Yoga, 6,* 4–10.

TWELVE

Resilience Training as a Complementary Treatment for PTSD

ROBIN L. TOBLIN AND AMY B. ADLER

Although there are several different definitions of resilience, probably the most useful definitions refer to resilience as a process. The American Psychological Association (2016), for example, defines resilience as

> the process of adapting well in the face of adversity, trauma, tragedy, threats or even significant sources of stress—such as family and relationship problems, serious health problems, or workplace and financial stressors. It means "bouncing back" from difficult experiences.

Other definitions focus on resilience as a trait (e.g., hardiness [Maddi, 2005]) or as an outcome trajectory, such as when individuals respond to a specific traumatic event without symptoms or with symptoms that dissipate quickly (Bonanno, Rennicke, & Dekel, 2005). Yet, thinking of resilience as a process of adaptation conveys specific advantages. When resilience is conceptualized as a process, the focus is on behaviors or attitudes that can lead to a positive outcome in the face of a significant or traumatic stressor. Individuals can be trained in these adaptive processes, and thus resilience can be enhanced.

RESILIENCE TRAINING FROM A PUBLIC HEALTH PERSPECTIVE

We conceptualize resilience training from a public health perspective. Public health models describe three levels of prevention: (1) primary prevention, or an intervention given universally because the negative outcomes are likely for the whole group (e.g., smoking prevention); (2) secondary prevention, or programs targeting groups at high risk for a negative outcome (e.g., acceptance skills for military personnel exposed to significant levels of combat); and (3) tertiary programs, or programs that treat conditions after they have begun and prevent it from getting worse (e.g., rehabilitation after an injury). Resilience training can be applied at all three levels. In this chapter, we discuss how primary and secondary prevention resilience training programs can be adapted for use as a complement to treatment for PTSD, a tertiary intervention.

EVIDENCE THAT RESILIENCE TRAINING WORKS

Indeed, there are well-established resilience-building programs designed to train individuals in resilience skills. One of the most studied is the Penn Resiliency Program (PRP) (Gillham & Reivich, 1999), which began as a school-based initiative designed to prevent the development of depression of at-risk adolescents. The training program focuses on a series of skills designed to build competencies such as optimism, emotional awareness, self-regulation, and flexibility. The PRP material essentially operationalizes the basics of cognitive behavioral therapy (CBT), in which individuals are taught how their beliefs or thoughts about a particular event influence their emotions and behaviors. Other evidence-based resilience factors are woven into the PRP curriculum, including problem solving, the building of close relationships, and effective communication.

Results from randomized trials demonstrate the PRP training is effective. In a meta-analysis of the PRP, Brunnwasser, Gillham, and Kim (2009) reported 17 randomized trials and found, in general, the PRP was associated with better mental health, although this effect was based on studies with survey-only comparison conditions, rather than active control conditions, and the effect sizes were small, as would be expected from universal interventions (Bliese, Adler, & Castro, 2011; Vanhove, Herian, Perez, Harms & Lester, 2015). Other resilience training programs with a basis in CBT have also been validated empirically (Masten & Reed, 2002; Shochet et al., 2001).

These kinds of resilience training materials have also been adapted for use with high-risk occupations. For example, a study of resilience training with police officers (Arnetz, Arble, Backman, Lynch, & Lublin, 2013; Arnetz, Nevedal, Lumley, Backman, & Lublin, 2009) randomized 75 police cadets to 10 weeks of training that emphasized progressive and cue-controlled relaxation methods and CBT skills compared with a standard training program. Eighteen months later, those who received the CBT skills did better in terms of health outcomes and problem-based coping.

The military has also studied the impact of this kind of training on mental health and performance. In a study during basic training within the Navy, 801 Navy recruits were assigned randomly to either a 9-week mental health/resilience training program (BOOTSTRAP) or an active control that provided education about other topics, such as swimming skills (Williams et al., 2004). The BOOTSTRAP training focused on increasing social connection (e.g., being assigned the task of talking to a shipmate, not criticizing, listening) and decreasing cognitive distortions. By the end of basic training, recruits in BOOTSTRAP had better well-being, performance, and graduation rates than those in the comparison condition. Another study also found psychoeducation centered on CBT skills to be associated with better mental health outcomes in soldiers going through basic training (Cohn & Pakenham, 2008).

In contrast, studies have found that brief interventions (e.g., two sessions) emphasizing CBT skills do not result in improved outcomes for soldiers (Adler, Williams, McGurk, Moss, & Bliese, 2016) or airmen (Cigrang, Todd, & Carbone, 2000) in basic training. These negative findings may be associated in part with the brief nature of the intervention. In contrast to these brief interventions, Adler, Bliese, Pickering, et al. (2015) found platoons assigned randomly to 8 hours of performance psychology training (e.g., goal setting, attention management, energy management) distributed across a 10-week basic training cycle had better mental skills and performance outcomes on challenging training events than platoons assigned to an active comparison condition during which soldiers received 8 hours of military history, despite soldiers in the comparison condition being more likely to report the information being important. Besides studies with service members in basic training, other studies have been conducted with soldiers in operational units. For example, the PRP was adapted for use in the Army (Reivich, Seligman, & McBride, 2011), and brigade training in these techniques generally had better mental health outcomes than other brigades (Harms, Herian, Krasikova, Vanhove, & Lester, 2013; Lester, Harms, Herian, Krasikova, & Beal, 2011). Similarly, psychoeducation emphasizing CBT techniques and reframing was effective in reducing levels of PTSD symptoms in soldiers with high levels of combat experiences (Adler, Bliese, McGurk, Hoge, & Castro, 2009) relative to an active comparison condition of standard stress management. A second trial conducted with soldiers postdeployment confirmed such training was associated with lower PTSD symptoms compared with a survey-only control condition (Castro, Adler, McGurk, & Bliese, 2012).

Taken together, these findings demonstrate resilience training can be effective in improving the mental health and performance of individuals. In particular, studies with individuals at risk for PTSD demonstrate the positive impact resilience training can have on reducing symptom levels. The question then emerges: Could resilience training be a useful adjunct to PTSD treatment? Although validated PTSD treatments exist, such treatments are effective for a portion of the patient population only (Feldner, Monson, & Friedman, 2007) and are associated with a substantial dropout rate (Schottenbauer, Glasss, Arnkoff, Tendick, & Gray, 2008). In looking to improve the efficacy of and commitment to treatment, one option is to institute resilience training as an adjunct to traditional PTSD treatments.

RESILIENCE TRAINING AS AN ADJUNCT TO PTSD TREATMENT

Although we are unaware of any systematic attempt to study the utility of resilience training as an adjunct to PTSD treatment, the potential benefit of resilience training can be informed by the existing literature on universally-applied and targeted early intervention programs with high-risk individuals. These studies, cited earlier, demonstrate resilience training can be effective. We note, however, the actual content of this training varies from program to program, and thus it is unclear which specific components of training should be included. Still, the consistent threads across these programs are related to CBT, arousal reduction, and social support. Although traditional therapy may address these same points, there are reasons why providing this information in a more education-based format might be reasonably expected to potentiate the effect of traditional treatment. By providing the material in a training format, rather than a traditional therapy format, the training may be more acceptable and accessible to those individuals who prefer self-management (Adler, Britt, Riviere, Kim, & Thomas, 2015) and may cast a wider net for improving the quality of daily life that might be missed by PTSD therapies focused on traumatic events. Providers equipped with multiple delivery options may also be better able to "meet the patient where he or she is at" with regard to obtaining informed consent and establishing the ongoing rapport necessary for continued treatment.

First, research with a range of populations has determined there are significant concerns about seeking help for mental health problems, and these underlying attitudes may be driving the relatively high dropout rates from traditional treatment. Although studies have found substantial rates of concerns about stigma (Gould et al.,

2010; Hoge et al., 2004), these concerns are not necessarily linked to decisions to seek mental health care (and, thus, presumably to remain in treatment). Instead, individuals tend to report their preference is to manage symptoms on their own ((Adler, Britt, Riviere, Kim, & Thomas, 2015); Mojtabai et al., 2011). This preference for self-management is not necessarily negative; it implies a sense of self-efficacy, an optimistic belief in one's ability to manage one's own reactions. Similarly, evidence suggests that negative attitudes toward mental health providers may also be linked to treatment-seeking behavior (Kim, Britt, Klocko, Riviere, & Adler, 2011), just as positive attitudes toward mental health providers may be linked to increased likelihood of seeking care (Adler, Britt, Riviere, Kim, & Thomas, 2015). If resilience training can be communicated easily as a method of self-management, and can be seen as immediately beneficial through a focus on skills for enhancing daily living, then perhaps resilience training can not only be a positive influence on mental health, but also may encourage individuals to stay engaged in treatment.

We note, however, that not all individuals will necessarily react positively to this concept of self-management. There may be a distinct difference between the degree of symptomatology and acceptance of the resilience training concept. For some individuals, their symptoms and degree of functional impairment may be so profound that the idea of learning resilience skills feels overwhelming or irrelevant. They may be more compelled to experience symptom relief and to have someone in an expert role treat the symptoms causing them significant distress. For other individuals, the idea of learning resilience skills that can enhance life quality may be an attractive addition to entering a system of medical care. This distinction in terms of who might be a good fit for resilience training needs to be considered in terms of individual difference variables (e.g., personality, symptom levels). Moreover, it may be possible to examine a patient's readiness to change in identifying individuals who might be ready to accept the resilience skills training approach, particularly because evidence suggests that being ready to change one behavior makes one ready to change another (i.e., "coaction") (Paiva et al., 2012).

In addition, resilience training is oriented toward building fundamental skills that go beyond the specific set of symptoms and problems that are typically the target of treatment for PTSD. This training can distill important resilience concepts into teachable forms and enable at-risk individuals to learn resilience skills that randomized trials have demonstrated to be effective. Evidence-based treatments (EBTs), such as cognitive processing therapy (CPT) (Resick, Monson, & Chard, 2007) and prolonged exposure (Foa, 2011), are trauma-focused therapies. Resilience training focuses on a broader array of reactions to everyday situations and skills to achieve successful work, relationship, health, and personal satisfaction outcomes. Discussions within a resilience framework include how to capitalize on positive personal characteristics, how to use daily activities to bolster one's outlook, and how to focus on goal achievement in decision making. By focusing on skills and positive characteristics, it may help individuals with PTSD to feel more hopeful and have greater self-efficacy, both of which may contribute to their willingness to engage in the homework and self-examination required by the EBTs. Resilience training may also increase the potential for posttraumatic growth (PTG) by providing lifelong skills that individuals can use well after they complete the main course of the EBT. In addition, resilience training may help lessen symptoms of other disorders that are often comorbid with PTSD, such as depression or generalized anxiety disorder (Kaufman & Charney, 2000; Kessler, Chiu, Demler, Merikangas, & Walters, 2005; Kilpatrick et al., 2003).

Moreover, some of these resilience skills, such as goal setting, energy management, and attention control, can be used to enhance functioning and not just reduce symptoms. Thus, the training can be useful across the mental health spectrum, not just for individuals labeled as "sick." This broader reach may lead to small changes in behavior that can have a cumulative effect on the adjustment of individuals with PTSD. By integrating these fundamental resilience skills into daily life, outside the traditional care environment (e.g., hospital ward, clinic office), the message is clear: the individual's experience is more than the trauma. This broadening, in and of itself, can be a significant message for individuals with PTSD because of the tendency for PTSD to result in an intense focus on the traumatic event and attendant symptoms.

RESILIENCE TRAINING: CATEGORIES AND CONTENT

Although there are many topics that can be included in a resilience training curriculum, we summarize key areas here. These topics are drawn from the CBT, positive psychology, and sports psychology subdisciplines and include (1) optimism, (2) relationship building, (3) cognitive skills, (4) energy management, (5) emotional regulation, and (6) PTG. Each category is described, and ideas for activities are suggested. It is less important that the training cover each concept than that the training follow an overarching model, that the skills be easy to use and quick to implement, and that the training itself be engaging and involve hands-on practice (Castro & Adler, 2011).

Optimism

For individuals with PTSD, optimism is easy to teach, but often difficult to operationalize (Peterson, 2000). With patients with PTSD, the rationale for focusing on optimism is particularly crucial because it is often perceived as being fake, dismissed by some as an unrealistic combination of "rainbows and puppies." It is, therefore, important to clarify that, in this case, optimism is defined as being realistic, identifying what can be changed, and seeking out the positive events and situations occurring even during difficult times. The framework of hope and gratitude seems to be effective in this population (Wood, Froh, & Geraghty, 2010). Describing the negativity bias (i.e., the proclivity to focus on negative events and minimize positive events) is also a concept with which participants can identify easily.

One activity to enhance optimism is to reflect on positive experiences throughout the day, especially small ones, such as a good cup of coffee or a pleasant exchange with a neighbor. At the end of each day, individuals are asked to write down positive things that happened during the day and to reflect how they can make this kind of positive moment happen again (Reivich et al., 2011). This activity ensures the positive experiences continue and build. The act of recording the event and reflecting on it also helps individuals process the event and gives them something to look back on when they are feeling down. This is akin to the validated "hope box" in which suicidal patients place mementos of good memories and events in their life they can return to when feeling hopeless (Ghahramanlou-Holloway, Cox, & Greene, 2012). The individual and provider should collaborate to determine an appropriate number of positive events written each evening, and the provider should help the individual complete several items to help stimulate what kinds of topics can be used for "good" events. Sharing these events as part of a resilience training group can also be useful in demonstrating how this kind of activity can be accomplished and in sharing optimism among group members.

Relationship Building

Another key category associated with resilience is building relationships with others. For individuals with PTSD, relationship building is a big challenge because they may struggle with feeling interpersonally withdrawn and disconnected. Individuals with PTSD may feel as though they are burdening others with their concerns or that no one understands them. They may also be deeply angry. The combination of disconnection and anger can undermine close relationships—an essential factor in maintaining resilience.

One activity focuses on assertive communication. This technique involves practicing using words that identify feelings. For example, when discussing a difficult topic, individuals can practice beginning a sentence with the phrase "I feel ___ when you ____" or using the sentence construction, "When you do [insert specific behavior], I feel [insert emotion word]." Identifying feelings may be a specific challenge for individuals with PTSD because they often report emotional numbing. Other activities include naming as many emotion words as possible or completing sentences with a range of emotion words to facilitate using assertive communication in more difficult scenarios.

In addition, as a result of the symptoms of withdrawal and emotional numbing, individuals sometimes report difficulty being genuine, and expressing interest and excitement over someone else's good news; this lack of response can undermine those connections that can help boost resilience. Thus, another activity is to practice responding to the good news of close others with constructive interest when they engage in capitalization, or the act of sharing good news with others (Reivich et al., 2011). By communicating that interest, the person making the capitalization attempt feels validated and understood, and the relationship is enhanced. For homework, individuals can be asked to identify how they normally respond (e.g., with disinterest, switching the topic, discussing the negative aspects of the other person's good news) and to practice responding in alternative, encouraging ways (e.g., asking follow-up questions, paying active attention).

Although this skill is designed to rebuild relationships made vulnerable by withdrawal and emotional numbing, it is this very symptom of PTSD that can make demonstrating constructive interest a challenge. Providers may need to address individuals' reluctance to practice constructive interest by emphasizing how this skill can strengthen relationships, which in turn may help reduce the numbing. In our experience, the skill itself is reinforced quickly by the positive response of the person with the good news, and thus even small attempts to demonstrate this skill may strengthen an individual's willingness to practice it.

Cognitive Skills

Many concepts used in resilience programs, such as the PRP, involve changing people's cognitions to be more realistic. These concepts borrow heavily from CBT (Reivich & Shatte, 2002; Seligman, Steen, Park, & Peterson, 2005). CBT techniques can be used to increase awareness of the negativity bias and how thoughts can influence emotions and behaviors.

For individuals receiving prolonged exposure treatment for PTSD, these cognitive techniques can be useful adjuncts, particularly if they are framed in simple and easy-to-learn terms. For individuals receiving CPT, providers of resilience training do not need to duplicate concepts already addressed via CPT. For example, using ABC sheets and exploring deeply held beliefs and cognitive distortions are an integral part of CPT, so it would not be necessary to include them in a resilience training program. We address some "cognitive skills"—an umbrella term for identifying several related skills typical of resilience training programs—in the following sections. We review three types of cognitive skills that do not overlap with CPT: reshaping thoughts, self-talk, and goal setting.

Reshaping Thoughts

With this approach, the goal is to have individuals identify the power their thoughts have to influence their emotions and behaviors. Resilience training can include exercises that identify thoughts that occur in response to typical triggering events. The training can then focus on how these thoughts influence emotions and behaviors. After identifying the typical triggering events and how thoughts can influence emotions and behaviors, resilience training activities can also be used to identify patterns in thinking or consistent distortions of biases. Common biases can be explained in the training and supplemental worksheets used to help practice identifying these distortions (Human Performance Resource Center, 2016). Through these activities, individuals can become more aware of their unhelpful thoughts. With awareness, comes the opportunity to practice challenging those thoughts. If a patient or group is engaged in CPT or has previously engaged in CBT, the previously mentioned activities could be truncated.

Within resilience training, there are some helpful ways to challenge unhelpful cognitions that are packaged and described somewhat differently than standard CPT/CBT and provide a helpful adjunct to those treatments. For example, sentence starters focus on the lack of evidence for the negative thought ("I'm not factoring in that . . ."), being optimistic ("A more pleasant way of viewing this is . . ."), and trying to find perspective by looking on the whole situation ("That may be true, but at least it isn't . . .").

Because individuals with PTSD find searching for evidence against their pessimistic thoughts to be difficult, another method to help search for alternative evidence is to ask questions that challenge the assumption underlying the pessimism, such as: How important is this? Am I being realistic? What can I control? Am I missing something? These questions then help the individual "talk back" to their distortions. The provider can help individuals with PTSD practice in session so patients are then prepared to use realistic thinking outside the clinic. In general, by talking about these fundamental skills (e.g., identifying how emotions can affect thoughts, cognitive distortions) and applying these concepts to daily life, individuals with PTSD can gain confidence in using these skills and see how the skills can be useful for addressing problems beyond the focus on the trauma.

Self-talk Interventions

Another CBT technique focuses on self-talk, or coaching oneself with positive words to promote adaptation and success. Within the sports psychology literature, self-talk has been found to facilitate learning, enhance performance, and increase resilience (Hatzigeorgiadis, Zourbanos, Galanis, & Theodorakis, 2011). Self-talk is rooted in self-instructional training (Meichenbaum, 1977) and is associated with enhancing attentional focus, increasing confidence, regulating effort, controlling cognitive and emotional reactions, and triggering automatic execution of tasks (Theodorakis, Hatzigeorgiadis, & Chroni, 2008). Self-talk can comprise different approaches, but effective cue words can be as simple as one word or a phrase. There is instructional self-talk, which is associated with executing a task by focusing on a instructing on directing attention ("see the finish line"), technique ("high elbow"), strategy ("push"), or form ("land softly"); and motivational self-talk, which is characterized by talk that increases enthusiasm ("Let's do this"), builds confidence ("I can do it"), and creates positive moods ("I'm awesome"). Studies have found that self-talk is especially helpful when embarking on novel tasks and when the tasks require high levels of concentration and precision. Most important, studies have found that training in using self-talk is beneficial (Hatzigeorgiadis et al., 2011).

By including self-talk in a resilience training program, providers can teach the simple skill of being one's own coach. For the symptom of emotional withdrawal, for example, individuals could start feeling greater connection to others by using the word *smile*. Or, if they are trying to incorporate deep breathing to prevent getting angry, they can say the word *breathe*. Being one's own coach is consistent with the self-management approach and may help engage individuals reluctant to participate in formal therapies. Like other skills, it is likely that self-talk will benefit from practicing the skill (Hatzigeorgiadis et al., 2011) and emphasizing the adherence to homework in future sessions.

Goal Setting

Goal setting is an easily accessible skill borrowed from the organizational psychology literature and is based on the idea that setting goals motivates action (Locke & Latham, 2002). Individuals with PTSD are often overwhelmed by tasks they have to accomplish and often stop pursuing those things they used to enjoy because of inertia and the energy required to initiate activity. Using structured goal setting can allow individuals with PTSD to overcome this inertia by helping them maintain a long-term vision and short-term motivation.

This balance between vision and motivation can be achieved by identifying a long-term goal (such as be able to spend meaningful time with children or graduate from college) and developing structured plans with both action steps and motivational statements to push the individual to accomplish the action steps. Goals within an individual's control (e.g., beat one's personal record for run time, increase frequency of social interaction) are more likely to succeed, and this success can be reinforcing for individuals rather than goals that depend on the behavior of others (e.g., win a race) or external events outside an individual's control (e.g., don't be traumatized again). After defining the larger goal, the individual then creates smaller, more manageable subgoals. For example, if an individual wanted to go to college, he would need to identify a college, determine how to pay for it, get accepted, complete the first course, and so on. This plan would then call for specific action steps to achieve those subgoals. These steps need to be "SMART," which is an acronym for specific, measurable, action-oriented, realistic, and time bound.[1] An example of a SMART step in pursing the goal of identifying a college is as follows: By the end of next week, I will identify two colleges in my city by going online and by phoning my friend, John, who just graduated. Individuals can motivate themselves to accomplish SMART steps by pairing a goal with a motivational statement (described in the self-talk section). In this case, "achieve," "success," "one step at a time," or "make my family proud" could all be appropriate motivational statements.

If delivered in a group setting, participants can review each other's goals and practice making SMART goals; likewise, a provider could work with a service member to set up SMART goals. Coming up with motivational statements can be turned into an activity. Another activity is to identify how individuals can be reminded of their goal every day to sustain their focus (e.g., write a note to themselves and put it on the bathroom mirror, set up an automatic reminder on their phone).

Providers should follow up with individuals to see if they are having success, discuss how to resolve barriers that have gotten in the way, and adjust steps as needed, emphasizing that being flexible is a part of ultimately achieving goals. Encouraging the pursuit of goals can provide a feeling of self-efficacy and control that can be elusive for individuals with PTSD.

Energy Management

Energy management refers to a category of skills derived from both sports psychology and mindfulness practices that help people think clearly and respond with control while minimizing the effects of stress. There are a variety of skills

---

[1] Sometimes there are different words used to explain the acronym. For example, A is sometimes identified as standing for *attainable* and R as *relevant*.

included in this category and individuals with PTSD are encouraged to test each of the skills and find which are most effective in helping to respond with control. Skills associated most commonly with energy management include controlled breathing, progressive muscle relaxation, meditation, positive imagery, and mental games.

Given that some of these topics are explored elsewhere in this volume, we highlight the concept of mental games here. Used to encourage distraction from unproductive cognitions and physiological arousal, to be effective, these games must require full attention and be hard, but fun, and something that can be completed within a few minutes. The goal is to move one's mind from the intense emotion to something else that will enable a person to calm down. A few examples of these games are counting backward from 1000 by sevens, pairing the alphabet with some kind of common theme (e.g., famous people, foods), naming as many athletes as possible in 2 minutes, reciting the lyrics to an upbeat song, or repeating the alphabet backward. A recent study found that playing the game Tetris helped prevent PTSD flashbacks presumably because the game required a high cognitive load and distracted individuals in the same way mental games can provide distraction (Holmes, James, Kilford, & Deeprose, 2010). These games can be added to cellular phones and other portable computers. If individuals are too distracted to participate in mental games they have to initiate and sustain, playing a computer-generated game may be easier. It is important to remind individuals these mental games, like all the techniques reviewed here, require practice to be most beneficial.

Emotional Regulation

Individuals with PTSD may have difficulty with emotional regulation—feeling numb, angry, and/or hyperaroused. Although traditional treatments address these concerns, resilience training can be used to enhance emotion regulation skills, considered a key characteristic of resilient people (Everly, McCormack, & Strouse, 2012). For example, mindfulness exercises can be integrated into training, and regular practice can become a part of the training sessions. Mindfulness exercises can focus on noticing physical reactions to situations, becoming aware and slowing breathing, and focusing on the here-and-now by cuing into physical sensations, thoughts, and emotional reactions.

During resilience training, several activities can be the focus of sessions on emotion regulation. Although covered elsewhere in this book, mindful breathing can be a very powerful tool to calm the body and the mind. Our experience with active-duty combat soldiers was they found mindful breathing novel and relaxing. The idea of pacing one's breath and focusing attention is an active strategy that resulted in their perception that they had gained physiological control. After learning this technique, they requested to have extra sessions of mindful breathing. Another activity that can be taught easily during a single session is the focus on all sensations, thoughts, and emotions related to a single, simple task, such as eating a raisin (Hasson, 2013). Providers should keep the context in mind before selecting the task for this activity. For example, in a military context, the common mindfulness activity of opening a small chocolate wrapped in foil had sexual connotations unbeknown to the provider.

Studies on mindfulness have found improved emotional well-being and cognitive performance (Chambers, Lo, & Allen, 2008; Weinstein, Brown, & Ryan, 2009), and the abilities to focus attention and enhance emotion regulation are fundamental building blocks of resilience skills. Although we use the term *mindful breathing* here, we recognize that briefly introducing the concept of mindfulness in the context of a larger resilience training program is not comparable with the mindfulness provided in validated training programs such as mindfulness-based stress reduction (Grossman, Niemann, Schmidt, & Wallach, 2004). The mindfulness activities presented are small samples of what could be obtained through practice at home (Carmody & Baer, 2008) and formal mindfulness courses (Grossman et al., 2004). It is compelling to note that even in a brief introduction to these kinds of mindfulness tasks, individuals with PTSD have reported feeling better, and this kind of improvement may reinforce their interest in resilience training, therapy, and pursuing additional mindfulness experiences.

Posttraumatic Growth

One topic not typically addressed in established resilience training programs (Brunwasser et al., 2009) is posttraumatic growth (PTG). PTG was coined in 1995 (Tedeschi & Calhoun, 1995) and has been defined as "positive personal changes that result from the struggle to deal with trauma and its psychological consequences" (Tedeschi & McNally, 2011, p. 19). PTG is not typically discussed in current resilience training programs because they do not usually focus on trauma. However, because the resilience training proposed here is for individuals with PTSD, there is a natural opportunity to address the concept. In addition, recent definitions of resilience have included words such as *grow* and *thrive* (Carver, 1998), dovetailing with the concept of posttraumatic growth.

Although there are no studies identifying exactly how to promote PTG, cross-sectional studies have found that PTG can buffer the impact of traumatic experiences on mental health. Tedeschi and McNally (2011) emphasize that it helps for individuals with PTSD to understand the normal reactions to trauma before they can learn about PTG. They then suggest that individuals with PTSD construct a narrative of the positive posttraumatic changes they have experienced or hope to experience using the five domains of PTG: personal strength, enhanced relationships with others, spiritual change, appreciation of life, and new opportunities. This narrative can be turned into a training activity by having individuals think about a personal example for each of these five domains or a goal to develop each domain in the future.

TAILORING CONTENT FOR INDIVIDUALS WITH PTSD

Most of resilience training is designed for a universal or primary prevention audience to enhance their current healthy functioning. When modifying content for a population with PTSD, the provider must be aware of how certain concepts may resonate with this population. For example, in one primary prevention curriculum, the discussion of resilience addresses companionship and an example describes one friend walking up to the other from behind and saying something comforting. In a healthy population, this example might not be noteworthy, but in a PTSD population, the concept of companionship and support might get lost in a discussion of one's startle response being activated by being approached from behind. Likewise, if the discussion about defining resilience focuses on toughness and success, individuals with PTSD might equate that with their own sense of failure. Similarly, convincing individuals with PTSD to accept the importance of optimism may require extra work, because the individuals' assumptions about the world, the benevolence of others, and the world being just and safe have been damaged (Janoff-Bulman, 1989, 1992). Providers have to ensure they avoid presenting optimism as an unrealistic goal given the pervasive pessimism that can accompany PTSD. Optimism should be presented as an achievable reality.

In addition to tailoring content, the provider must also be aware of the symptoms of PTSD and be prepared for individuals to dissociate, have flashbacks, have difficulty concentrating, or be triggered so that they leave the group in anger or distress. In a group setting, providers must have contingency plans to deal with these reactions, such as having a backup provider who can pull the individual away from the group or who can help find the rest of the group another location to continue the session. In general, providers must be keenly aware of which topics might be a trigger or upsetting for individuals with PTSD, particularly when discussing concepts such as PTG or optimism.

IMPLEMENTATION ISSUES

As mentioned earlier, although most of the research on resilience training has been conducted with resilience training as a primary and secondary prevention, resilience training can also be given after a person has developed PTSD as an adjunct to EBTs (tertiary prevention). In our own work, we've implemented different types of resilience training targeting training units (primary prevention) and at-risk operational units (secondary prevention), and in a military hospital system serving individuals with PTSD in a day-treatment setting (tertiary prevention). The following implementation considerations are based on these experiences as well as the literature.

Models of Delivery

Resilience training could be implemented as an adjunct to PTSD treatment using a group or individual delivery model. Group sessions for individuals with PTSD can focus on a different resilience skill each group session, allowing time for discussion among group members. Individual training encounters could be added to the end of an individual therapy session during the course of an EBT for PTSD, much like a personal trainer can help individuals with weight control outside of efforts with a dietitian. Alternately, the sessions could stand on their own as booster-type sessions following completion of an EBT.

There are numerous issues to consider when implementing a resilience training program. The following considerations are reviewed in terms of implementing a group training program, although several of these concerns might also apply to individual modalities: (1) screening, (2) open versus closed groups, (3) size of the group, (4) attendance requirements, (5) length of sessions, (6) number of sessions, and (7) incorporating homework. We'll address each issue in the following sections.

Screening

The first consideration is how members are selected for resilience training. Optimally, the provider meets each individual in person for a screening to determine suitability for group training. This screening may include assessment of motivation, severity of illness, and commitment and ability to attend the sessions. Because resilience is thought to be a set of skills that can be learned, no previous knowledge is necessary to participate in the group.

The screening session may also serve to prepare group members for what they will encounter in the group, and to establish some rapport between the potential group members and the provider. Although a screening is optimal, depending on the setting, it may not be feasible. In a group setting, skipping the screening process is not ideal because the provider has to try to establish a rapport quickly with new group members while conducting the group. If the group is an open group, there may be an imbalance, with the provider already having a rapport with some participants but not the new members.

Open Versus Closed Groups

Closed groups do not accept new members after they begin and often meet for a predetermined number of sessions whereas open groups allow new members to join, with the number of sessions less likely to be determined ahead of time. Closed groups may allow members to get to know one another better, which may increase openness and disclosure. They also allow providers to follow a curriculum or treatment plan without having to review and educate new members each week. However, closed groups are also at risk of having too few members as other obligations and barriers lead to dropout; groups do not function optimally if there are too few members. Furthermore, people will have to wait until a new group begins to receive training.

Open groups allow group members immediate access, but the nature of open groups may cause the group size to fluctuate, make it easier for group members to skip a session, lead to less commitment to the group, and cause the dynamic to change unpredictably from week to week, depending on who is in the group. This dynamic may alter participation from one week to the next. Thus, there are pros and cons to each kind of group.

When it comes to resilience training, the information tends to be psychoeducational and skill based in nature, with accompanying homework assignments and a finite number of sessions. In a group such as this, particularly if the length of the session is brief, it is ideal not to have to recap the previous weeks' topics for new members or go over homework assignments that do not hold much meaning for a new member (i.e., in an open group). Furthermore, topics often build on one another, so a new member coming in at week 3 might not understand as much as a new member who happens to arrive at week 1. Thus, if feasible, we recommend resilience groups be closed groups. This seems most possible when training is offered as an adjunct treatment to outpatient therapy. In day treatment or inpatient treatment settings, closed groups may not be possible and providers will have to adjust by shortening the length of time spent on discussion, making homework review briefer and trying to make each week a self-contained skill or topic. In this way, missing a week or arriving in the middle of the rotation of sessions is not disruptive.

Group Size

Yalom (1995) suggests that seven to eight group members is optimal, with outer limits of five to 10. He suggests that fewer than five group members leads to diminished member interaction, more one-to-one interactions that do not involve the other group members, passive participation, and lack of group cohesion. Having more than 10 participants may lead to individuals not having enough time to participate meaningfully, may allow more forceful members to dominate, and may lead to cliques that make others feel excluded, which would be particularly problematic for someone who is already having problems with trust and emotional attachment. Longer sessions may alleviate how much time each group member has to participate, but would not resolve the other concerns.

For a resilience group that is more didactic and skill based, the group may be able to tolerate more group members. However, the meaningful group interactions will decrease and the session will be led mostly by the provider, and thus some of the benefits of group therapy (e.g., broad validation, being able to analyze one's interactions with others) may be lost. For closed groups, the provider might choose to enroll more group members as a result of expected dropout. For an open enrollment group, the provider can still limit the group size. Nevertheless, if there are handouts, providers should be prepared for more group members and may have to alter activities to match the number—by "pairing" three people for activities, for example. In general, a group that can stay closer to the seven or eight ideal espoused by Yalom (1995) is still optimal, even with the more skills-based approach in resilience training.

Attendance Requirements

Providers need to decide whether group members can miss sessions or whether they need to attend a certain percentage to remain in the group. To the extent each of the resilience topics builds on each other, group members need to attend as many sessions as possible to get benefit from the material. This is particularly the case if only a few key topics are being highlighted because of a limited number of sessions being presented to the group members. In addition, group cohesion is much greater if all the members are committed to attending and get to know the other group members. Depending on the setting, group members may have a number of other medical appointments to attend to or may have emotional difficulty with some of the topics and find they are unable to handle the session. However, we recommend emphasizing session attendance without making attendance mandatory.

Frequency and Length of Session

The frequency of sessions is typically once or twice a week, which provides enough time to process the information but not forget the material. This pace is also less demanding on the group member's time—an important consideration for members trying to incorporate training into their work week. Typically, resilience work is relatively upbeat and easy to comprehend, so twice-weekly sessions would not demand too much of the group members' cognitive or emotional load.

The length of the session is a very important group characteristic. Common wisdom in the therapeutic community says 80 to 90 minutes is the ideal length for a group and provides time to warm up, get to the meat of the session, and then see the discussion through (Yalom, 1995). In a group that focuses on resilience, there will be review of homework assignments, a didactic portion that involves discussion, and a practice portion. The 90-minute session seems best suited for all the information to be processed fully for this type of group. This time length is especially true if the group is open in its enrollment so that the topics of the group must be reintroduced each week or if the group is large so that all participants need time to share homework and in-session activity responses. However, the reality of many clinics is that group therapy sessions must fit into other programming and are, therefore, often 50 to 60 minutes long, similar to an individual session. With this format, the provider has to keep only the most relevant didactic points and make sure the group does not stray too far in discussions. The provider also has to ensure the activity given to the group can be completed in sufficient time so group members feel they are able to master the skill. One possible schedule for these condensed sessions is to allot 10 minutes for homework and reviewing concepts, 20 to 30 minutes for didactic presentation and discussion, and 20 minutes for activities and practice.

Number of Sessions

The number of training sessions depends on a number of factors. When developing a resilience training program, the provider has to decide how many topics to cover. This number may depend in part on how much time is available to work with patients. In outpatient settings, there could be 12 sessions: one a week over a 3-month period. As Yalom (1955) noted, group members typically cannot be retained for more than 12 sessions. Patients may only be present in an inpatient or day-treatment setting for 1 month or less, so a four-session model may be more appropriate. Ideally,

TABLE 12.1 Curriculum for 12 60-Minute Sessions

Session	Topic	Description	Sample Activity
1	Defining Resilience	Introduce concept; list examples in literature, news	Read poems that focus on different aspects of resilience
2	Optimism	Define optimism, identify situations for gratitude	Use journal to reflect on positive daily experiences with first day completed in session
3	Relationship Building—Genuine Care	Understand how to respond to good news (capitalization)	In pairs, act out modes of responding to an ordinary situation and highlight the most productive type
4	Relationship Building—Assertive Communication	Learn to communicate without aggression or loss of needs	Name as many emotions as possible or complete sentences with a range of emotions
5	Cognitive Techniques—Reshaping Thoughts	Use questions to challenge assumptions and "talk backs" to cognitive distortions	Use sentence starters such as "A more optimistic way to view this is . . ."
6	Cognitive Techniques—Self-talk	Identify key phrases and situations for self-talk	Choose a mantra or motivator such as "I've got this" or "This, too, shall pass"
7	Cognitive Techniques—Goal Setting	Identify a long-term goal, choose SMART action steps	Write out the SMART action steps in session
8	Energy Management—Mental Games	Discuss goal of and options for mental games	Have group members share favorite mental games such as "going on a picnic" or counting backward by seven
9	Emotion Regulation—Deep Breathing	Introduce deep breathing, add mindful breathing component	Have provider lead a 5-minute mindful breathing meditation
10	Emotion Regulation—Mindfulness	Practice awareness of the here-and-now	Use script to eat a raisin
11	Posttraumatic Growth	Identify the five domains of posttraumatic growth	Have participants write out what they hope to achieve in each domain
12	Conclusions	Review all skills	Identify the three top skills to put into regular use

SMART, specific, measurable, action-oriented, realistic, and time bound.

The first four sessions can be used as a short form of training if time with patients is limited.

resilience training is eight 90-minute sessions or 12 60-minute sessions. Table 12.1 provides a template schedule for a 12-week course with 60-minute sessions, because of the likelihood that providers will have 60 minutes allotted for each session rather than the traditional 90 minutes suggested by group therapists.

Trainers

Another implementation issue is who should provide the resilience training. In typical primary and secondary resilience training, trainers have not been limited to licensed mental health providers (Adler et al., 2009; Gillham, Reivich, et al., 2006; Reivich et al., 2011). However, in this case, depending on the intensity of the symptoms, using licensed mental health providers as trainers may be the more prudent option. For some institutions, the use of licensed mental health providers may be a requirement.

It is also important to remind the provider to use a training approach focused on discussing skills, rather than a therapy/treatment approach when delivering the material. The approach should help ensure the provider stays true to the original goals of the training and avoids duplicating treatment. Yet, despite the goal of establishing a training type of context, there will be moments when the group will want to process a particular point or comment on one another's contributions. Given that larger goals in resilience training include connecting to individuals and emotional awareness, such comments are not actually counterproductive. The challenge is maintaining a balance. Furthermore, although the topics in resilience training will be familiar to mental health providers, the names and concepts applied within this format might not be. In the Army's master resilience training model, the providers first experience the training as students, and are then trained to teach the material (Reivich et al., 2011). This approach enables providers to apply the material to their own lives, demonstrating the relevance of such material for a broad range of contexts. Although organizations may not be able to afford providers so much training time, if such training can be provided in a condensed format with continuing education credits, then it may be cost-effective and efficient.

Also, if a patient has different providers for individual PTSD treatment and resilience training, it is important also to offer individual therapy providers a brief course (with continuing education credits if possible) in the language, techniques, and approach of resilience training so that providers can become familiar and the information can be reinforced and integrated across session type. We have developed such a course for behavioral health providers.

Homework

Completing the homework is critical for mastering resilience training skills (Yalom, 1995). The amount of homework given may depend on how much other treatment the group member is receiving and the amount and intensity of homework from those other treatment modalities. For example, a group member who is receiving concurrent prolonged exposure or cognitive processing therapy will have significant daily homework critical to the effectiveness of those therapies. Thus, it would be important to keep homework assignments in the resilience training group short. Another consideration is the concentration and memory difficulties associated with PTSD. The provider may suggest that group members put a reminder for homework into their planner/smartphone for that evening. The treatment team may also be able to work together such that the providers can remind group members about the homework as well.

Resilience Training as an Adjunct to EBTs

Resilience training as an adjunct to individual EBT can be implemented either at the end of a session or as a mini session held at another time. The former could be very brief (e.g., 5–10 minutes) and skills based. As mentioned previously, given the amount and importance of the homework to the EBT, resilience training homework should be something people can do during the course of their day (e.g., practice mental games or self-talk) or that takes minimal time at home (e.g., write down one positive event each day).

Another possibility is to integrate resilience training into the follow-up/booster sessions typical of many EBTs. Resilience training could be added to those sessions, and the frequency of follow-up/booster sessions could be increased to incorporate the training. The follow-up period could be a particularly opportune time to introduce concepts of optimism and growth, given that individuals will likely have stronger self-efficacy in terms of their belief in the ability to change, and a renewed belief that things can improve. Follow-on sessions would also allow providers to assign more homework because they would not be competing with intensive homework from the EBT.

FUTURE DIRECTIONS

There are a number of open research questions with regard to resilience training as an adjunct to traditional PTSD treatment. First: Is resilience training helpful for individuals with PTSD? Thus far, results have shown that resilience training has modest effects and is most effective with those who have symptoms, and is effective in the short term (Adler et al., 2009; Gillham, Hamilton, Freres, Patton, & Gallop, 2006). Thus, it seems likely that patients with PTSD would be good candidates for training that could enhance treatment effects. Studies should examine whether there is a benefit to receiving resilience training over the long term and whether resilience training is best provided before, during, or after treatment for PTSD. Study outcomes should focus on traditional PTSD outcomes, comorbid symptomatology, and a broader array of resilience markers such as life satisfaction, interpersonal connection, and self-efficacy. Studies should also assess treatment motivation and dropout rates.

Other research topics are to determine which resilience skills are most effective and whether the efficacy varies by type of trauma (e.g., natural disaster, combat, rape). Given the limited time providers have with individuals with PTSD, it is important to know which skills should be the focal point of resilience training.

And finally: In what manner should the information be best presented: groups or individuals? Within or outside traditional sessions? Although EBTs have a significant research base to provide a rationale for individual therapy, we expect the group format is optimal for resilience training because hearing the experiences of others in using skills might be more convincing and authentic than having the provider explain the concepts.

In summary, resilience training offers a new accompaniment to traditional treatment for PTSD while potentially providing unique benefits—an immediate sense of efficacy, tools for self-management, a focus beyond trauma-specific material for a more whole-person approach to mental health, and training skills that can enhance coping and growth. With an emphasis on positive attributes, day-to-day functioning, and how to grow and thrive in the face of trauma, we believe that incorporating resilience training can complement evidence-based treatments and help to rebuild a meaningful life (Table 12.1).

KEY POINTS

- When resilience is conceptualized as a process, the focus is on behaviors or attitudes that can lead to a positive outcome in the face of a significant or traumatic stressor.
- Resilience training focuses on a broad array of reactions to everyday situations and skills to achieve successful work, relationship, health, and personal satisfaction outcomes.

- Resilience training is typically based on cognitive–behavioral models of behavior change.

- Universal and targeted resilience training programs (e.g., primary and secondary prevention programs) can be adapted for use as a complement to treatment for PTSD, which is a tertiary intervention.

- By focusing on skills and positive characteristics, resilience training may help individuals with PTSD to feel more hopeful and have greater self-efficacy, which may contribute to their willingness to engage in the homework and self-examination required by EBTs.

- Resilience topics that seem especially fitting as an adjunct for PTSD treatment are (1) optimism, (2) relationship building, (3) cognitive skills, (4) energy management, (5) emotional regulation, and (6) PTG.

- When modifying content designed for a primary prevention audience for a population with PTSD, the provider must consider how concepts may resonate with this population.

- For resilience groups, several implementation considerations apply: (1) screening, (2) open versus closed groups, (3) size of the group, (4) attendance requirements, (5) length of sessions, (6) number of sessions, and (7) incorporating homework.

- Resilience training as an adjunct to individual EBT can be implemented either at the end of a session or as a mini session held at another time.

- Future studies should examine the timing of resilience training relative to trauma-focused treatment, whether it varies by trauma type, and which modalities are optimal.

REFERENCES

Adler, A. B, Bliese, P. D., McGurk, D., Hoge, C. W., & Castro, C. A. (2009). Battlemind debriefing and battlemind training as early interventions with soldiers returning from Iraq: Randomization by platoon. *Journal of Consulting and Clinical Psychology*, *77*(5), 928–940.

Adler, A. B., Bliese, P. D., Pickering, M. A., Hammermeister, J., Williams, J., Harada, C., Holliday, B., Ohlson, C. (2015). Mental skills training with basic combat training soldiers: A group-randomized trial. *Journal of Applied Psychology, 100*(6), 1752–1764.

Adler, A. B., Britt, T. W., Riviere, L. A., Kim, P. Y., & Thomas, J. L. (2015). Longitudinal determinants of mental health treatment-seeking by US soldiers. *The British Journal of Psychiatry*, *207*(4), 346–350.

Adler, A. B., Williams, J., McGurk, D., Moss, A., & Bliese, P. D. (2015). Resilience training with soldiers during basic combat training: Randomisation by platoon. *Applied Psychological Health and Well Being*, *7*(1), 85–107.

American Psychological Association (2016). The Road to Resilience. *Psychology Help Center*. Retrieved from: http://www.apa.org/helpcenter/road-resilience.aspx.

Arnetz, B. B., Arble, E., Backman, L., Lynch, A., & Lublin, A. (2013). Assessment of a prevention program for work-related stress among urban police officers. *International Archives of Occupational and Environmental Health*, *86*(1), 79–88.

Arnetz, B. B., Nevedal, D. C., Lumley, M. A., Backman, L., & Lublin, A. (2009). Trauma resilience training for police: Psychophysiological and performance effects. *Journal of Police and Criminal Psychology*, *24*, 1–9.

Bliese, P. D., Adler A. B., & Castro, C. A. (2011). The deployment context: Psychology and implementing mental health interventions. In: Adler, A. B., Bliese, P. D., & Castro, C. A. (Eds.), *Deployment Psychology: Evidence-Based Strategies to Promote Mental Health in the Military* (pp. 103–124). Washington, DC: American Psychological Association.

Bonanno, G. A., Rennicke, C., & Dekel, S. (2005). Self-enhancement among high-exposure survivors of the September 11th terrorist attack: Resilience or social maladjustment? *Journal of Personality and Social Psychology*, *88*(6), 984–998.

Brunwasser, S. M., Gillham, J. E., & Kim, E. S. (2009). A meta-analytic review of the Penn Resiliency Program's effect on depressive symptoms. *Journal of Consulting and Clinical Psychology*, *77*(6), 1042–1054.

Carmody, J., & Baer, R. A. (2008). Relationships between mindfulness practice and levels of mindfulness, medical and psychological symptoms and well-being in a mindfulness-based stress reduction program. *Journal of Behavioral Medicine*, *31*(1), 23–33.

Carver, C. S. (1998). Resilience and thriving: Issues, models, and linkages. *Journal of Social Issues*, *54*(2), 245–266.

Castro, C. A., & Adler, A. B. (2011). Military mental health training: building. In Southwick, S. M., Litz, B. T., Charney, D., & Friedman, M. J. (Eds.). *Resilience and Mental Health: Challenges Across the Lifespan* (pp. 323–339). Cambridge, UK: Cambridge University Press.

Castro, C. A., Adler, A. B., McGurk, D., & Bliese, P. D. (2012). Mental health training with soldiers four months after returning from Iraq: Randomization by platoon. *Journal of Traumatic Stress*, *25*(4), 376–383.

Chambers, R., Lo, B. C. Y., & Allen, N. B. (2008). The impact of intensive mindfulness training on attentional control, cognitive style, and affect. *Cognitive Therapy and Research*, *32*(3), 303–322.

Cigrang, J. A., Todd, S. L., & Carbone, E. G. (2000). Stress management training for military trainees returned to duty after a mental health evaluation: Effect on graduation rates. *Journal of Occupational Health Psychology*, *5*(1), 48–55.

Cohn, A., & Pakenham, K. (2008). Efficacy of a cognitive–behavioral program to improve psychological adjustment among soldiers in recruit training. *Military Medicine*, *173*(12), 1151–1157.

Everly, G. S., McCormack, D. K., & Strouse, D. A. (2012). Seven characteristics of highly resilient people: Insights from Navy SEALs to the "Greatest Generation." *International Journal of Emergency Mental Health*, *14*(2), 137–143.

Foa, E. B. (2011). Prolonged exposure therapy: Past, present, and future. *Depression and Anxiety*, *28*(12), 1043–1047.

Feldner, M. T., Monson, C. M., & Friedman, M. J. (2007). A critical analysis of approaches to targeted PTSD prevention: Current status and theoretically derived future directions. *Behavior Modification*, *31*(1), 80–116.

Ghahramanlou-Holloway, M., Cox, D. W., & Greene, F. N. (2012). Post-admission cognitive therapy: A brief intervention for psychiatric inpatients admitted after a suicide attempt. *Cognitive and Behavioral Practice*, *19*, 233–244.

Gillham, J. E., Hamilton, J., Freres, D. R., Patton, K., & Gallop, R. (2006). Preventing depression among early adolescents in the primary care setting: A randomized controlled study of the Penn Resiliency Program. *Journal of Abnormal Child Psychology*, *34*(2), 195–211.

Gillham, J. E., & Reivich, K. J. (1999). Prevention of depressive symptoms in schoolchildren: A research update. *Psychological Sciences*, *10*(5), 461–462.

Gillham, J. E., Reivich, K. J., Freres, D. R., Lascher, M., Litzinger, S., Shatté, A., et al. (2006). School-based prevention of depression and anxiety symptoms in early adolescence: A pilot of a parent intervention component. *School Psychology Quarterly*, *21*(3), 323.

Gould, M., Adler, A., Zamorski, M., Castro, C., Hanily, N., Steele, N., et al. (2010). Do stigma and other perceived barriers to mental health care differ across Armed Forces? *Journal of the Royal Society of Medicine, 103*(4), 148–156.

Grossman, P., Niemann, L., Schmidt, S., & Walach, H. (2004). Mindfulness-based stress reduction and health benefits: A meta-analysis. *Journal of Psychosomatic Research, 57*(1), 35–43.

Harms, P. D., Herian, M. N., Krasikova, D. V., Vanhove, A., & Lester, P. B. (2013). The Comprehensive Soldier and Family Fitness program evaluation report #4: Evaluation of resilience training and mental and behavioral health outcomes. Arlington, VA: Department of Defense.

Hasson, G. (2013). *Mindfulness: Be Mindful: Live in the Moment.* Chichester, UK: Capstone Publishing Ltd (A Wiley Company).

Hatzigeorgiadis, A., Zourbanos, N., Galanis, E., & Theodorakis, Y. (2011). Self-talk and sports performance: A meta-analysis. *Perspectives on Psychological Science, 6*(4), 348–356.

Hoge, C. W., Castro, C. A., Messer, S. C., McGurk, D., Cotting, D. I., & Koffman, R. L. (2004). Combat duty in Iraq and Afghanistan, mental health problems, and barriers to care. *New England Journal of Medicine, 351*(1), 13–22.

Holmes, E. A., James, E. L., Kilford, E. J., & Deeprose, C. (2010). Key steps in developing a cognitive vaccine against traumatic flashbacks: Visuospatial Tetris versus verbal pub quiz. *PLoS One, 5*(11), e13706.

Human Performance Resource Center. (2016). Reframe your "thinking traps" for peak performance. Retrieved from: http://hprc-online.org/total-force-fitness/performance-boosters/reframe-your-201cthinking-traps201d-for-peak-performance).

Janoff-Bulman, R. (1989). Assumptive worlds and the stress of traumatic events: Applications of the schema construct. *Social Cognition, 7*(2), 113–136.

Janoff-Bulman, R. (1992). *Shattered Assumptions: Towards a New Psychology of Trauma.* New York, NY: Free Press.

Kaufman, J., & Charney, D. (2000). Comorbidity of mood and anxiety disorders. *Depression and Anxiety, 12*(Suppl. 1), 69–76.

Kessler, R. C., Chiu, W. T., Demler, O., Merikangas, K. R., & Walters, E. E. (2005). Prevalence, severity, and comorbidity of 12-month DSM-IV disorders in the National Comorbidity Survey Replication. *Archives of General Psychiatry, 62*(6), 617–627.

Kilpatrick, D. G., Ruggiero, K. J., Acierno, R., Saunders, B. E., Resnick, H. S., & Best, C. L. (2003). Violence and risk of PTSD, major depression, substance abuse/dependence, and comorbidity: Results from the National Survey of Adolescents. *Journal of Consulting and Clinical Psychology, 71*(4), 692–700.

Kim, P. Y., Britt, T. W., Klocko, R. P., Riviere, L. A., & Adler, A. B. (2011). Stigma, negative attitudes about treatment, and utilization of mental health care among soldiers. *Military Psychology, 23*(1), 65–81.

Lester, P. B., Harms, P. D., Herian, M. N., Krasikova, D. V., & Beal, S. J. (2011). The Comprehensive Soldier Fitness program evaluation report #3: Longitudinal analysis of the impact of master resilience training on self-reported resilience and psychological health data. Arlington, VA: Department of Defense.

Locke, E. A., & Latham, G. P. (2002). Building a practically useful theory of goal setting and task motivation: A 35-year odyssey. *American Psychologist, 57*(9), 705–717.

Maddi, S. R. (2005). On hardiness and other pathways to resilience. *American Psychologist, 60*(3), 261–262.

Masten, A. S., Cutuli, J. J., Herbers, J. E., & Reed, M. G. J. (2002). Resilience in development. In C. R. Snyder & S. J. Lopez (Eds.), *Handbook of positive psychology* (pp. 74–88). New York, NY: Oxford University Press.

Meichenbaum, D. H. (1977). *Cognitive Behavior Modification: An Integrative Approach.* New York, NY: Plenum.

Mojtabai, R., Olfson, M., Sampson, N. A., Jin, R., Druss, B., Wang, P. S., et al. (2011). Barriers to mental health treatment: Results from the National Comorbidity Survey Replication. *Psychological Medicine*, *41*(8), 1751–1761.

Paiva, A. L., Prochaska, J. O., Yin, H. Q., Rossi, J. S., Redding, C. A., Blissmer, B., et al. (2012). Treated individuals who progress to action or maintenance for one behavior are more likely to make similar progress on another behavior: Coaction results of a pooled data analysis of three trials. *Preventive Medicine*, *54*(5), 331–334.

Peterson C. (2000). The future of optimism. *American Psychologist*, *55*(1), 44–55.

Reivich, K. J., Seligman, M. E. P., & McBride, S. (2011). Master resilience training in the US Army. *American Psychologist*, *66*(1), 25–34.

Reivich, K., & Shatte, A. (2002). *The Resilience Factor: 7 Keys to Finding Your Inner Strength and Overcoming Life's Hurdles*. New York, NY: Broadway Books.

Resick, P. A., Monson, C. M., & Chard, K. M. (2007). *Cognitive Processing Therapy Veteran/Military Version*. Boston, MA: National Center for PTSD.

Schottenbauer, M. A., Glass, C. R., Arnkoff, D. B., Tendick, V., & Gray, S. H. (2008). Nonresponse and dropout rates in outcome studies on PTSD: Review and methodological considerations. *Psychiatry*, *71*(2), 134–168.

Seligman, M. E., Steen, T. A., Park, N., & Peterson, C. (2005). Positive psychology progress: Empirical validation of interventions. *American Psychologist*, *60*(5), 410–421.

Shochet, I. M., Dadds, M. R., Holland, D., Whitefield, K., Harnett, P. H., & Osgarby, S. M. (2001). The efficacy of a universal school-based program to prevent adolescent depression. *Journal of Clinical Child Psychology*, *30*(3), 303–315.

Tedeschi, R. G., & Calhoun, L. G. (1995). *Trauma & Transformation: Growing in the Aftermath of Suffering*. Thousand Oaks, CA: Sage Publications.

Tedeschi, R. G., & McNally, R. J. (2011). Can we facilitate posttraumatic growth in combat veterans? *American Psychologist*, *66*(1), 19–24.

Theodorakis, Y., Hatzigeorgiadis, A., & Chroni, S. (2008). Self-talk: It works, but how? Development and preliminary validation of the functions of Self-Talk Questionnaire. *Measurement in Physical Education and Exercise Science*, *12*(1), 10–30.

Vanhove, A. J., Herian, M. N., Perez, A. L. U., Harms, P. D., & Lester, P. B. (2015). Can resilience be developed at work? A meta-analytic review of resilience-building programme effectiveness. *Journal of Occupational and Organizational Psychology*, 1–30. doi: 10.1111/joop.12123

Wood, A. M., Froh, J. J., & Geraghty. A. W. A. (2010). Gratitude and well-being: A review and theoretical integration. *Clinical Psychology Review*, *30*(7), 890–905.

Weinstein, N., Brown, K. W., & Ryan, R. M. (2009). A multi-method examination of the effects of mindfulness on stress attribution, coping, and emotional well-being. *Journal of Research in Personality*, *43*(3), 374–385.

Williams, A., Hagerty, B. M., Yousha, S. M., Horrocks, J., Hoyle, K. S., & Liu, D. (2004). Psychosocial effects of the boot strap intervention in Navy recruits. *Military Medicine*, *169*(10), 814–820.

Yalom, I. D. (2005). *The Theory and Practice of Group Psychotherapy (5th ed.)*. New York: Basic Books.

PART
4

ALTERNATIVE
DELIVERY METHODS

THIRTEEN

Virtual Reality Exposure Therapy for PTSD

MICHAEL J. ROY, ALBERT RIZZO, JOANN DIFEDE, AND BARBARA O. ROTHBAUM

EXPERT TREATMENT GUIDELINES AND CONSENSUS STATEMENTS IDENTIFIED imaginal exposure therapy as a first-line treatment for posttraumatic stress disorder (PTSD) more than a decade ago (Ballenger et al. 2000; Foa et al. 1999; Rothbaum et al. 2000b). Subsequently, an Institute of Medicine report concluded that cognitive–behavioral therapy with exposure therapy is the *only* therapy with sufficient evidence to recommend it for PTSD (Berg et al. 2008). Imaginal exposure has been the most widely used exposure approach. It requires the patients to recall and narrate repeatedly their traumatic experience in progressively greater detail, both to facilitate the therapeutic processing of related emotions and to decondition the learning cycle of the disorder via a habituation–extinction process. Prolonged exposure (Foa & Kozak 1986; Jaycox et al. 2002), one of the best-evidenced forms of exposure therapy, incorporates psychoeducation, controlled breathing techniques, in vivo exposure, prolonged imaginal exposure to traumatic memories, and processing of traumatic material, typically for 9 to 12 therapy sessions of about 90 minutes each. However, avoidance of reminders of the trauma is a defining feature of PTSD, so it is not surprising many patients are unwilling or unable to visualize effectively and recount traumatic events repeatedly. Some studies of imaginal exposure have reported 30% to 50% dropout rates before completion of treatment (Rauch, King, Abelson, et al. 2015; Schnurr, Friedman, Engel, et al. 2007; Yehuda, Pratchett, Elmes, et al. 2014). Adding to the challenge, some patients have an aversion to "traditional" psychotherapy as well as to pharmacotherapy, and may find alternative approaches more appealing. Younger individuals in particular may be attracted to virtual reality-based therapies.

Virtual reality exposure therapy (VRET) represents a particularly promising method for delivering exposure therapy, during which provocative stimuli can be introduce in real time and controlled precisely. Virtual reality researchers emphasize that the technology enables delivery of specific, consistent, evocative, and controllable multisensory stimuli that serve as conditioned stimuli, and the success of several clinical applications has been documented (Glantz et al. 2003; Rizzo & Kim 2005; Rizzo et al. 2004; Rose, Brooks, & Rizzo 2005). Virtual reality has been defined as "a way for humans to visualize, manipulate, and interact with computers and extremely complex data" (Aukstakalnis & Blatner 1992, p. 2). Such advanced human–computer interaction is facilitated by the integration of computers, real-time graphics, visual displays, body tracking sensors, and specialized interface devices that serve to immerse a participant in a simulated world that changes in a natural way with head and body motion.

Virtual reality environments typically display computer graphics in a motion-tracked head-mounted display, which can be augmented by vibration platforms, localizable three-dimensional sounds, physical props such as rifles, and scent delivery technology, to facilitate a multisensory immersive experience for participants. This approach engenders a strong sense of presence, or "being there," for those immersed in the virtual environment. This immersion can enable clinical assessment and intervention options beyond what is possible with traditional methods (Rizzo et al. 1998, 2004). Similar to an aircraft simulator that tests and trains pilots under various controlled conditions, virtual reality provides context-relevant simulated environments that can assess and treat cognitive and emotional conditions. The clinician can use virtual reality to deliver precisely and systematically complex, dynamic, and ecologically relevant stimuli, reinforced by behavioral tracking, performance recording, and physiological monitoring to foster sophisticated interaction.

Diverse virtual environments have been developed and have shown efficacy in several psychiatric disorders. Among the most salient applications are fear reduction in a wide range of phobias, including claustrophobia (Botella et al. 1998, 2000), fear of flying (Botella et al. 2004; Rothbaum et al. 1996, 2000a, 2002, 2006; Smith et al. 1999; Wiederhold & Wiederhold 2002), acrophobia (Emmelkamp et al. 2001; Rothbaum et al. 1995), arachnophobia (Carlin et al. 1997; Garcia-Palacios et al.

2002), and fear of driving after an automobile accident (Beck et al. 2007; Walshe et al. 2003). The use of virtual reality in the treatment of simple phobias has been well summarized (Parsons & Rizzo 2008; Powers & Emmelkamp 2008). Virtual reality has also demonstrated utility for body image disturbances in patients with eating disorders (Riva 2011), and for the assessment and rehabilitation of attention, memory, spatial skills, and other cognitive functions in both clinical and unimpaired populations (Brooks et al. 1999; Brown et al. 1998; Matheis et al. 2007; Parsons, Rizzo 2008; Pugnetti et al. 1995; Rizzo et al. 2006; Rose et al. 2005). Virtual reality has utility in social anxiety disorder (Anderson et al. 2003; Klinger et al. 2005), other anxiety disorders (Krijn et al. 2004; Powers & Emmelkamp 2008; Rothbaum & Hodges 1999), addiction (Bordnick et al. 2005), and acute pain reduction (Gold et al. 2005). Most notably, several studies have shown efficacy for virtual reality treatment of PTSD (Difede et al. 2002, 2007; Roy et al. 2010, Rothbaum et al. 2010, Reger et al. 2011, 2013; Rothbaum et al. 2001), which are described in more detail in the following sections.

VIRTUAL VIETNAM

The first application of VRET to PTSD occurred in 1997, when Georgia Tech and Emory University researchers used a Virtual Vietnam environment with Vietnam veterans (Rothbaum et al. 2001). The study population had chronic PTSD, with persistent impairment evident in mental health, overall functional status, and quality of life, despite the application of various traditional PTSD treatment methods throughout the decades since the Vietnam War. The virtual environment delivered via the head-mounted display featured rice fields, riverbanks, and perspectives from the inside and outside of a military helicopter, supplemented by visual and auditory stimuli such as machine gun fire, rockets, explosions, and shouting. An initial case study of a 50-year-old male Vietnam veteran with PTSD (Rothbaum & Hodges 1999) documented posttreatment improvement on all measures of PTSD, and maintenance of these gains 6 months later—a 34% decrease in clinician-rated symptoms and a corresponding 45% decrease in self-reported symptoms of PTSD. In a subsequent open clinical trial, in which 16 male Vietnam veterans with PTSD participated in an average of 13 exposure therapy sessions over 5 to 7 weeks, Rothbaum et al. (2001) reported a significant reduction in PTSD and related symptoms. The degree of immersion was evidenced by patients who reported seeing things, such as enemy soldiers and burning vehicles, which were not in the virtual environment but were, in fact, part of their own memories.

VIRTUAL WORLD TRADE CENTER

Difede and Hoffman (2002) treated a World Trade Center (WTC) survivor of the 9/11/2001 attack with VRET, effecting a complete remission. The virtual environment included 9/11 audio recordings made by a national news network as well as virtual humans (avatars) who, for example, could be seen falling from the burning WTC towers. In a subsequent clinical trial, WTC survivors who completed VRET treatments demonstrated statistically and clinically significant decreases on the Clinician-Administered PTSD Scale (CAPS) relative to pretreatment and to the wait-list control group, with a between-group posttreatment effect size of 1.54 (Difede et al. 2006, 2007). Nine of 10 completers in the virtual reality group had clinically and statistically significant improvement in symptoms, including seven who achieved remission of their PTSD. None of the wait-list control subjects achieved remission. Treatment gains in completers were maintained at the 6-month follow-up. Also noteworthy, 5 of the 10 virtual reality patients had participated previously in imaginal exposure treatment with no clinical benefit. In a follow-up randomized controlled trial (RCT) comparing virtual reality exposure (VRE) enhanced with d-cycloserine (DCS) with VRE with placebo in 25 participants (a full description is provided later in the chapter), participants in both VRE conditions showed a significant decrease in PTSD symptoms posttreatment and at the 6-month follow-up (Difede et al. 2014). These results suggest that virtual reality warrants further study as a potentially useful treatment option for terrorism-related PTSD.

THE EVOLVING USE OF VIRTUAL SIMULATIONS TO TREAT PTSD FOLLOWING WAR OR TERRORISM

VRET may have distinct advantages for military personnel or combat veterans. Studies addressing treatment failures with imaginal exposure have shown that an inability to engage emotionally is the best predictor of a poor treatment outcome (Cardena & Spiegel 1993; Foa et al. 1995; Jaycox et al. 1998; Koopman et al. 1994). In particular, the emotional detachment often necessary for success on the battlefield may pose a significant obstacle to therapy requiring repeated acknowledgment of fears and emotions. Although VRET does not obviate the need for such disclosures, a vivid, attractive medium may facilitate recall and expression. VRET offers a way to circumvent natural avoidance by delivering multisensory contextual cues directly that evoke the trauma. VRET can facilitate recall of traumatic events and related feelings and reactions, thus enabling a therapist to identify and ameliorate disabling symptoms more quickly, especially for patients who are more avoidant or alexithymic.

VRET offers an appealing, nontraditional treatment approach that may be perceived with less stigma by "digital generation" service members and veterans who are often reluctant to participate in traditional talk therapies. A sophisticated and realistic virtual environment may enhance treatment credibility and may be especially appealing to service members who have shown distrust and reluctance toward traditional mental health services. Service members, particularly those returning with their units rather than alone, attach significantly greater stigma to psychological issues than to medical problems, suggesting that subjective norms influence stigma perceptions (Britt 2000). The challenges inherent in emotionally engaging with fear structures, as required in exposure therapies, and the stigma associated with traditional "talk therapies" pose significant barriers to optimizing access to care that might be addressed more effectively through VRET. Although service-wide efforts have reduced modestly some of the more commonly cited obstacles to seeking mental health care, these barriers nevertheless remain highly prevalent (Hoge et al. 2004; Warner et al. 2008). Even if the efficacy of VRET is no greater than for imaginal exposure, the novelty or appeal alone may be sufficient to attract greater numbers of service members and veterans to engage in treatment. This potential increased treatment reach could reduce the morbidity of PTSD significantly.

Studies of several virtual environments to treat PTSD in survivors of war and terrorist attacks have been reported. A case series by Wood et al. (2009) identified significant improvement in PTSD symptoms in 9 of 12 Iraq War service members using virtual reality combined with meditation and attentional refocusing. However, the report did not include statistical analyses, and the mean pretreatment PTSD Checklist–Military Version (PCL-M) score was 47.3 points, which is less than the conservative cutoff score of 50 points that best identifies PTSD (Weathers et al. 1993). A report from Gamito et al. (2010) identified modest improvement with VRET for male retired service members of the Portuguese Colonial Wars in Africa compared with wait-list control subjects and imaginal exposure. As with Virtual Vietnam, PTSD symptoms in this population had been present for decades, which could be expected to diminish the magnitude and frequency of response.

Virtual Iraq/Afghanistan

The University of Southern California's Institute for Creative Technologies has spearheaded the development of a highly sophisticated virtual reality environment: Virtual Iraq/Afghanistan. The original environment was based on Full Spectrum Warrior, a commercially successful Xbox game, which in turn had been adapted from a U.S. Army–funded combat tactical simulation trainer. The virtual environment has undergone progressive evolution, with the application of both existing and novel art and technology assets in response to feedback from patients and therapists.

The second version of Virtual Iraq/Afghanistan features a Middle Eastern–themed city and desert road scenarios (Figures 13.1–13.23) intended to resemble the environments most service members encounter during deployment to Iraq or Afghanistan. An 18-square-block city setting includes a marketplace, desolate streets, old buildings, ramshackle apartments, warehouses, mosques, shops, and dirt lots strewn with junk. Access to building interiors and rooftops is available, and the backdrop creates the illusion of being immersed in a desert city. Virtual vehicles and animated pedestrians (civilian and military) can be inserted or removed from scenes, and helicopters can be made to take off, fly overhead, and land. A desert road scenario incorporates expansive sand dunes interspersed with palm trees and other vegetation, intact and dilapidated structures, bridges, battle wreckage, a checkpoint, debris, and virtual human figures that create ambushes. The patient can be positioned as the driver, as a passenger, or in the turret of a Humvee, traveling alone or within a convoy; fellow passengers or passengers in other vehicles may suffer visible wounds. A subsequent adaptation incorporates such elements as snow-capped mountains to imitate more closely the landscape of Afghanistan rather than Iraq. The most recent version allows the patient to exit the Humvee and proceed on foot, expanding the realism and array of options available.

A new version of the Virtual Iraq/Afghanistan system, now referred to as the *BRAVEMIND system* has recently been developed. This newer version expands the diversity of scenario content and functionality. The expansion was informed by patient and clinician feedback acquired during clinical use of the initial Virtual Iraq/ Afghanistan clinical application. Built on the Unity software platform, the system was designed to provide a flexible software architecture that allows for new content to be built on top of the existing assets more easily, based on future feedback from both patients and clinicians. The BRAVEMIND system has completed beta testing successfully and offers the therapist 14 distinct scenarios from which to choose (compared with four in the previous version), with widely expanded clinician controls (Figure 13.24) to enhance the realism and experiential options, and to facilitate the tailoring of the exposure to each individual patient. In addition, the development effort has allowed for the reuse of many of the simulation assets to expand the VRET system for use to address the therapeutic needs of combat medics/corpsmen (Rizzo et al. 2013). These tools are also being tested for use in resilience training

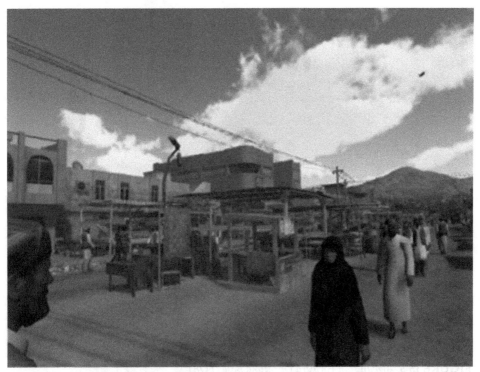

FIGURE 13.1 *Afghanistan City Market*

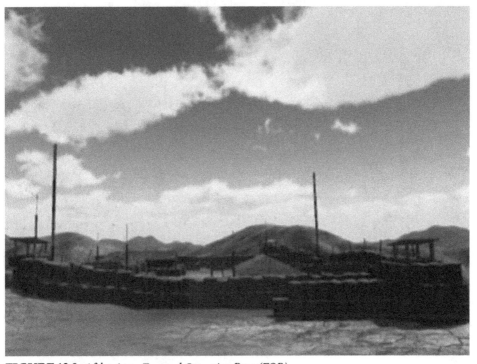

FIGURE 13.2 *Afghanistan Forward Operating Base (FOB)*

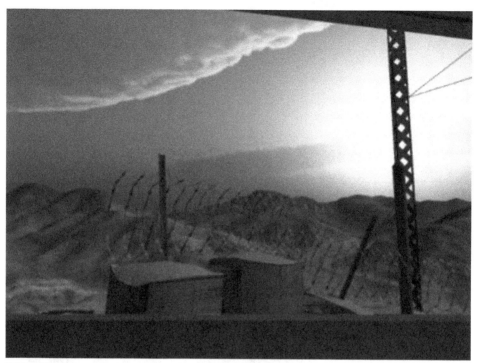

FIGURE 13.3 *Afghanistan Forward Operating Base (FOB)*

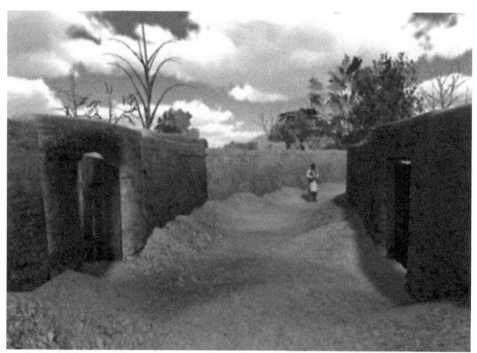

FIGURE 13.4 *Afghanistan Rural Village*

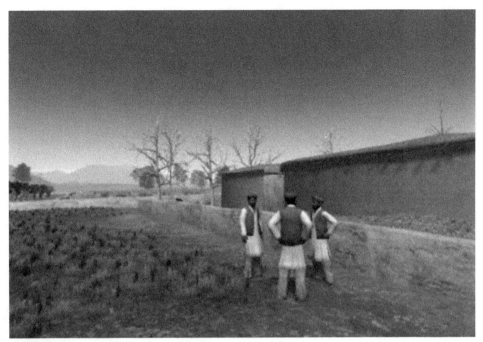

FIGURE 13.5 *Afghanistan Rural Village*

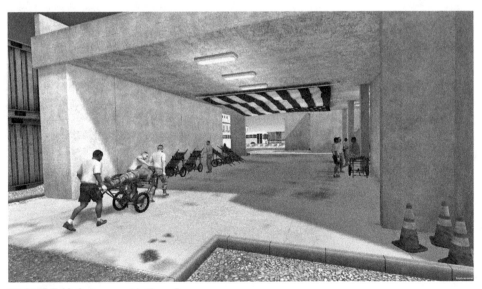

FIGURE 13.6 *Bagram Air Force Base*

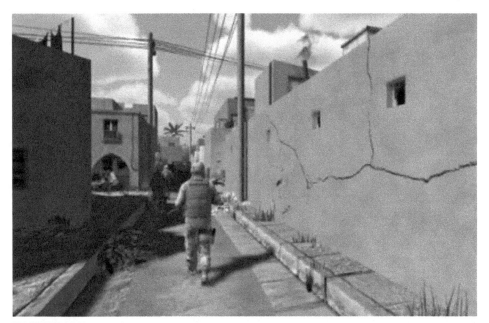

FIGURE 13.7 *Iraq City*

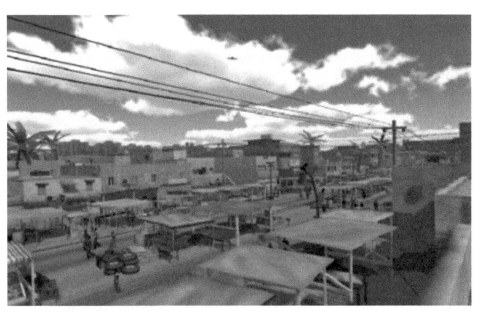

FIGURE 13.8 *Iraq City*

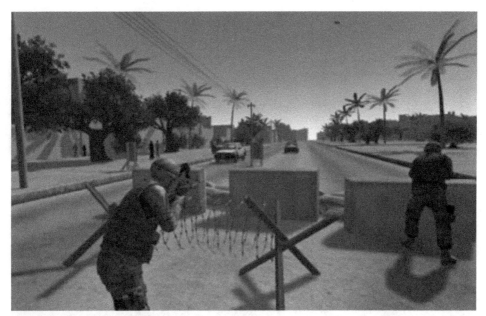

FIGURE 13.9 *Checkpoint Zone*

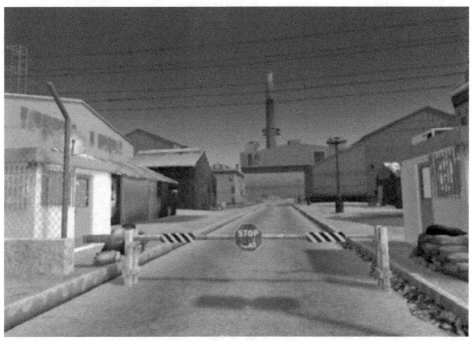

FIGURE 13.10 *Industrial Zone*

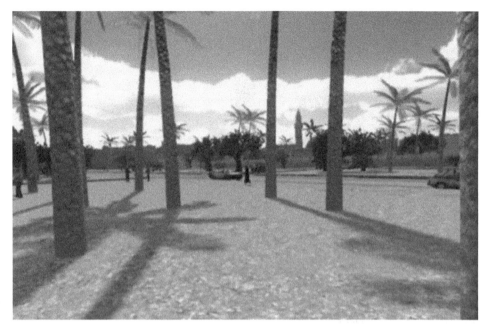

FIGURE 13.11 *Palm Grove Resident Zone*

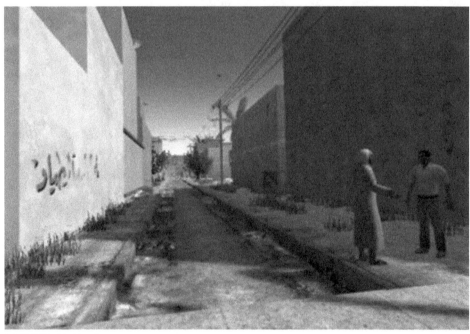

FIGURE 13.12 *Slum Zone*

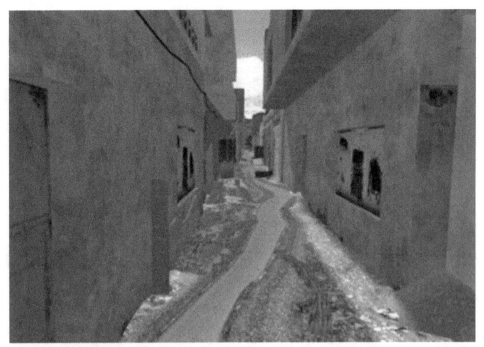

FIGURE 13.13 *Slum Zone*

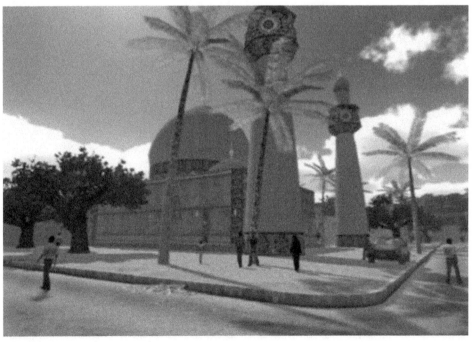

FIGURE 13.14 *Mosque Resident Zone*

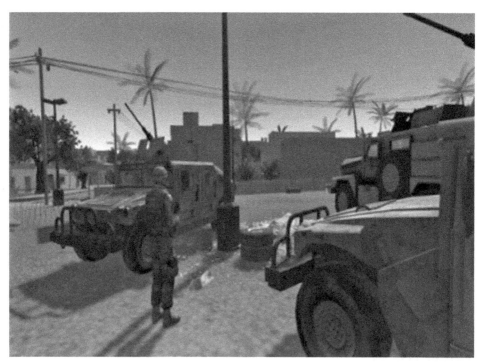

FIGURE 13.15 *Safe Zone*

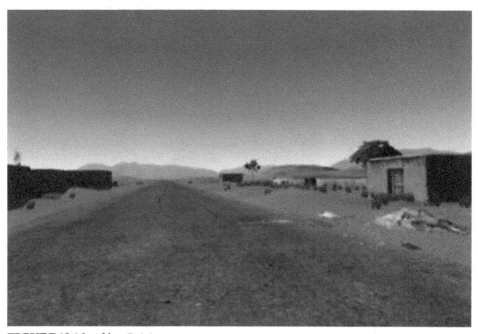

FIGURE 13.16 *Afghan Driving*

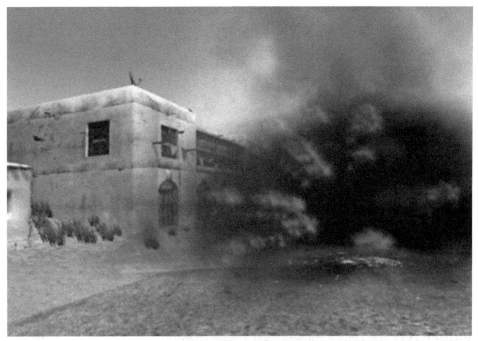

FIGURE 13.17 *Afghan Driving (Improvised Explosive Device)*

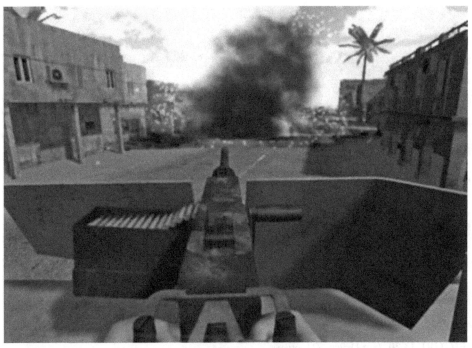

FIGURE 13.18 *Iraq Driving (Improvised Explosive Device)*

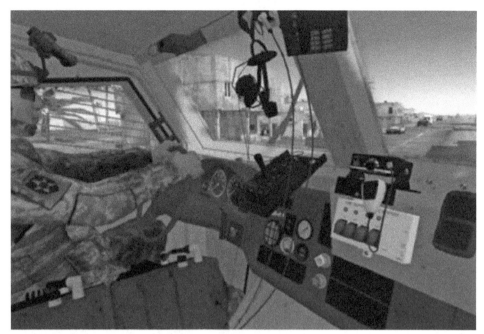

FIGURE 13.19 *Iraq Driving (Mine-Resistant Ambush Protected)*

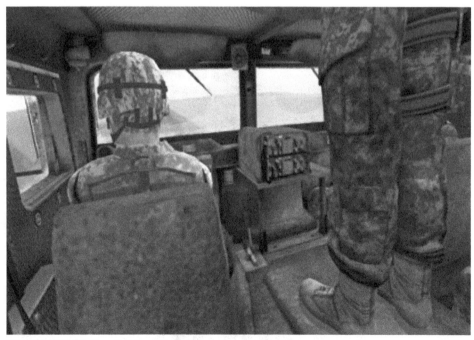

FIGURE 13.20 *Iraq Driving (Humvee)*

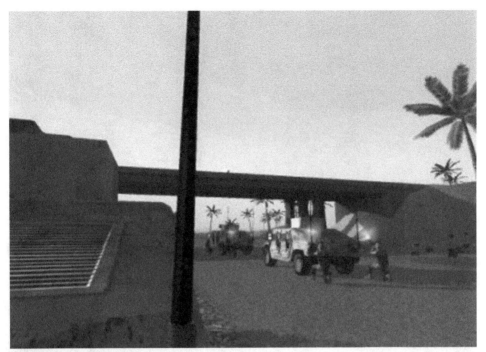

FIGURE 13.21 *Iraq Bridge Attack*

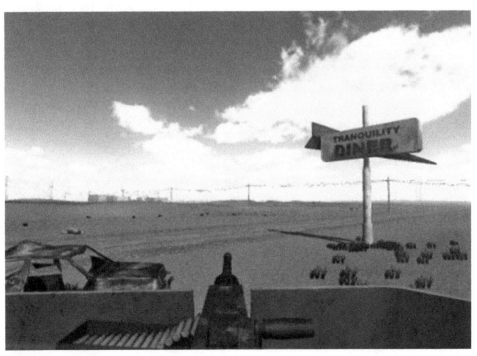

FIGURE 13.22 *USA Desert Driving*

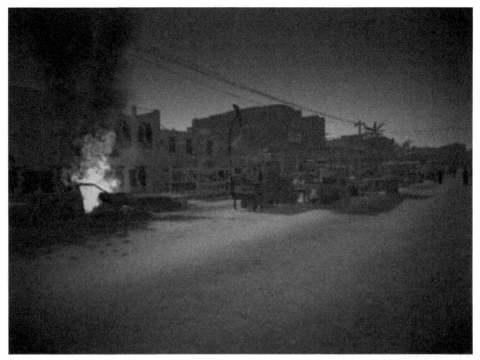

FIGURE 13.23 *Night Vision Setting*

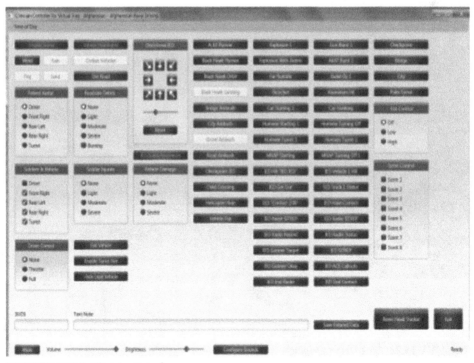

FIGURE 13.24 *Clinician Interface*

TABLE 13.1 Fourteen Scenarios Available in the BRAVEMIND Beta System

1. Afghanistan city	Dismounted patrol
2. Afghanistan Forward Operating Base (FOB)	Dismounted patrol
3. Afghanistan rural village	Dismounted patrol
4. Afghanistan Bagram Air Force Base	Dismounted patrol
5. Iraq city	Dismounted patrol
6. Hybrid Mid-East city checkpoint	Dismounted patrol
7. Hybrid Mid-East city industrial zone	Dismounted patrol
8. Hybrid Mid-East city palm grove	Dismounted patrol
9. Hybrid Mid-East city slum zone	Dismounted patrol
10. Hybrid Mid-East city mosque/residential zone	Dismounted patrol
11. Hybrid Mid-East city safe zone	Dismounted patrol
12. Rural roadway/village Afghanistan	Driving/dismounted patrol
13. Rural roadway/village Iraq desert	Driving/dismounted patrol
14. Rural roadway United States	Driving/dismounted patrol

(Buckwalter et al. 2011; Rizzo et al. 2013). The 14 scenarios currently available in the beta system are listed in Table 13.1.

Within the 14 scenarios, the therapist can adjust the time of day or night, level of illumination, and weather conditions (e.g., sandstorm, rain), and can insert a night vision perspective or ambient sounds (e.g., wind, motors, city noise, prayer call) via the use of the Clinician Interface (Figure 13.24). Clinicians can insert (or teleport) users into a variety of starting locations within each virtual scenario based on their perception of patient need at that point in time. Patients can drive the Humvee or mine-resistant ambush-protected vehicle with a standard gamepad controller and can walk through the dismounted foot patrol scenarios with either the gamepad or a "thumb-mouse" controller mounted on a replica of an M4 rifle. The visual stimuli presented via the head-mounted display can be supplemented by directional three-dimensional audio, vibrotactile, and olfactory stimuli. The therapist has the "Wizard of Oz" capability to introduce and remove each stimulus with the click of a mouse on a computer screen, while being in full audio contact with the patient, which enables an individually customized approach, taking into account the patient's past experience and treatment progress. In addition to the Southwest Asia environments, an American roadway is also available within the system for those who may wish to experience and familiarize themselves with the virtual reality environment in a relatively safe context before exposure to more provocative scenarios.

The high prevalence of PTSD in service members returning from Iraq and Afghanistan, coupled with the relatively low cost of the system, has led to widespread use of Virtual Iraq/Afghanistan as a research tool for the treatment of PTSD in studies across the United States (Rizzo et al. 2013). The system has been used for a variety of PTSD-related investigations with active-duty service members and veterans at multiple military, Veterans Affairs and civilian sites, including the Naval Medical Center–San Diego (NMCSD), Madigan Army Medical Center, Camp Pendleton, Emory University, Walter Reed National Military Medical Center (formerly Walter Reed Army Medical Center), and the Weill Medical College of Cornell University. User-centered tests with early prototypes of the Virtual Iraq application were conducted at the NMCSD, as well as within an Army Combat Stress Control team in Iraq. This informal feedback provided essential information on the content, realism, and usability of the initial "intuitively designed" system.

EVALUATION OF VIRTUAL REALITY EXPOSURE THERAPY WITH VIRTUAL IRAQ/AFGHANISTAN

To date, three case studies, two open trials, and two RCTs have been reported involving the Virtual Iraq/Afghanistan environment in the treatment of PTSD. The first case report, published from Emory University, documented a 56% reduction in the CAPS score for a veteran of Operation Iraqi Freedom (OIF) with PTSD, representing a significant decrease in clinical severity (Gerardi et al. 2008). Similar results were reported in other early case studies reported using this system (Reger & Gahm 2008; Rizzo et al. 2008).

An open clinical trial was conducted with active-duty service members recently returned from Iraq and diagnosed with PTSD at NMCSD and Camp Pendleton. Participants in this study were service members who had achieved no benefit from a previous course of conventional PTSD treatment such as group therapy, prolonged exposure, and selective serotonin reuptake inhibitors. The participants consented to a protocol featuring an average of 90- to 120-minute sessions twice weekly for 5 weeks. The actual number and frequency of sessions were adjusted to meet individual needs. Because this was an initial feasibility trial, if the client was showing improvement, they were allowed to continue past the standard 10 sessions, or 5 weeks. Analyses of the first 20 treatment completers (19 male, 1 female; mean age, 28 years; age range, 21–51 years) showed a significant decrease in mean PCL-M score from a baseline of 54.4 ± 9.7 (standard deviation) points to 35.6 ± 17.4 points after treatment ($t = 5.99$, $df = 19$, $p < .001$). Sixteen of 20 completers no longer met (American Psychiatric Association 1994), criteria for PTSD at posttreatment. Scores on the Beck Anxiety Inventory decreased significantly from 18.6 ± 9.5 points to 11.9 ± 13.6 points after treatment ($t = 3.37$, $df = 19$, $p < .003$), and scores on the nine-item Patient Health Questionnaire-9 for depression decreased from 13.3 ± 5.4 points to 7.1 ± 6.7 points

($t = 3.68$, $df = 19$, $p < .002$). The average number of sessions for this sample was just under 12. Following this study, another open clinical trial with active-duty soldiers ($N = 24$) produced significant pre-/postreductions in PCL-M scores and a large treatment effect size (Cohen's $d = 1.17$) (Reger et al. 2011). After an average of seven sessions, 45% of those treated no longer screened positive for PTSD and 62% had reliably improved.

This work was followed by a small randomized trial comparing VRET versus treatment as usual, with the latter receiving approaches including pharmacotherapy, imaginal exposure, cognitive processing therapy, and eye movement desensitization and reprocessing. Seven of 10 randomized to VRET were reported to have achieved a 30% reduction in CAPS scores compared with only one of nine control subjects (McLay et al. 2011). Although these results are limited by small size, lack of blinding, a single therapist, and comparison with a relatively uncontrolled usual care condition, these findings have added to the incremental evidence suggesting virtual reality to be a safe and effective treatment for combat-related PTSD.

We conducted the Virtual Reality Therapy and Imaging in Combat Veterans trial at Walter Reed Army Medical Center, assigning active duty service members randomly to VRET or to prolonged exposure. Each arm featured 12 to 20 90-minute sessions over approximately 6 weeks, with half the time during VRET sessions spent in the Virtual Iraq environment (the remainder of the time involved preparation for the virtual reality element, and debriefing and processing after the virtual reality), starting with the fourth session. The primary outcome measure was the score on CAPS, administered by a trained, blinded assessor at the end of treatment and at the end of a 12-week follow-up compared with the baseline CAPS score. Secondary measures included the PCL-M, the Beck Depression Inventory to assess depression, the Beck Anxiety Inventory to assess anxiety, and the 36-Item Short Form Health Survey and the World Health Organization Disability Assessment Schedule II to assess functional status. Nineteen participants completed treatment, 9 VRET and 10 prolonged exposure. Mean age was 33 years in each arm, and all but one were male. Those assigned to the VRET arm had clinically significant improvements (defined as a decrease in CAPS score of 10 points or more), with a mean decline in the CAPS score from 80 points to 64 points, whereas those assigned to prolonged exposure had a less than clinically significant change, with CAPS scores declining from 71 points to 65 points (Roy et al. 2014). However, study therapists reported similar improvements for both arms, as measured on the Clinical Global Impression scale, with a mean improvement score of 2.4 points for each treatment group, where 2 points is much improved and 3 points is minimally improved. Moreover, baseline CAPS scores were higher in the group randomized to VRET, so the greater improvement identified by CAPS may have been more a result of this than the form of treatment. Study participants in both arms reported subjectively to their study therapists decreased avoidant behavior, such as using the subway and attending restaurants, sporting events, and movie theaters. Although the numbers in this study were not sufficient to determine definitively whether prolonged exposure or VRET improved brain function more than the other, the most compelling finding from this study was that, when functional magnetic resonance imaging (fMRI) for the two arms was combined, exposure therapy resulted in significant improvements in each of the three brain region associated closely with PTSD: the amygdala, hippocampus, and anterior cingulate cortex (Roy et al. 2010). We recently published further data demonstrating that postdeployment military service members without PTSD who underwent fMRI 3 months apart showed no significant fMRI changes in these brain regions, confirming the changes were, in fact, the result of the treatment and not merely a practice effect (Roy et al. 2014).

Three RCTs are currently in progress, and another has recently been published (Rothbaum et al. [2014]; see the section on DCS later in this chapter for a full description), using the Virtual Iraq/Afghanistan system with service members and veteran populations. One RCT is comparing treatment efficacy between VRET and prolonged exposure (Reger & Gahm 2008), another compares VRET alone versus VRET plus a supplemental care approach (Beidel et al. 2011), and the third compares VRE with exposure therapy with and without DCS in an double-blind RCT design in active-duty and veterans of OIF, Operation Enduring Freedom (OEF), and Operation New Dawn (https://clinicaltrials.gov/ct2/show/NCT01352637, re-accessed the link April 22, 2016). Department of Defense (DoD) funding support for these RCTs underscore the interest that the DoD/Veterans Affairs (VA) has in exploring this innovative approach for delivering exposure therapy using virtual reality.

The reluctance of service members with mental disorders to seek mental health care has been well documented (Hoge et al. 2004), and VRET could play a future role in addressing this problem. In particular, consideration could be given to embedding some form of VRET within the debriefing and retraining elements that occur immediately postdeployment, which would have the added benefit of decreasing perceived stigma associated with seeking behavioral health treatment.

From the perspective of the clinician, virtual reality systems have the potential to enhance the array of options they can provide to patients, maximizing benefit in the context of overall care delivered by a thoughtful professional cognizant of the complexity of PTSD. Virtual reality systems are intended for use by professionals with appropriate training in the conduct of exposure therapy, not as "self-help" tools or in an automated treatment protocol.

SYSTEMATIC REVIEWS OF VRET

A systematic review identified 10 published studies on VRET for PTSD (Goncalves et al. 2012), including the previously described reports, noting that seven of them reported superiority to wait-list control subjects, although none documented superiority over another form of exposure therapy. A more recent systematic review (Canadian Agency for Drugs and Technologies in Health 2014) identified one additional RCT (Roy et al. 2014), and the authors were not able to draw appreciably different conclusions than the earlier review. There are methodological limitations to many of the identified studies, with only 5 of 11 representing randomized trials, two were controlled without randomization, and four were not controlled. The studies included small numbers, with only 10 to 20 participants each, and blinded outcomes measurements and intent-to-treat analyses were frequently lacking. In summary, VRET appears to have promise as a treatment approach, but larger and better-quality studies are needed.

AUGMENTATION OF VIRTUAL REALITY WITH DCS

DCS was approved by the U.S. Food and Drug Administration more than 50 years ago for the treatment of tuberculosis and urinary tract infections, and has documented safety in humans. It is related to quinolone antibiotics such as ciprofloxacin. DCS was found in animal studies to facilitate the extinction of learned fear and to produce generalized extinction (Davis et al. 2006). DCS is thought to act as a partial agonist at N-methyl-D-aspartate glutamate receptors thought to be important in short-term learning and memory. As a result, DCS has been incorporated in studies using exposure therapy to determine whether it can enhance synergistically the action of glutamate released into synapses in response to psychotherapy.

The first clinical application was a randomized, double-blind, placebo-controlled trial of DCS in conjunction with VRET for 28 patients with acrophobia (Ressler et al. 2004). Those receiving DCS had significantly greater improvement on multiple outcome measures compared with those receiving placebo, both posttreatment after only two sessions and 3 months later. Two studies found that, compared with placebo, 50 mg DCS administered 1 hour before exposure therapy sessions for treatment of social phobia induced a higher response rate (Guastella et al. 2008; Hofmann et al. 2006). Several studies have also assessed the efficacy of DCS in conjunction with exposure therapy for obsessive–compulsive disorder. The two studies with positive findings used 100 mg DCS 1 hour before each of 10 exposure sessions (Wilhelm et al. 2008) and 125 mg 2 hours before 10 exposure sessions (Kushner et al. 2007). The only study to find no advantage to adjunctive DCS used 250 mg 4 hours before each of 12 90-minute sessions (Storch et al. 2007). Rothbaum (2008) postulated several possible explanations for the negative trial of Storch et al. (2007): (1) DCS may have been given too early; (2) the dose may have been too high, resulting in more antagonistic action, given that DCS is a partial agonist; and (3) because more and longer sessions were used in both arms, the response rate was so high in the comparison group that it made a distinction between DCS and placebo difficult to discern. Factors such as these suggest that additional studies are needed to clarify the benefit of DCS in clinical practice. The first RCT of DCS (50 mg 1 hour before therapy sessions) augmentation of prolonged exposure therapy for PTSD did not identify a significant difference in remission rates as measured by the gold standard CAPS, but 19 of the 67 study participants were allowed to end the study early because they took at least one dose of study medication (DCS or placebo) and achieved remission. However, an intent–to-treat analysis did find that those receiving DCS were three times more likely to have a clinically significant response (reduction in CAPS score of 10 points or more). Moreover, for those completing the full course of treatment, those receiving DCS were four times more likely to have a response and were nine times more likely to have this response sustained at the 3-month follow-up assessment. de Kleine et al. (2012) also found that, for subjects who completed all study sessions, those receiving DCS had a higher response rate as measured by CAPS, although there was not a difference in remission rates. A smaller controlled trial randomized 26 veterans with PTSD after the Iraq and Afghanistan wars to a more brief six sessions of exposure therapy with either DCS (50 mg 30 minutes before sessions 2 through 5) or placebo (Litz et al. 2012). That study likewise found no difference in remission rates between those receiving DCS and placebo. The initial target number for the study was 68, but because of enrollment difficulties, only 26 initiated the study and then six participants dropped out during the brief course of treatment. However, the response rates (CAPS score decrease of 10 points or more) were in contrast to those seen by de Kleine et al. (2012), with 7 of 11 who received placebo achieving a response compared with only three of nine who received DCS. This was a small study with a very brief treatment course. In contrast, in a randomized, blinded, placebo controlled clinical trial comparing VRE enhanced with DCS with virtual reality and placebo for WTC-related PTSD (Difede et al. 2014) found that 69% of those in the VR + DCS group were in remission, as defined by a CAPS score of less than 20 points and no or minimal functional impairment 6 months after treatment. A 100-mg dose of DCS was administered 90 minutes before the psychotherapy session. These positive results may be explained in part by differences in dose (100 mg vs. 50 mg in the other DCS studies), timing of medication (90 minutes before treatment vs. 30 minutes in the other studies), and treatment population (terrorism vs. combat exposure). Finally, prior DCS studies used imaginal exposure, and it is possible that DCS enhancement was facilitated by the standardized sensory stimuli available in the virtual reality scenarios. Convergent evidence for the efficacy of DCS enhancement of VRE is provided by the recently published randomized controlled study by Rothbaum et al. (2014) using VRE combined with medication (DCS, alprazolam, or placebo), which found VRE successful in the treatment of OEF and OIF veterans with PTSD. This trial showed the benefit of DCS on startle response and cortisol measures after treatment, but not on the overall report of PTSD symptoms (Rothbaum et al. 2014). Thus, although DCS may have the potential to enhance the response to psychotherapy, further study is clearly needed to determine the optimal target population, timing and dosage of medication, and type and duration of therapy.

EMERGING APPLICATIONS OF VIRTUAL IRAQ AND AFGHANISTAN ENVIRONMENTS

Virtual reality simulations of OIF/OEF combat environments were used initially in the treatment of psychiatric disorders, but other applications have been explored subsequently. The assessment of physiological responses to the virtual environment during VRET therapy can help therapists adjust the pace and direction of the exposure. Such assessments also allow for nontreatment uses, such as screening for PTSD as well as prevention or stress inoculation. With regard to the latter, individual or group virtual training before deployment could enable soldiers to practice their duties in a simulated, stressful war environment, providing greater preparation and confidence for performance "under fire." This sort of training might do particularly well in addressing factors that have been associated strongly with risk for PTSD, including perceived preparedness for duties and unit cohesion. It might even be possible to monitor the success of training by measuring physiological responses.

Several efforts have been initiated along these lines (Cosic et al. 2010; Ilnicki et al. 2012; Rizzo et al. 2012). One of these in particular which is currently is in progress is STRIVE (STress Resilience In Virtual Environments). This project has taken the approach of recycling parts of the BRAVEMIND simulations to create emotionally challenging combat situations as contexts for experiential learning of cognitive–behavioral emotional coping and other psychological resilience strategies in service members before deployment (Rizzo et al. 2013). The process involves immersing and engaging service members within a variety of virtual "missions." Service members are confronted with the emotionally challenging situations inherent in a combat environment. Interaction by service members within such emotionally challenging scenarios aims to provide a more meaningful context in which to learn and practice psychoeducational and cognitive coping strategies. These strategies play a role in the psychological preparation for combat deployment. To accomplish this, STRIVE has been designed as a multiepisode interactive narrative in virtual reality that spans a typical deployment cycle. At the end of each of the graded 10-minute episodes, an emotionally challenging event occurs, designed in part from feedback provided by service members undergoing PTSD VRET (e.g., seeing/handling human remains, direct threat to safety via an improvised explosive device attack in a vehicle, moral challenges resulting from culturally relativistic events, the death of a civilian child, death of a squad member, grief processing in-theatre). At that point in the episode, the virtual world "freezes in place" and an interactive virtual human "mentor" emerges from the midst of the chaotic virtual reality scenario to guide the user through stress-related psychoeducational and self-management tactics, as well as provides rational restructuring exercises for appraising and processing the virtual experience. The resilience training component is drawing on evidence-based content that has been endorsed as part of standard classroom-delivered DoD resilience training programs, as well as content that has been applied successfully in nonmilitary contexts (e.g., humanitarian worker training, sports psychology). In this fashion, STRIVE provides a digital "emotional obstacle course" that can be used as a tool for providing context-relevant learning of emotional coping strategies under very tightly controlled and scripted simulated conditions. Training in this format is hypothesized to improve generalization to real-world situations via a state-dependent learning component (Godden & Baddeley 1980) and further supports resilience by leveraging the learning theory process of latent inhibition. Latent inhibition refers to the delayed learning that occurs as a result of preexposure to a stimulus without a consequence (Feldner et al. 2007; Lubow & Moore 1959). Thus, the exposure to a simulated combat context is believed to decrease the likelihood of fear conditioning during the real event (Sones et al. 2011).

Similarly, elements of BRAVEMIND have been tailored for use in conjunction with psychophysiological assessments to facilitate risk stratification of service members for the development of PTSD following their deployment. We have documented that physiological responses, most notably heart rate, correlate with PTSD symptom severity in recently returned service members, but further research is needed to determine whether physiological responses to the virtual environment can be used to help determine who warrants intervention for PTSD and which intervention would be most efficacious. We monitored multiple physiological responses to three unique 2-minute virtual reality scenarios taken from the Virtual Iraq simulation in a cohort of 81 U.S. military service members—who did not meet criteria for

PTSD, depression, or postconcussive syndrome—within 2 months after their return from Iraq or Afghanistan (Roy et al. 2013). Two of the sequences were presented from the perspective of a Humvee in a convoy confronted with improvised explosive devices and ambushes (convoy 1, gunner position and convoy 2, cabin of a Humvee), whereas the third featured a foot patrol through a village marketplace replete with explosions and terrorists firing rocket-propelled grenades (city). We used serial univariate and multivariate regression analyses to demonstrate a significant association between heart rate response to all three virtual reality sequences and overall PTSD symptoms as measured by the self-administered PCL-M, with heart rate explaining 14% of the variance in PCL-M score. HR and skin conductance together were more potent in explaining the variance in the gold standard CAPS total score (21% of variance) as well as Cluster D symptoms (20%), whereas heart rate alone correlated best with Cluster B symptoms (23%) and Cluster D PTSD symptoms (32% of variance). Subthreshold PTSD symptoms have been linked previously to significant functional impairment and risk for developing full PTSD (Cukor 2010), so the ability to distinguish them physiologically could prove helpful in enabling targeted intervention. This study identifies a novel additional application for virtual reality: helping to define the severity of symptoms and providing important insight into the utility of using multimodal tools of assessment. Other investigators have also been examining whether immersion in a virtual environment before deployment, or other stressors, for that matter, might be beneficial (Cosic, Popovic, Kulolja, Horvat, & Dropuljic, 2010; Ilnicki, Wiederhold, Maciolek, et al. 2012; Rizzo et al. 2012). Demonstration of benefit is likely to require relatively large numbers, though, because most will not develop PTSD even in the absence of intervention.

CONCLUSION

VRET has become a viable option for the treatment of PTSD during the past decade, although current and future studies will help to define more completely how well it compares with alternatives and whether there is a way to identify those most likely to benefit from this approach.

This work can also be viewed in a larger context when considering the impact of war on driving innovation in behavioral health care and thinking, If one reviews the history of war's impact on advances in clinical care, it could be suggested that the use of new technologies such as virtual reality to address clinical challenges may be an idea whose time has come. For example, during World War I, the Army Alpha/Beta Classification Test emerged from the need for better cognitive ability assessment; that innovative development later set the stage for the civilian intelligence testing movement during the early to mid 20th century. In addition, the birth of clinical psychology as a treatment-oriented profession was borne from the need to provide care for the many veterans returning from World War II with "shell shock." This led to the formation of the VA psychology internship program in 1946, which was instrumental in advancing the field of clinical psychology. Moreover, the National Institute of Mental Health was founded in 1948, and was charged by President Truman to address the problems of soldiers and veterans with "combat neurosis" (Insel, 2013). More recently, the Vietnam War drove the recognition of PTSD as a definable and treatable clinical health condition. In a similar fashion, one of the clinical "game-changing" outcomes of the OIF/OEF conflicts could derive from the DoD's/VA's support for research and development in the area of new technologies for the delivery and wider dissemination of care. New technologies seen in the form of mobile applications, teletherapy systems, Web-based systems, and virtual reality are changing the military behavioral health landscape and are being investigated at a pace that might not have occurred within a peacetime civilian context. The DoD/VA research programs that have support technology-based behavioral health systems in general, and virtual reality specifically, could be the driver of increased recognition and adoption within the civilian sector and may lead to quantum advances in clinical outreach and outcomes. As we have seen throughout history, innovations that emerge in military health care, driven by the urgency of war, typically have a lasting influence on civilian health care long after the last shot is fired. Thus, although much of the work with VRET to date has been done in a military population, there is no reason to believe that it will not be applicable to civilian populations as well, but further study is needed to expand on the work done with 9/11-related PTSD to demonstrate this. Some have expressed concerns that civilian trauma may be more diverse and difficult to replicate, or that virtual reality may be more problematic to apply to some common causes of PTSD, such as rape. However, BRAVEMIND has a wide variety of user-friendly features available to enable therapists to recreate cogent elements of patients' traumas, and it should not be more difficult to do the same for civilians. Furthermore, a recent addition to BRAVEMIND incorporates elements to address victims of military sexual trauma specifically and, although it has yet to be validated, this is evidence that palatable virtual environments can be developed to address a considerable range of trauma. It is likely that VRE interventions for PTSD will continue to drive novel research, which will help to address the significant clinical and social welfare challenges that exist in those who have experienced trauma.

At this juncture, it is important to demonstrate positive efficacy and cost–benefit outcomes from research with these military-based virtual reality applications. As in all areas of new technology design and development, it is easy for one to get caught up in the excitement that surrounds the potential for innovative clinical opportunities, while casting a blind eye to the pragmatic challenges that exist for building and disseminating useful and usable applications. Thus far, rational minds have prevailed among clinical virtual reality developers and clinicians, most of whom have approached this area with an honest measure of enthusiastic vision, good science, and healthy skepticism. This has led to a growing interest in virtual reality within the healthcare community because clinical tests are demonstrating incrementally that virtual reality can be implemented safely, at a reasonable cost, and that it has now begun to yield clinical outcomes that are at the least equivalent to, and sometimes more effective than, more traditional approaches. Thus, any rush to adopt virtual reality should not disregard principles of evidence-based and ethical clinical practice. In the end, technology is really no more than a tool. The technology, in and of itself, does not "fix" anybody. Rather, these systems are designed either to train or to extend the skills of a well-trained clinician. These systems, although providing treatment options not possible until recently, will most likely produce therapeutic benefits when administered within the context of appropriate care via a thoughtful and professional appreciation of the complexity of these important behavioral healthcare challenges.

KEY POINTS

- VRET provides an alternative to imaginal exposure therapy for PTSD, which may be particularly appealing to younger, more technologically savvy patients.
- To date, there is more experience with VRET in combat-related PTSD than with civilian trauma.
- BRAVEMIND represents a particularly robust, adaptable, and sophisticated virtual environment for addressing combat-related PTSD.
- Psychophysiological responses to VRE appear to be proportionate to PTSD symptom severity and may afford a risk stratification method in the aftermath of trauma.
- Virtual environments may also be used to promote resilience in advance of traumatic exposure, such as combat.
- Low-dose DCS augmentation of VRET sessions may enhance response rates.

- Further study is required to define more completely the potential benefits of VRET and to determine whether there are particular subsets of the population with PTSD for whom it may be most effective.

DISCLAIMER

The views expressed herein are solely the views of the authors and do not necessarily represent those of Uniformed Services University, the DoD, or the U.S. government.

DISCLOSURE

Dr. Rothbaum is a consultant to and owns equity in Virtually Better, Inc., which is developing products related to virtual reality research. However, Virtually Better did not create the Virtual Iraq environment described in this chapter. The terms of this arrangement have been reviewed and approved by Emory University in accordance with its conflict-of-interest policies.

REFERENCES

American Psychiatric Association: *Diagnostic and Statistical Manual of Mental Disorders, Fourth Edition*. Washington, D.C.: American Psychiatric Association, 1994.

Anderson P, Rothbaum BO, Hodges LF: Virtual reality exposure in the treatment of social anxiety: two case reports. Cogn Behav Pract 10:240–247, 2003.

Aukstakalnis S, Blatner D: The art and science of virtual reality. Berkeley, CA, Peachpit Press, 1992.

Ballenger JC, Davidson JR, Lecrubier Y, et al.: Consensus statement on posttraumatic stress disorder from the International Consensus Group on Depression and Anxiety. J Clin Psychiatry 61:60–66, 2000.

Beck JG, Palyo SA, Winer EH, Schwagler BE, Ang EJ: Virtual reality exposure therapy for PTSD symptoms after a road accident: an uncontrolled case series. Behav Ther 38(1):39–48, 2007.

Beidel DC, Frueh BC, Uhde TW, Wong N, Mentrikowski JM: Multicomponent behavioral treatment for chronic combat-related posttraumatic stress disorder: a randomized controlled trial. J Anxiety Disord 25:224–231, 2011.

Berg AO, Breslau N, Lezak MD, et al.: Treatment of posttraumatic stress disorder: an assessment of the evidence. Washington, DC, National Academies Press, 2008.

Bordnick P, Graap K, Copp H, et al.: Virtual reality cue reactivity assessment in cigarette smokers. Cyberpsychol Behav 8:487–492, 2005.

Botella C, Banos RM, Perpiná C, Villa, H, Alcaniz, M, Rey, A: Virtual reality treatment of claustrophobia: a case report. Behav Res Ther 36:239–246, 1998.

Botella C, Banos RM, Villa H, et al.: Virtual reality in the treatment of claustrophobic fear: a controlled, multiple-baseline design. Behav Ther 33:583–595, 2000.

Botella C, Osma J, Garcia-Palacios A, et al.: Treatment of flying phobia using virtual reality: data from a 1-year follow-up using a multiple baseline design. Clin Psychol Psychother 11:311–323, 2004.

Britt TW: The stigma of psychological problems in a work environment: evidence from the screening of service members returning from Bosnia. J Appl Physiol 30:1599–1618, 2000.

Brooks BM, Attree EA, Rose FD, Clifford BR, Leadbetter AG: The specificity of memory enhancement during interaction with a virtual environment. Memory 7:65–78, 1999.

Brown DJ, Standen PJ, Cobb SV: Virtual environments special needs and evaluative methods. Stud Health Technol Inform 58:91–102, 1998.

Buckwalter JG, Rizzo AA, John BS, et al. Analyzing the impact of stress: A comparison between a factor analytic and a composite measure of allostatic load. Proceedings of the Interservice/Industry Training, Simulation and Education Conference. 2011. Accessible online at http://ntsa.metapress.com/link.asp?id=69725r5332425l33.

Canadian Agency for Drugs and Technologies in Health: Virtual reality exposure therapy for adults with post-traumatic stress disorder: a review of the clinical effectiveness. Ottawa, ON, Canadian Agency for Drugs and Technologies in Health, 2014.

Cardena E, Spiegel D: Dissociative reactions to the San Francisco Bay Area earthquake of 1989. Am J Psychiatry 150:474–478, 1993.

Carlin AS, Hoffman HG, Weghorst S: Virtual reality and tactile augmentation in the treatment of spider phobia: a case report. Behav Res Ther 35:153–158, 1997.

Cosic K, Popovic S, Kulolja D, Horvat M, Dropuljic B: Physiology-driven adaptive virtual reality stimulation for prevention and treatment of stress related disorders. Cyberpsychol Behav Soc Netw 13:73–78, 2010.

Cukor J, Wyka K, Javasinghe N, Difede J: The nature and course of subthreshold PTSD. J Anxiety Disord 24:918–923, 2010.

Davis M, Ressler K, Rothbaum BO, et al.: Effects of D-cycloserine on extinction: translation from pre-clinical to clinical work. Biol Psychiatry 60:369–375, 2006.

de Kleine RA, Hendriks JG, Kusters WJ, Broekman TG, van Minnen A: A randomized placebo-controlled trial of D-cycloserine to enhance exposure therapy for posttraumatic stress disorder. Biol Psychiatry 71:962–968, 2012.

Difede J, Cukor J, Jayasinghe N, et al.: Virtual reality exposure therapy for the treatment of posttraumatic stress disorder following September 11, 2001. J Clin Psychiatry 68:1639–1647, 2007.

Difede J, Cukor J, Patt I, et al.: The application of virtual reality to the treatment of PTSD following the WTC attack. Ann N Y Acad Sci 1071:500–501, 2006.

Difede J, Cukor J, Wyka K, Olden M, Hoffman H, Lee FS, Altemus M: D-cycloserine augmentation of exposure therapy for post-traumatic stress disorder: a pilot randomized clinical trial. Neuropsychopharmacology 39:1052–1058, 2014.

Difede J, Hoffman HG: Virtual reality exposure therapy for World Trade Center posttraumatic stress disorder: a case report. Cyberpsychol Behav 5:529–535, 2002.

Difede J, Hoffman H, Jaysinghe N: Innovative use of virtual reality technology in the treatment of PTSD in the aftermath of September 11. Psychiatr Serv 53:1083–1085, 2002.

Emmelkamp PM, Bruynzeel M, Drost L, et al.: Virtual reality treatment in acrophobia: a comparison with exposure in vivo. Cyberpsychol Behav 4:335–339, 2001.

Feldner MT, Monson CM, Friedman MJ: A critical analysis of approaches to targeted PTSD prevention: current status and theoretically derived future directions. Behav Modification 31:80–116, 2007.

Foa EB, Kozak MJ: Emotional processing of fear: exposure to corrective information. Psychol Bull 99:20–35, 1986.

Foa EB, Davidson RT, Frances A: Expert Consensus Guideline Series: treatment of posttraumatic stress disorder. J Clin Psychiatry 60:5–76, 1999.

Foa EB, Riggs DS, Massie ED, et al.: The impact of fear activation and anger on the efficacy of exposure treatment for PTSD. Behav Ther 26:487–499, 1995.

Gamito P, Oliveira J, Rosa P, et al.: PTSD elderly war veterans: a clinical controlled pilot study. Cyberpsychology Behavior and Social Networking 13:43–48, 2010.

Garcia-Palacios A, Hoffman H, Carlin A, et al.: Virtual reality in the treatment of spider phobia: a controlled study. Behav Res Ther 40:983–993, 2002.

Gerardi M, Rothbaum BO, Ressler K, et al.: Virtual reality exposure therapy using a Virtual Iraq: case report. J Trauma Stress 21:209–213, 2008.

Glantz K, Rizzo AA, Graap K: Virtual reality for psychotherapy: current reality and future possibilities. Psychotherapy: Theory, Research, Practice, Training 40:55–67, 2003.

Godden DR, Baddeley AD: When does context influence recognition memory? British Journal of Psychology 71:99–104, 1980.

Gold JI, Kim SH, Kant AJ, Joseph, MH, Rizzo, AA: Virtual anesthesia: the use of virtual reality for pain distraction during acute medical interventions. Semin Anesth Periop Med Pain 24:203–210, 2005.

Goncalves R, Pedrozo AL, Coutinho ESF, Figueira I, Ventura P: Efficacy of virtual reality exposure therapy in the treatment of PTSD: a systematic review. PLoS One 7(12):e48469, 2012.

Guastella AJ, Richardson R, Lovibond PF, et al.: A randomized controlled trial of D-cycloserine enhancement of exposure therapy for social anxiety disorder. Biol Psychiatry 63:544–549, 2008.

Hofmann SG, Meuret AE, Smits JA, et al.: Augmentation of exposure therapy with D-cycloserine for social anxiety disorder. Arch Gen Psychiatry 63:298–304, 2006.

Hoge CW, Castro CA, Messer SC, et al.: Combat duty in Iraq and Afghanistan, mental health problems, and barriers to care. N Engl J Med 351:13–22, 2004.

Ilnicki S, Wiederhold BK, Maciolek J, et al.: Effectiveness evaluation for short-term group predeployment VR computer-assisted stress inoculation training provided to Polish ISAF soldiers. Stud Health Technol Inform 181:113–117, 2012.

Insel T: NIMH director's blog. August 13, 2013. Accessible online at http://www.nimh.nih.gov/about/director/2013/healing-invisible-wounds-an-action-plan.shtml.

Jaycox LH, Foa EB, Morral AR: Influence of emotional engagement and habituation on exposure therapy for PTSD. J Consult Clin Psychol 66:185–192, 1998.

Jaycox LH, Zoellner L, Foa EB: Cognitive–behavior therapy for PTSD in rape survivors. J Clin Psychol 58:891–906, 2002.

Klinger E, Bouchard S, Legeron, S, Roy, S, Lauer, F, Chemin, I, Nugues, P: Virtual reality therapy versus cognitive behaviour therapy for social phobia: a preliminary controlled study. Cyberpsychol Behav 8:76–88, 2005.

Koopman C, Classen C, Spiegel D: Predictors of posttraumatic stress symptoms among survivors of the Oakland/Berkeley, Calif, firestorm. Am J Psychiatry 151:888–894, 1994.

Krijn M, Emmelkamp PM, Olafsson RP, et al.: Virtual reality exposure therapy of anxiety disorders: a review. Clin Psychol Rev 24:259–281, 2004.

Kushner MG, Kim SW, Donahue C, et al.: D-cycloserine augmented exposure therapy for obsessive–compulsive disorder. Biol Psychiatry 62:835–838, 2007.

Litz, BT, Salters-Pedneault K, Steenkamp MM, Hermos JA, Bryant RA, Otto MW & Hofmann S. A randomized placebo-controlled trial of D-cycloserine and exposure therapy for posttraumatic stress disorder. J Psychiatr Research 46, 1184–1190, 2012.

Lubow RE, Moore AU: Latent inhibition: the effect of non-reinforced exposure to the conditioned stimulus. J Comp Physiol Psychol 52:415–419, 1959.

Matheis RJ, Schultheis MT, Tiersky LA, DeLuca J, Millis SR, Rizzo A: Is learning and memory different in a virtual environment? Clin Neuropsychol 21:146–161, 2007.

McLay RN, Wood DP, Webb-Murphy JA, Spira JL, Wiederhold MD, et al.: Randomized, controlled trial of virtual reality-graded exposure therapy for post-traumatic stress disorder. Cyberpsychol Behav and Soc Netw14:223–229, 2011.

Morrow K, Docan C, Burdea G, Merians, A: Low-cost virtual rehabilitation of the hand for patients post-stroke. IEEE Explore, 2006, pp. 6–10 Available at: http://ieeexplore.ieee.org/xpl/login.jsp?tp=&arnumber=1707518&url=http%3A%2F%2Fieeexplore.ieee.org%2Fxpls%2Fabs_all.jsp%3Farnumber%3D1707518

Parsons TD, Rizzo AA: Initial validation of a virtual reality environment for assessment of memory function: virtual reality cognitive performance assessment test. Cyberpsychol Behav 11:17–25, 2008.

Powers MB, Emmelkamp PM: Virtual reality exposure therapy for anxiety disorders: a meta-analysis. J Anxiety Disord 39:250–261, 2008.

Pugnetti L, Mendozzi L, Molta A, Cattaneo A, Barbieri E, Brancotti A: Evaluation and retraining of adults' cognitive impairment: which role for virtual reality technology? Comput Biol Med 25:213–217, 1995.

Rauch SA, King AP, Abelson J, et al.: Biological and symptom changes in posttraumatic stress disorder treatment: a randomized clinical trial. Depress Anxiety 32:204–212, 2015.

Reger GM, Gahm GA: Virtual reality exposure therapy for active duty soldiers. J Clin Psychol 64:940–946, 2008.

Reger GM, Holloway KM, Candy C, Rothbaum BO, Difede J, Rizzo AA, Gahm GA: Effectiveness of virtual reality exposure therapy for active duty soldiers in a military mental health clinic. J Trauma Stress 24:93–96, 2011.

Ressler KJ, Rothbaum BO, Tannenbaum L, et al.: Cognitive enhancers as adjuncts to psychotherapy: use of D-cycloserine in phobic individuals to facilitate extinction of fear. Arch Gen Psychiatry 61:1136–1144, 2004.

Riva G. The key to unlocking the virtual body: virtual reality in the treatment of obesity and eating disorders. J Diabetes Sci Technol 5:283–292, 2011.

Rizzo AA, Bowerly T, Buckwalter JG, Mitura R, Parsons TD: A virtual reality scenario for all seasons: the virtual classroom. CNS Spectr 11:35–44, 2006.

Rizzo AA, Buckwalter JG, Forbell E, Difede J, Rothbaum BO, Lange B, Koenig S, Talbot B: Virtual reality applications to address the wounds of war. Psychiatr Ann 43:123–138, 2013.

Rizzo A, Buckwalter JG, John B, Newman B, Parsons T, Kenny P, Williams J: STRIVE: Stress Resilience in Virtual Environments: a pre-deployment VR system for training emotional coping skills and assessing chronic and acute stress responses. Stud Health Technol Inform 173:379–385, 2012.

Rizzo AA, Difede J, Rothbaum BO, Johnston S, McLay RN, Reger G, Gahm G, Parsons T, Graap K, Pair J: VR PTSD Exposure Therapy Results with Active Duty Iraq War Combatants. Stud Health Technol Inform 132:420–425, 2008.

Rizzo AA, Kim G: A SWOT analysis of the field of virtual rehabilitation and therapy. Presence Teleoperators Virtual Environ 14:1–28, 2005.

Rizzo AA, Schultheis MT, Kerns K, et al.: Analysis of assets for virtual reality applications in neuropsychology. Neuropsychol Rehabil 14:207–239, 2004.

Rizzo AA, Wiederhold M, Buckwalter JG: Basic issues in the use of virtual environments for mental health applications. In Virtual reality in clinical psychology and neuroscience. Edited by Riva G, Wiederhold B, Molinari E. Amsterdam, The Netherlands, IOS Press, 1998, pp 21–42.

Rose FD, Brooks BM, Rizzo AA: Virtual reality in brain damage rehabilitation: review. Cyberpsychol Behav 8:241–262, 2005.

Rothbaum BO: Critical parameters for D-cycloserine enhancement of cognitive–behavioral therapy for obsessive–compulsive disorder. Am J Psychiatry 165:293–296, 2008.

Rothbaum BO, Anderson P, Zimand E, et al.: Virtual reality exposure therapy and standard (in vivo) exposure therapy in the treatment of fear of flying. Behav Ther 37:80–90, 2006.

Rothbaum BO, Hodges LF: The use of virtual reality exposure in the treatment of anxiety disorders. Behav Modif 23:507–525, 1999.

Rothbaum BO, Hodges L, Anderson PL, et al.: Twelve-month follow-up of virtual reality and standard exposure therapies for the fear of flying. J Consult Clin Psychol 70:428–432, 2002.

Rothbaum BO, Hodges LF, Kooper R, et al.: Effectiveness of virtual reality graded exposure in the treatment of acrophobia. Am J Psychiatry 152:626–628, 1995.

Rothbaum BO, Hodges LF, Ready D, et al.: Virtual reality exposure therapy for Vietnam veterans with posttraumatic stress disorder. J Clin Psychiatry 62:617–622, 2001.

Rothbaum BO, Hodges L, Smith S, et al.: A controlled study of virtual reality exposure therapy for the fear of flying. J Consult Clin Psychol 68:1020–1026, 2000a.

Rothbaum BO, Hodges L, Watson BA, et al.: Virtual reality exposure therapy in the treatment of fear of flying: a case report. Behav Res Ther 34:477–481, 1996.

Rothbaum BO, Meadows EA, Resick P, et al.: Cognitive–behavioral treatment position paper summary for the ISTSS Treatment Guidelines Committee. J Trauma Stress 13:558–563, 2000b.

Rothbaum BO, Price M, Jovanovic T, Norrholm S, Gerardi M, Dunlop B, Davis M, Bradley B, Duncan EJ, Rizzo A, Ressler K: A randomized, double-blind evaluation of D-cycloserine or alprazolam combined with virtual reality exposure therapy for posttraumatic stress disorder (PTSD) in OEF/OIF war veterans. Am J Psychiatry 171: 640–648, 2014.

Rothbaum BO, Rizzo AS, Difede J: Virtual reality exposure therapy for combat-related posttraumatic stress disorder. Ann NY Acad Sci 1208:126–132, 2010.

Roy MJ, Costanzo M, Jovanovic T, Leaman S, Taylor P, Norrholm SD, Rizzo AA: Heart rate response to fear conditioning and virtual reality in subthreshold PTSD. Stud Health Technol Inform 191:115–119, 2013.

Roy MJ, Costanzo M, Blair J, Rizzo A: Compelling evidence that exposure therapy for PTSD normalizes brain function. Stud Health Technol Inform 199:61–65, 2014.

Roy MJ, Francis J, Friedlander J, Banks-Williams L, Lande RJ, Taylor P, Blair J, McLellan J, Law WA, Tarpley VK, Patt I, Yu H, Mallinger A, Difede J, Rizzo A, Rothbaum BO: Improvement in cerebral function with treatment of posttraumatic stress disorder. Ann N Y Acad Sci 1208:142–149, 2010.

Schnurr PP, Friedman MJ, Engel CC, et al.: Cognitive behavioral therapy for posttraumatic stress disorder in women: a randomized controlled trial. JAMA 297:820–830, 2007.

Smith SG, Rothbaum BO, Hodges L: Treatment of fear of flying using virtual reality exposure therapy: a single case study. Behav Therap 22:154–158, 1999.

Sones HM, Thorp, SR, Raskind M: Prevention of posttraumatic stress disorder. Psychiatr Clin North Am 34:79–94, 2011.

Storch EA, Merlo LJ, Bengtson M, et al.: D-cycloserine does not enhance exposure–response prevention therapy in obsessive–compulsive disorder. Int Clin Psychopharmacol 22:230–237, 2007.

Walshe DG, Lewis EJ, Kim SI, et al.: Exploring the use of computer games and virtual reality in exposure therapy for fear of driving following a motor vehicle accident. Cyberpsychol Behav 6:329–334, 2003.

Warner CH, Appenzeller GN, Mullen K, et al.: Soldier attitudes toward mental health screening and seeking care upon return from combat. Mil Med 173:563–569, 2008.

Weathers FW, Litz BT, Herman DS, et al.: The PTSD Checklist (PCL): reliability, validity, and diagnostic utility [abstract]. International Society for Traumatic Stress Studies. October 1993. Accessible online at http://www.pdhealth.mil/library/downloads/pcl_sychometrics.doc.

Wiederhold BK, Wiederhold MD: Three-year follow-up for the treatment of fear of flying: a controlled investigation. J Consult Clin Psychol 70:1112–1118, 2002.

Wilhelm S, Buhlman U, Tolin DF, et al.: Augmentation of behavior therapy with D-cycloserine for obsessive–compulsive disorder. Am J Psychiatry 165:335–341, 2008.

Wood DP, Murphy JA, McLay R, Koffman R, Spira J, et al.: Cost-effectiveness of virtual reality graded exposure therapy with physiological monitoring for the treatment of combat related post traumatic stress disorder. Stud Health Technol Inform 144:223–229, 2009.

Yehuda R, Pratchett LC, Elmes MW, et al.: Glucocorticoid-related predictors and correlates of posttraumatic stress disorder treatment response in combat veterans. Interface Focus 4:20140048, 2014.

FOURTEEN

Internet and Computer-Based Treatments for the Management of PTSD

BRADLEY E. BELSHER, DANIEL P. EVATT, MICHAEL C. FREED, AND CHARLES C. ENGEL

A RAPID EXPANSION IN THE DEVELOPMENT OF TELEHEALTH TREATMENTS HAS OC-curred during the past several decades, with a growing body of evidence supporting online therapies for behavioral health disorders (Andrews, Cuijpers, Craske, McEvoy, & Titov, 2010; Cuijpers et al., 2009; Hedman, Ljotsson, & Lindefors, 2012; Reger & Gahm, 2009; Spek et al., 2007). These online interventions have focused primarily on the treatment of depression, panic disorder, social phobia, and generalized anxiety disorder (Andrews et al., 2010). More recently, and with the relative success of the previous Web-based treatments, several online treatments for posttraumatic stress disorder (PTSD) have emerged. This chapter provides an overview of Internet and computer-based treatments (ICTs) for PTSD. The chapter begins with a general discussion of computerized treatments followed by a review of specific ICTs that have been developed and tested for PTSD. In the second half of the chapter, some of the critical issues surrounding ICTs are explored, and an example of how online treatments can be incorporated into a larger care model is presented. The chapter concludes with a brief discussion on the use of mobile health applications to augment treatment.

The views expressed in this article are those of the authors and do not necessarily represent the views of the Department of Defense, the US Government, or any other organization or agency, public or private.

Telemental health refers to behavioral health services that use communication technology for assessment, treatment, and consultative purposes (Field, 1996). Telemental health can use a variety of technologies to improve care, including video teleconferencing technology, virtual reality, and Internet- and computer-based technology. Although all media of telehealth technology offer specific advantages, the versatility of ICTs are appealing in terms of their potential to increase treatment reach. With four of five people in the United States owning a computer or enjoying Internet access (Miniwatts Marketing Group, 2015a), ICTs can, theoretically, reach a large population of individuals regardless of geographic location or logistical barriers. ICTs are accessible by patients at any time of day or night without the need to coordinate a specific time with a supporting clinician. Certain ICTs can be delivered without therapist support or with minimal and remote guidance, reducing healthcare costs and freeing up system resources. Based on these advantages, ICTs have gained popularity as a potential solution to improve care access for patients with PTSD.

The majority of individuals with PTSD do not receive adequate care (Hoge et al., 2004; Jaycox, Marshall, & Schell, 2004; Kimerling & Calhoun, 1994; Spoont, Murdoch, Hodges, & Nugent, 2010; Trusz, Wagner, Russo, Love, & Zatzick, 2011; Zatzick, 2003). The consequences of inadequate treatment for PTSD are considerable. Left untreated, PTSD may develop into a chronic condition that engenders significant social and functional impairment (Davidson, Stein, Shalev, & Yehuda, 2004; Ormel et al., 2008). From a societal perspective, the economic burden of PTSD is high. For instance, in the Military Health System alone, the 2-year estimated costs associated with untreated PTSD and depression ranges from $4 billion to $6 billion (Jaycox et al., 2004). Common treatment barriers that trauma survivors endorse include stigma concerns, treatment access issues, limited resources, and a desire to handle problems on one's own (Hoge et al., 2004; Jaycox et al., 2004; Kim, Thomas, Wilk, Castro, & Hoge, 2010; Ouimette et al., 2011; Trusz et al., 2011). ICTs have the potential to overcome many of these treatments barriers by delivering evidence-informed care directly to patients at their home or other private location.

Several ICTs for PTSD have been developed. These treatments are designed for preventive and treatment purposes. Preventive ICTs target members of an identified population who may be at greater risk for developing posttraumatic symptoms (e.g., disaster survivors). Treatment-oriented ICTs often complement or substitute for in-person care for patients with PTSD. Although preventive ICTs often consist of psychoeducation and skills training, treatment-oriented ICTs typically offer sequenced elements of evidence-based psychotherapy on par with clinical interventions.

ICTs often differ based on the degree of human support required. At one end of the spectrum are therapist-driven online interventions that require intensive specialist

TABLE 14.1 Defining Characteristics of Internet and Computer-Based Treatments

Integration Model

Stand-alone Model	Virtual Clinic	Integrated Care	Stepped Care
Treatments are available to consumers via online searches and advertisements.	Treatment is delivered over the Internet and is managed by mental health professional via phone and Internet.	Treatment is implemented and integrated in the context of healthcare practice.	Patients are matched to Internet and computer-based treatments based on preferences, symptoms, and treatment response.

Support Needed

None	Minimal	Moderate	High	Full
Self-help.	Limited guidance by a technician to remind patients to complete work.	More intensive support that may include e-mail, instant messaging, and telephone calls.	Greater support that can include face-to-face appointments and reliance on providers to deliver components of therapy	Treatment is fully dependent on the clinician and the Internet is used solely as a medium of communication.

Expertise Required

None	Low	Moderate	High
No requirement for support.	Technicians typically serve to remind patients to complete work and do not need knowledge of psychotherapeutic principles.	Some level of training is required, as is experience working within the mental health field and a familiarity with psychotherapeutic principles.	A high degree of specialization and familiarity with evidence-based principles of psychotherapy are required.

involvement throughout therapy; pure self-help treatments requiring no clinician involvement are at the other end of the spectrum. Research suggests that most patients prefer some therapist involvement (Casey, Joy, & Clough, 2013). Treatment adherence and outcomes may be better with this involvement (Gellatly et al., 2007; Hirai & Clum, 2006; Lewis, Pearce, & Bisson, 2012), and support by a nonclinician may be just as effective (Robinson et al., 2010; Titov, Andrews, Davies, et al., 2010). One meta-analysis found that online treatments with therapist support obtained large effect sizes whereas those without this support demonstrated small effect sizes (Spek et al., 2007). Clinician involvement in ICTs (i.e., whether to include, by whom, and how much) must be understood within the context of the purpose of the ICT. For instance, if the goal of an online treatment is wide dissemination for prevention purposes, requirements for intensive clinician involvement may tax resources unnecessarily and limit reach.

ICTs for PTSD also vary in the degree to which they are integrated into the larger healthcare system. Stand-alone ICTs are typically identified by consumers through online searches or outside provider recommendations. Other ICTs may be integrated more seamlessly into a system of care to replace, augment, or precede traditional mental health care. Notably, these distinctions can become arbitrary, such as when a stand-alone treatment becomes incorporated into a specialty or primary care setting. Table 14.1 distinguishes how ICTs may differ based on the relevant characteristics described.

ETHICAL AND LEGAL CONSIDERATIONS

Professional practice organizations and regulatory agencies have attempted to keep pace with the rapid advancements in telehealth-based interventions by developing legal and ethical guidelines surrounding the delivery of treatments. Telehealth treatments in general, and online treatments specifically, introduce a range of new ethical considerations surrounding patient care. Although many of the general standard ethics apply, online therapies introduce unique considerations regarding competency, informed consent, privacy and confidentiality, appropriateness of treatment, online assessment and diagnosis, boundaries, and crisis intervention. Professionals who plan to use online therapies should become familiar with the telehealth guidelines developed by their specific professional organizations, the laws and regulations within their jurisdiction, and the local institutional guidelines of their practice. For a more in-depth review on this topic, we encourage you to review Hilgart, Thorndike, Pardo, and Ritterband (2012). As with all clinical interventions, specific care delivery guidelines are context and population dependent and there remains a duty to ensure care is delivered safely and in ways that are consistent with local laws and regulatory constraints. Providers, patients, administrators, and policymakers alike should determine whether specific ICTs for PTSD are appropriate based on the peer-reviewed literature, best practices guidelines, and patient preferences. The following section reviews the available research on ICTs for PTSD.

EVIDENCE REVIEW ON PTSD ICTs

Extant PTSD treatment trials vary considerably in study design, population evaluated, inclusion/exclusion criteria, and outcomes measured. Given the heterogeneity across these investigations, general conclusions are relatively limited and it is useful to evaluate individual trials to glean more informative data. The treatments reviewed here comprise ICTs for PTSD identified through a comprehensive literature search. Treatments evaluated specifically in community samples are first described, followed by online therapies developed for military and veteran service members. Within each section, the randomized controlled trials (RCTs) are described before ICTs evaluated in less rigorous research designs (e.g., open trials). A breakdown of these treatments is listed in Table 14.2.

General Population

Interapy

The first controlled trials evaluating an ICT for PTSD emerged from the Netherlands in 2001 with Interapy (Lange et al., 2003; Lange, van de Ven, Schrieken, & Emmelkamp, 2001). Interapy for PTSD consists of a 5-week protocol that requires high levels of therapist involvement throughout the treatment. Patients complete a structured online writing assignment twice a week over a 5-week period. The writing assignments aim to promote exposure and habituation to traumatic memories, and encourage cognitive restructuring of problematic beliefs. The assigned therapist reviews the narratives regularly, presents tailored feedback, and provides guidance on how to proceed with the next writing assignment (all via the secured website). Therapists dedicate around 14 hours per patient throughout the course of treatment (Marks et al., 2009). In the Netherlands, Interapy is currently a fee-based, closed-access treatment offered through virtual clinics and reimbursable by insurance. Virtual clinics operate from a centralized location and provide online treatments for a range of mental health disorders.

Three RCTs conducted on Interapy for PTSD demonstrated that treatment completers experience significant reductions in PTSD symptoms compared with patients in a wait-list control group (Knaevelsrud & Maercker, 2007; Lange et al., 2001; Lange et al., 2003). The improvements were maintained up to 18 months posttreatment in

TABLE 14.2 Research Trials on ICT for PTSD

Reference	ICT	RCT	CG Used	N	Sample	AR (%)	ES[a]
Lange et al. (2001)	Interapy	Yes	Wait list	30	Netherlands students	13	1.49–1.97
Lange et al. (2003)	Interapy	Yes	Wait list	184	Netherlands civilians	36	1.28–1.39
Knaevelsrud and Maercker (2007)	Interapy	Yes	Wait list	96	German Civilian	16	0.98–1.41
Litz et al. (2007)	DE-STRESS	Yes	Online placebo	45	U.S. military	30	0.41–0.95
Engel et al. (2015)	DESTRESS-PC	Yes	TAU	80	U.S. military	13	0.08–0.47
Ivarrson et al. (2014)	Guided ICBT for PTSD	Yes	Online placebo	62	Netherlands civilian	13	1.25
Craske et al. (2011)	CALM Tools for Living	Yes	TAU	1004	U.S. primary care	20	0.29–0.48
Spence et al. (2011)	The PTSD Program	Yes	Wait list	42	Australian civilian	8	0.47
Possemato et al. (2011)	Written Emotional Disclosure	Yes	Online placebo	31	U.S. military veterans	0	None reported
Hirai and Clum (2005)	Self-help for Traumatic Consequences	Yes	Wait list	33	U.S. students	28	0.62–0.80
Brief et al. (2013)	VetChange	Yes	Wait list	617	U.S. veterans	66	None reported
Hobfoll et al. (2015)	VETS PREVAIL	Yes	Wait list	303	U.S. military veterans	34	0.30
Klein et al. (2010)	PTSD Online	No	N/A	22	Australian civilians	27	N/A
Ruggiero et al. (2006)	Treatment for disaster-affected populations	No	N/A	285	New York residents	44	N/A
Bush et al. (2014)	Afterdeployment.org	No	N/A	11	College veterans	0	N/A
Belsher et al. (2015)	Afterdeployment.org	No	N/A	24	PTSD specialty clinic	50	N/A

AR, attrition rate; CALM, Coordinated Anxiety and Learning Management; CG, comparison group; DE-STRESS, Delivery of self training and education for stressful situations; DE-STRESS-PC, Delivery of self training and education for stressful situations - primary care; EF, effect size; ICT, Internet and computer-based treatments; N/A, not applicable; PTSD, posttraumatic stress disorder; RCT, randomized control trial; TAU, treatment as usual.

[a]Effect size (between treatment arms) based on Cohen's D. Ranges indicate different effect sizes at different assessment points.

one study (Knaevelsrud & Maercker, 2010). Participants also reported significant reductions in other psychopathology, including depression, anxiety, somatization, and sleeping problems. Interapy has been evaluated primarily on younger females who have experienced traumas occurring 9 to 10 years before treatment, limiting the generalizability of the findings to other groups. In one trial, dropout rates were high, with more than one-third of participants dropping from treatment (Lange et al., 2003). Emotional distress and technical problems were the primary reasons reported by participants for dropping out of treatment (Knaevelsrud & Maercker, 2007; Lange et al., 2003). Interapy demonstrates promising findings, although high attrition rates and intensive clinician involvement must be taken into account when considering this intervention.

The PTSD Program

The PTSD Program (Spence et al., 2011) is a cognitive–behavioral therapy (CBT)-based intervention that consists of seven online sessions. Therapist assistance is included in the treatment via several media (telephone, e-mail, online forums). Clinicians perform diagnostic interviews initially over the phone and then encourage eligible participants to initiate the online treatment. There is homework for each session and participants are encouraged to engage in an online discussion forum moderated by a clinical psychologist who posts comments. The clinician calls and e-mails patients on a weekly basis to monitor symptoms, provide support, and clarify any questions about the online materials.

An RCT conducted on an Australian community sample ($N = 42$) demonstrated that participants who engaged in The PTSD Program experienced significant reductions in PTSD, depression, and generalized anxiety symptoms compared with a wait-list condition (Spence et al., 2011). The participants evaluated in this trial were primarily educated females with moderate to high PTSD symptoms related to physical or sexual assault and/or transportation accidents. The treatment outcomes were not related to pretreatment PTSD severity or number of comorbid conditions. Adherence rates were high and more than 90% of the treatment group completed all the modules. In a subsequent trial, it was determined that The PTSD Program without the exposure component was equally efficacious as the original intervention (Spence et al., 2014).

Guided ICBT for PTSD

Guided ICBT for PTSD consists of eight CBT-based modules accompanied by written homework assignments reviewed by a therapist on a weekly basis. Participants gain access to subsequent modules only if they complete current homework assignments. The therapist communicates with patients through a secured website to guide participants through the intervention, encourage completion of the modules, and provide individual feedback on completed assignments. Providers spend on average 28 minutes/week per patient (Ivarsson et al., 2014).

Guided ICBT for PTSD was evaluated among 62 Netherlands citizens who were diagnosed with PTSD through standardized measures (Ivarsson et al., 2014). The treatment was compared with a control condition in which participants were offered online information on general well-being. Typical participants were middle-age, educated woman reporting partner abuse or a life-threatening disease. Results of the trial indicated that participants in the treatment arm experienced significant reductions in PTSD and depressive symptoms relative to the control group. Posttreatment, 81.5% ($n = 22$) of the treated participants no longer met the criteria for PTSD compared with 38.9% ($n = 14$) in the control group. Results further suggested that treatment gains were maintained at the 1-year follow-up. Participants completed an average of 5.1 modules (standard deviation, 3.2), with 39% of participants completing all of the modules.

CALM Tools for Living

CALM Tools for Living is a computer-assisted CBT intervention developed to support clinicians' delivery of evidence-based therapy. The CALM intervention relies on intensive involvement by a clinician who views the online work with the patient, typically in-person. CALM was developed to be used with novice clinicians who get prompted by the online tool to help patients engage in specific tasks. CALM contains four different anxiety modules based on the patient's primary concern: PTSD, generalized anxiety disorder, social anxiety disorder, and panic disorder. Each module is eight sessions and includes two generic sessions focused on symptom monitoring and breathing retraining (shared by all the modules), followed by disorder-specific sessions that focus on exposure work and cognitive restructuring.

The CALM Tools for Living treatment was implemented and evaluated in a large effectiveness trial as part of a collaborative care intervention (Craske et al., 2011; Roy-Byrne et al., 2010). This trial enrolled more than 1000 primary care patients who were randomized to the collaborative care treatment or usual care. Patients randomized to the active intervention were offered the computer-assisted treatment, psychotropic medication, or both. Patient symptoms were monitored through a Web-based outcomes system to determine whether they achieved clinically significant improvement or required more intensive care. Of this large sample, one-third of patients chose and were treated exclusively with the ICT. Close to 90% of patients completed at least six modules. Patients reported high engagement in the treatment, and attrition rates were minimal across the trial. However, participants engaged in the online PTSD module did not experience statistically significant reductions in PTSD symptoms, possibly because of the small sample of patients treated for PTSD (6% of entire sample). Nevertheless, this large effectiveness trial demonstrates that computerized interventions can be implemented feasibly within larger care models and offered as one form of care.

Self-help for Traumatic Event-Related Consequences

Self-help for Traumatic Event-Related Consequences was developed and evaluated as a computerized CBT intervention that limits therapeutic contact to brief e-mail reminders to complete assignments (Hirai & Clum, 2005). The intervention consists of an 8-week program that includes modules on psychoeducation, relaxation training, cognitive restructuring, and exposure. In a study of university and community participants ($N = 33$), 5 of the 18 participants (28%) randomized to the active intervention dropped out. Analyses of the treatment completers indicated the treatment resulted in significant reductions in trauma-related avoidance and intrusion frequency, and improvements in coping efficacy, compared with the wait-list control group (Hirai & Clum, 2005). Participants were primarily female and most met subthreshold PTSD criteria only. Individuals with a history of childhood sexual abuse or combat-related trauma were excluded from the study.

PTSD Online

PTSD Online is a clinician-supported PTSD intervention evaluated in a small open trial with an Australian community sample ($N = 22$). The treatment includes modules on relaxation training, cognitive restructuring, exposure work, and relapse prevention (Klein et al., 2009; Klein et al., 2010). The online treatment is 10 weeks and users complete weekly modules and communicate with their therapist through e-mail. Results from the open trial indicated that treatment completers reported significant decreases in PTSD symptoms posttreatment and at 3 months (Klein et al., 2010). Future studies on PTSD Online that include a larger sample size and validated measures, and use a comparison group are required to establish the efficacy of this intervention.

Online Treatment for Disaster-Affected Populations

Ruggiero et al. (2006) evaluated an anonymous, preventive ICT developed for survivors of major disasters. The program uses a filtering process to tailor treatments based on presenting concerns and includes different modules for trauma survivors: PTSD/Panic, Depression, Alcohol, Marijuana, Drug, Smoking, and Worry. The modules are brief and consist of a single session only that takes about 20 minutes to complete. As part of a larger study on survivors of the 9/11 terrorist attacks, 1035 New York residents were invited to participate in the online intervention 2 years after the attack. Approximately one-third of individuals agreed to participate in the online work. Among those who were enrolled into the PTSD module, about half actually completed it. Although the authors report that participants appeared to report increased knowledge after completing the modules, no outcome data were collected on symptom changes (Ruggiero et al., 2006).

Military and Veteran Population

DE-STRESS

Delivery of Self-Training and Education for Stressful Situations (DE-STRESS) is a therapist-assisted, self-management intervention developed to treat U.S. military service members with PTSD (Litz, Bryant, Williams, Engel, & Wang, 2004). DE-STRESS is designed to promote an individualized approach to treatment by integrating a balance of therapist involvement to support engagement with the online intervention. Participants initially participate in a 2-hour face-to-face meeting with a clinician (nurse or master's level professional), at which time the therapist introduces the online treatment, generates an in vivo hierarchy with the patient, and teaches coping skills (e.g., relaxation exercises, basic cognitive restructuring techniques). Subsequent homework assignments are given online. The clinician conducts five scheduled calls during the 8 weeks in addition to sending weekly e-mail to participants. Patients are encouraged to log on to the website daily (Litz et al., 2004).

During the DE-STRESS trial (Litz, Engel, Bryant, & Papa, 2007), 45 U.S. military service members with PTSD were randomized to either DE-STRESS or an Internet-based supportive counseling intervention. Participants in both groups experienced significant reductions in PTSD and depressive symptoms across the treatment, with the DE-STRESS group reporting a sharper decline in symptoms compared with the online supportive counseling group. At the 6-month follow-up, DE-STRESS participants reported significantly fewer PTSD, depressive, and anxiety symptoms. In a subsequent trial, DE-STRESS (renamed DESTRESS-PC) was modified to be used as an integrated primary care intervention, with primary care nurses providing supportive telephone check-ins every other week. The amount of online work was also reduced for participants. Results from this trial ($N = 80$) demonstrated that participants in the DESTRESS-PC arm experienced significant reductions in PTSD at the 12-week assessment relative to a treatment-as-usual arm, with treatment differences between the study arms diminishing by week 18 (Engel et al., 2015). The authors suggest that DESTRESS may be one promising option for patients in need of PTSD treatment who may be unwilling or unable to engage in specialty care.

VetChange

VetChange is a Web-based, self-management tool designed for U.S. military veterans to treat alcohol misuse problems and PTSD (Brief, Rubin, Enggasser, Roy, & Keane, 2011). The ICT program is offered anonymously online and requires no therapist support. The eight modules (completed weekly) incorporate motivational and alcohol management strategies. Modules include tailored feedback to participants about drinking patterns and PTSD symptoms, motivational techniques to promote readiness to change, strategies to manage alcohol use, and CBT skills for stress management. Each module takes approximately 20 minutes, and participants receive automated feedback on each module regarding treatment progress (Brief et al., 2011).

VetChange was evaluated in a large study that randomized military veterans to the intervention or to a wait-list control condition (Brief et al., 2013). Using social media to advertise the treatment, 600 veterans were enrolled in the study within just a few months. Treatment completers reported significant reductions in drinking patterns and PTSD symptoms compared with the wait-list group, with gains maintained up to 3 months posttreatment. Although attrition rates were high (approximately 66%), one-third of this anonymous sample completed all the modules and experienced significant improvement in drinking behaviors and PTSD symptoms without support from a clinician (Brief et al., 2013).

VETS PREVAIL

VETS PREVAIL is an anonymous, online intervention targeting mild to moderate posttraumatic stress and depressive symptoms through the use of an interactive website design (Hobfoll, Blais, Stevens, Walt, & Gengler, 2015). The treatment consists of traditional CBT components (e.g., psychoeducation, behavioral activation, problem-solving skills training, goal-setting practice) but does not include trauma exposure work. Unique to this ICT, the intervention incorporates a gaming platform to encourage treatment adherence. For example, each lesson is presented as a "level," with the goal of earning reward points and advancing in "rank" within the online community network. Veterans can redeem their rewards points for financial incentives (up to $10 per user). The intervention also places an emphasis on social support by incorporating a 24-hour peer chat portal. Within this portal, users can interact with other veterans via online message boards or engage in real-time chats with certified peer counselors. The peer chat portal is managed by military veterans who are trained to provide supportive guidance and not offer official counseling.

In an RCT conducted from 2011 to 2013, 303 veterans were randomized to VETS PREVAIL or a wait-list comparison group. Participants were primarily male (81%) and white (70%) who were employed or students (79%). Close to three-quarters of participants randomized to the VETS PREVAIL arm completed at least five sessions. Participants in the active treatment arm experienced significant reductions in PTSD and depressive symptoms, with 31% of participants experiencing full PTSD symptom remission compared with 12% in the wait-list condition. There was evidence of a dose–response effect, with the completion of more lessons associated with a greater likelihood of symptom remission for both PTSD and depression. Although participant-specific data regarding use of the peer chat portal were not collected, Web estimates indicated a substantial amount of activity on the community message boards.

Written Emotional Disclosure

The Written Emotional Disclosure (WED) intervention aims to promote cognitive processing of trauma through three exposure-based writing assignments via an Internet program. Clinicians initially meet with patients in person and orient them to the Web-based materials. Therapists then contact patients by phone before each assignment to remind participants about the homework, assess safety concerns, and answer any questions. WED was evaluated on U.S. military veterans recruited out of primary care clinics and compared with an online time management course (Possemato, Ouimette, & Knowlton, 2011). All 15 participants randomized to the treatment intervention completed the WED treatment. WED participants did not report significant improvements on any outcomes when compared with the time management participants. The authors suggest that greater therapist involvement may result in better outcomes (Possemato et al., 2011).

Afterdeployment.org

Afterdeployment.org is an anonymous Department of Defense–funded online suite developed to address PTSD and other psychological health conditions experienced by U.S. service members and veterans (Bush et al., 2014). Afterdeployment is designed to be used without the need of therapist support and is organized into 21 topic areas relevant to service member, veterans, and their family members. The PTSD-specific self-help workshop, Adjusting to War Memories, contains eight sessions, with each session taking approximately 30 to 45 minutes to complete. In an open pilot trial, 11 college veterans with PTSD symptoms completed the Adjusting to War Memories workshop without any therapist support (Bush et al., 2014). There were no dropouts and participants

TABLE 14.3 Therapeutic Components of Specific ICTs for PTSD

System	Sessions	Skills/ Training	ME	Cognitive Work	Written Exposure	In Vivo Exposure	Therapist involvement
Interapy	10			X	X		High
CALM Tools for Living	8	X	X	X		X	High
DE-STRESS	18–56	X		X	X	X	Moderate to high
The PTSD Program	7	X		X	X	X	Moderate
Guided ICT for PTSD	8	X		X	X	X	Moderate
PTSD Online	10	X		X	X	X	Moderate
Written Emotional Disclosure	3				X		Moderate
Self-help for Traumatic Consequence	8	X		X	X		Low
Afterdeployment. org	8	X		X	X	X	None to low
VetChange	8	X	X	X			None
VETS PREVAIL	6	X	X			X	None
Treatment for disaster-affected populations	1	X	X				None

CALM, Coordinated Anxiety Learning and Management; DESTRESS, Delivery of self training and education for stressful situations; ICT, Internet and computer-based treatments; ME, Motivational enhancement strategy; N/A, not applicable; PTSD, posttraumatic stress disorder.

reported high satisfaction with the online tool. Five participants (45%) demonstrated statistically significant decreases in their PTSD symptoms. In a subsequent open trial, veterans with PTSD who declined traditional psychotherapy were invited to complete Adjusting to War Memories with brief, weekly telephone support. Results were similar to the previous study and suggest this online treatment is acceptable, feasible, and potentially helpful for military veterans with PTSD (Belsher et al., 2015).

In review, several ICTs for PTSD have been developed and tested during the past decade. Across the RCTs, the treatments evaluated against a wait-list control group were demonstrated to be efficacious in treating PTSD, and two treatments evidenced better outcomes when compared with a placebo control group (Ivarsson et al., 2014; Spence et al., 2011). As documented in Table 14.3, all the treatments evaluated were CBT-oriented and included treatment components such as psycho-education, coping skills training, trauma processing, in vivo exposure work, and cognitive restructuring exercises. Despite the common treatment orientation, the computerized treatments varied widely based on duration of treatment, popula-tion targeted, and methods to deliver and support treatment. Therapist involve-ment ranged across the treatments from high support to no support. The degree of professional expertise also varied among studies, depending on whether a techni-cian, nurse, peer, or psychologist supported treatment. In general, these prelimi-nary findings suggest that computerized treatments can be feasible and efficacious interventions for PTSD, although the specific format and context in which these interventions are delivered requires additional research. Along with the encourag-ing findings, however, these treatment trials also highlight several issues that need to be taken into consideration when determining how ICTs can be translated most effectively to standard practice. As discussed in the subsequent section, these con-cerns focus on the accessibility, adequacy, and acceptability of ICTs.

CONCERNS AND CONSIDERATIONS

Accessibility

A large proportion of the worldwide population does not have Internet access or use the Internet on a regular basis. Although the United States and western European countries boast the highest percentages of Internet access, other regions of the world report much lower access rates. As of 2012, less than 50% of the populations in Latin America, the Middle East, Africa, and Asia have Internet access, although these regions also demonstrate that highest increasing penetration of Internet usage (Miniwatts Marketing Group, 2015b). If Internet-based interventions are to be ac-cessible and seemingly helpful to the larger population, reliable Internet connections need to exist.

Despite the high accessibility of Internet use within the United States, a "digital divide" exists, with certain segments of the population less likely to have regular Internet access (Martin & Robinson, 2007). U.S. census data from 2011 indicate those with less education, lower socioeconomic states, older, and nonwhite are less likely to use the Internet on a regular basis (U.S. Census Bureau, 2013). These groups also tend to have less access to adequate treatments (Wang et al., 2005) and thus may benefit from alternative health delivery methods. This divide is well illustrated by the study by Ruggiero et al. (2006) on 9/11 disaster survivors in New York. Of 1832 residents screened, 33% ($n = 603$) did not have Internet access from home. These individuals were more likely to be women, black or Hispanic, older, unemployed, and less educated.

When ICTs can be accessed, guidance is needed for appropriate treatment selection. The credibility of many ICTs is questionable and specific interventions could potentially be harmful to the end user. Bremner, Quinn, Quinn, and Veledar (2006) found that 42% of online PTSD treatments identified through a basic online search provided inaccurate and potentially harmful information, with the majority of information not referencing any scientific data. Only 59% of sites used a mental health professional to develop the content of the treatment, with many of the websites developed by individuals with no specialized training in trauma (Bremner et al., 2006). Notably, the majority of the PTSD ICTs reviewed in this chapter are not available for public use, limiting their accessibility for patients, providers, and researchers.

Adequacy of Care

Concerns have been raised about whether ICTs are suitable for patients with severe symptoms and comorbid conditions, especially in light of the fact that individuals who seek Internet treatments report just as severe symptoms as those seeking face-to-face services (Titov, Andrews, Kemp, & Robinson, 2010). In general, the literature appears to support the use of ICTs for highly symptomatic patients who would otherwise not access standard care (e.g., Batterham, Neil, Bennett, Griffiths, & Christensen, 2008; Proudfoot et al., 2004). Some of the PTSD treatments studies reviewed earlier in the chapter are consistent with this finding and indicate that patients with high initial levels of PTSD benefit equally from treatment as those with less severe symptoms (Spence et al., 2011). Furthermore, two of the treatments treated patients with PTSD and other comorbid conditions effectively (Brief et al., 2011; Spence et al., 2011). As is typical with controlled trials, the majority of these studies excluded patients with high-risk concerns such as suicidal ideations, psychotic symptoms, and substance dependence. Therefore, implications from these trials cannot be generalized to these higher risk groups.

A pertinent issue may concern patients who experience increased symptoms during the online treatment and require a different level of care (Titov et al., 2013). For example, in the Interapy trial (Lange et al., 2003), a large proportion of participants dropped out of the intervention because of increased distress. In The PTSD Program trial (Spence et al., 2011), several participants required crisis management and assistance in seeking face-to-face treatment with their local mental health team during the intervention. This issue may go undetected in ICTs if the treatment protocol does not have adequate methods to track patients who drop out prematurely from care as a result of increased distress. Computerized treatments run the risk of doing more harm than good if the treatment exacerbates symptoms and there is minimal oversight by providers and a lack of alternative treatment option for patients. As discussed later in this chapter, one way to address these concerns is by embedding ICTs within comprehensive care systems that include ongoing symptom monitoring, care management, and alternative treatment options for patients as needed.

Acceptability

Low uptake and high attrition rates are one of the biggest concerns raised over the use of computerized treatments (Christensen, Griffiths, Korten, Brittliffe, & Groves, 2004; Eysenbach, 2005; Farvolden, Denisoff, Selby, Bagby, & Rudy, 2005). In clinical practice, the time and resources devoted to ICTs are unjustified if patients are unreceptive to this form of treatment, as indicated by an unwillingness even to begin treatment or a high likelihood of dropping out of treatment. Several controlled ICT trials report between 20% and 30% of seemingly appropriate participants decline an initial referral to an online treatment from the outset (Cavanagh, Seccombe, & Lidbetter, 2011; Marks et al., 2003; Proudfoot et al., 2003; Proudfoot et al., 2004). The PTSD studies described in this chapter often did not include a large proportion of participants, which may reflect some ambivalence toward computerized treatments in general. Many factors may influence this reluctance, including a lack of familiarity with online treatments, low expectations or misunderstandings about treatment, concerns over the lack of therapist support, reduced accountability, and a desire for a more individualized approach.

High dropout rates are a major limitation of ICTs. On average, about one-third of participants drop out of online treatments in tightly controlled research trials (Kaltenthaler et al., 2008). More strikingly, when ICTs are made available to the general public ("open"), a minority of users actually complete the treatment. Usage rates evaluated on a free depression ICT in a large community sample found that 85% of users dropped out after the first session and less than 1% of users completed the entire treatment (Christensen et al., 2004). Similar findings have been reported elsewhere on ICTs for anxiety disorders (Farvolden et al., 2005). These concerns have led to efforts to understand more fully facilitators of ICT adherence.

Research on demographic predictors of ICT dropout is mixed (Batterham et al., 2008; Christensen, Griffiths, & Farrer, 2009) and, in general, components of ICT packages may be more important in predicting treatment adherence over and beyond user characteristics. For example, participants referred to an online treatment by a mental health professional have a greater likelihood of engaging in the treatment (Batterham et al., 2008). Frequent and scheduled reminders for users to log on and complete the work are associated with greater adherence to the treatment (Fry & Neff, 2009; Tate, Jackvony, & Wing, 2006). Human support demonstrates a greater influence on treatment adherence than automated reminders (Spek et al., 2007; Tate et al., 2006), with support provided by a nonspecialized technician equally effective as clinician support for certain interventions (Robinson et al., 2010; Titov, Andrews, Davies, et al., 2010). Inclusion of these specific components into ICT packages, and within the context of the purpose and resources available for the intervention, is important. Future efforts should continue to focus on factors that contribute to ICT uptake and engagement so that treatments can be packaged to improve uptake and adherence rates (Christensen & Mackinnon, 2006; Eysenbach, 2005).

ICTs WITHIN COLLABORATIVE CARE FRAMEWORKS

The concerns raised in the previous section have prompted a rethinking of the scope and target of ICTs. Based on high attrition rates, ICTs may not be well suited to be the primary treatment option for the majority of patients. Rather, ICTs may serve as one treatment option among many based on patient preferences, symptom presentation, and treatment response. For the large percentage of patients who are unwilling to engage in computerized treatments, alternative options for care are needed. Furthermore, given that the majority of patients tend to complete only a few sessions of online treatments, ICTs may be delivered more efficiently as short-term interventions rather than full treatment packages on par with traditional treatments.

Collaborative care models may be particularly useful in the integration of new treatment technologies such as computerized treatments. Collaborative care models are comprehensive system-level interventions that integrate mental health services into primary care through the use of a care team that includes a care manager. Essential components of collaborative care models include routine screening for patients, ongoing care management to improve care continuity and treatment adherence, electronic health record to track symptoms and support clinical decision making, and stepped care treatment algorithms to match patient needs best with appropriate treatment (Von Korff, Gruman, Schaefer, Curry, & Wagner, 1997). Collaborative care approaches strive to achieve maximum effectiveness and efficiency through a balance of population- and individual-level interventions.

Within a collaborative care framework, ICTs may be delivered as short-term interventions (one to three sessions) that aim to improve population reach, point-of-care entry, and treatment preparedness for those in need of more intensive interventions (Christensen & Mackinnon, 2006; Graff, Kaoukis, Vincent, Piotrowski, & Ediger, 2012). In this comprehensive care system, ICT attrition and treatment nonresponse is counterbalanced by continuous symptom monitoring, ongoing care management, and the availability of stepped-up care as needed (Craske et al., 2009; Roy-Byrne et al., 2010). Patients not benefiting from treatment or who are at risk for dropping out of care can be identified and offered a different form of treatment.

From a public health perspective, patients who benefit adequately from a first-step ICT intervention free up system resources and improve care access for patients who may need face-to-face care. For example, an insomnia ICT implemented within a collaborative care system reduced the need for in-person consultations by 50% as a result of sleep improvements. Furthermore, wait times for in-person psychological treatment was reduced from 18 months to 2 to 4 weeks (Graff et al., 2012). Thus, ICTs may make a significant impact as early and first-line interventions within collaborative care systems, with the aim of treating subthreshold patients and identifying more symptomatic patients before their symptoms get worse. Within this framework, ICTs offer a unique contribution to the care continuum, rather than aiming to replicate traditional face-to-face care. Future research efforts should continue to evaluate ICT within comprehensive care frameworks that emphasize care continuity.

INNOVATIVE USE OF TECHNOLOGIES IN TREATMENT

With the growing sophistication of technology, new and innovative treatment tools are frequently emerging. mHealth, the use of mobile devices (e.g., smartphones) to support healthcare delivery, is a promising new development. Smartphones are an advanced expansion of mobile phones, enabling constant Internet access and the capacity to communicate real-time information continuously. Potential reach using mobile devices is a significant advantage. In 2013, there were almost as many mobile–cellular subscriptions as people in the world, with more than 460 million subscribers in the United States alone (International Telecommunication Union, 2013). Moreover, there are fewer sociodemographic differences between users and nonusers of mobile technology compared with stand-alone computers (Pew Research Center, 2015). Research supports the efficacy and feasibility of several mobile interventions, with the literature centered primarily on smoking cessation, weight loss, treatment adherence, and disease management (Riley et al., 2011). Although there has been substantial growth in mobile applications for other conditions (e.g., mood, anxiety, eating, sleep disorders), research on these products is only beginning to emerge (Luxton, McCann, Bush, Mishkind, & Reger, 2011).

mHealth applications for PTSD have been developed. PTSD Coach (U.S. Department of Veterans Affairs, 2015) is a mobile application designed for veterans and military service members that provides users with educational material, self-assessment tracking tools, self-management tools (e.g., relaxation exercises, anger management strategies), and direct links to support. Other mobile PTSD applications serve to support traditional face-to-face treatments, such as the PE Coach (prolonged exposure), the CPT Coach (cognitive processing therapy) and the Cognitive Behavioral Therapy—Insomnia (CBT-i) Coach (U.S. Department of Veterans Affairs, 2015). These applications aim to enhance conventional face-to-face treatments by improving accessibility of treatment materials, enabling patients to track symptoms on their phone, and storing the treatment materials centrally in the mobile application. The added benefit of these applications to standard treatments awaits evaluation. For an in-depth discussion see Chapter 15, "Mobile Apps to Improve Outreach, Engagement, Self-management, and Treatment for Posttraumatic Stress Disorder."

Outside of replicating and complementing standard PTSD treatments, technology may function to advance treatment beyond the current mind-set of the 50-minute treatment session. Computer-based interventions (e.g., eHealth and mHealth) have the potential to offer novel solutions to the treatment of mental health issues that are not possible or are not feasible using traditional face-to-face approaches. Perhaps the most promising aspect of computer-based interventions is that computer technologies permit symptom assessment, behavioral reminders, and communication in a variety of contexts during nearly any time of the day. Specific mHealth tools that can extend care outside the traditional paradigm include ecological momentary assessments to collect and communicate real-time symptoms, "push out" technologies that remind patients to complete assignments or assessments, physiological arousal measures that can be used during exposure exercises with biofeedback sensors, a global positioning system to track compliance with behavioral homework by identifying whether patients engage in exposure exercises, and facilitated communication with providers and support networks via text, audio, and video technologies. Treatment packages that integrate components of face-to-face care, online interventions, and mHealth tools optimally may prove to be acceptable and effective interventions that expand our current care delivery model. Research is needed in this evolving area to understand more completely the feasibility, acceptability, and clinical effectiveness of integrated telehealth interventions for PTSD.

CONCLUSION

Advances in Internet-based programming and the increasing accessibility of online services have prompted growth in computerized treatments for PTSD. ICTs for PTSD have significant appeal and are, theoretically, accessible to anyone at any time with a computer or mobile device. Within the context of controlled research trials, ICTs appear to be a promising tool to treat PTSD in certain populations. These findings represent initial steps in the gradual integration of computerized psychological treatments into standard clinical practice. Despite some of the unique advantages of ICTs, however, there are several concerns common across ICTs when compared with more traditional models of delivery, including availability of evidence-informed interventions, poor uptake and adherence rates, and a lack of care continuity. Future efforts need to continue to build on these initial trials to determine how computerized treatments can contribute optimally to and augment the healthcare continuum, taking into consideration these salient issues. Collaborative care frameworks, in which computerized treatments serve as first-line treatments, may present one context in which the advantages of ICTs can be optimized and their limitations minimized.

Although the research trials reviewed in this chapter represent essential steps in the validation of a novel treatment, the use of computerized treatments within the confines of the traditional care paradigm may be a limiting perspective. Innovation often necessitates new models of care, and in many ways ICTs (including eHealth and mHealth) have the potential to challenge and extend our traditional paradigm of care. Leveraging advancements in telehealth technology with established principles of behavioral science can, potentially, forge more efficient and effective care models for PTSD that have yet to be considered.

KEY POINTS

- A growing body of evidence demonstrates that online therapies may be effective for a range of behavioral health disorders, including depression, panic disorder, social phobia, and generalized anxiety disorder.
- Several ICTs for PTSD have been developed and tested.
- ICTs for PTSD present a number of advantages, most notably the potential to increase treatment access to a large population of individuals with PTSD who are not receiving adequate treatment.
- ICTs can differ based on whether they are for primarily preventive or treatment purposes, the level of therapist involvement required, the level of integration of the ICT into a larger healthcare system, and the degree of evidence that supports the intervention.

- The research on ICTs suggests most patients prefer some therapist involvement, and outcomes may be better with this support.

- Professionals who plan to use online therapies should become familiar with telehealth guidelines developed by their specific professional organizations, the laws and regulations within their jurisdiction, and the local institutional guidelines of the practice.

- Providers should determine whether specific online interventions are appropriate based on the peer-reviewed literature, best practices guidelines, and patient preferences.

- All the treatments identified in the peer-reviewed literature are CBT oriented and included treatment components such as psychoeducation, coping skills training, written trauma processing, in vivo exposure work, and cognitive restructuring exercises.

- Although the ICT PTSD treatment trials vary considerably, the current evidence on ICTs for PTSD is promising regarding the feasibility and efficacy of specific interventions.

- There are several concerns related to the practical implementation of ICTs, including issues related to accessibility, adequacy, and the acceptability of online treatments.

- Despite the high accessibility of Internet use, a "digital divide" exists, with certain segments of the population less likely to have regular Internet access, including those who are less educated, in lower socioeconomic status groups, older, and nonwhite.

- The credibility of many online ICTs is questionable, and specific interventions could potentially be harmful to the end user. Bremner et al. (2006) found that 42% of online PTSD treatments identified through a basic online search provided inaccurate and potentially harmful information, with the majority of information not referencing any scientific data. Only 59% of sites used a mental health professional to develop the content of the treatment, with many of the websites developed by individuals with no specialized training in trauma.

- A pertinent issue surrounding ICT use concerns patients who experience increased symptoms during the online treatment and require a different level of care. This issue may go undetected if the treatment protocol does not have adequate methods to track patients who drop out prematurely from care as a result of increased distress. Computerized treatments run the risk of doing more harm than good if the treatment exacerbates symptoms and there is minimal oversight by providers and a lack of alternative treatment option for patients.

- Low uptake and high attrition rates are one of the biggest concerns raised over the use of computerized treatments. When ICTs are made available to the general public ("open"), a minority of users actually complete the treatment. One trial demonstrated that 85% of users dropped out after the first session and less than 1% of users completed the entire treatment.

- Collaborative care frameworks are one model of care in which ICTs may be delivered optimally to counterbalance ICT attrition and treatment nonresponse. Collaborative care frameworks promote continuous symptom monitoring, ongoing care management, and the availability of stepped-up care as needed.

- Research supports the efficacy and feasibility of several mobile interventions, with the literature centered primarily on smoking cessation, weight loss, treatment adherence, and disease management. Although there has been substantial growth in mobile applications for other conditions (e.g., mood, anxiety, eating, sleep disorders), research on these products is only beginning to emerge.

REFERENCES

Andrews, G., Cuijpers, P., Craske, M. G., McEvoy, P., & Titov, N. (2010). Computer therapy for the anxiety and depressive disorders is effective, acceptable and practical health care: a meta-analysis. *PLoS One, 5*(10), e13196.

Batterham, P. J., Neil, A. L., Bennett, K., Griffiths, K. M., & Christensen, H. (2008). Predictors of adherence among community users of a cognitive behavior therapy website. *Patient Prefer Adherence, 2,* 97–105.

Belsher, B. E., Kuhn, E., Maron, D., Prins, A., Cueva, D., Fast, E., et al. (2015). A preliminary study of an Internet-based intervention for OEF/OIF veterans presenting for VA specialty PTSD care. *J Trauma Stress, 28,* 1–4.

Bremner, J. D., Quinn, J., Quinn, W., & Veledar, E. (2006). Surfing the Net for medical information about psychological trauma: an empirical study of the quality and accuracy of trauma-related websites. *Med Inform Internet Med, 31*(3), 227–236.

Brief, D. J., Rubin, A., Enggasser, J. L., Roy, M., & Keane, T. M. (2011). Web-based intervention for returning veterans with symptoms of posttraumatic stress disorder and risky alcohol use. *J Contemp Psychother, 41*(4), 237–246.

Brief, D. J., Rubin, A., Keane, T. M., Enggasser, J. L., Roy, M., Helmuth, E., et al. (2013). Web intervention for OEF/OIF veterans with problem drinking and PTSD symptoms: a randomized clinical trial. *J Consult Clin Psychol, 81*(5), 890–900.

Bush, N. E., Prins, A., Laraway, S., O'Brien, K., Ruzek, J., & Ciulla, R. P. (2014). A pilot evaluation of the AfterDeployment.org online posttraumatic stress workshop for military service members and veterans. *Psychol Trauma, 6*(2), 109–119.

Casey, L. M., Joy, A., & Clough, B. A. (2013). The impact of information on attitudes toward e-mental health services. *Cyberpsychol Behav Soc Netw, 16*(8), 593–598.

Cavanagh, K., Seccombe, N., & Lidbetter, N. (2011). The implementation of computerized cognitive behavioural therapies in a service user-led, third sector self help clinic. *Behav Cogn Psychother, 39*(4), 427–442.

Christensen, H., Griffiths, K. M., & Farrer, L. (2009). Adherence in Internet intervention for anxiety and depression: systematic review. *J Med Internet Res, 11*(2), 1–16.

Christensen, H., Griffiths, K. M., Korten, A. E., Brittliffe, K., & Groves, C. (2004). A comparison of changes in anxiety and depression symptoms of spontaneous users and trial participants of a cognitive behavior therapy website. *J Med Internet Res*, 6(4), e46.

Christensen, H., & Mackinnon, A. (2006). The law of attrition revisited. *J Med Internet Res*, 8(3), e20; author reply e21.

Craske, M. G., Rose, R. D., Lang, A., Welch, S. S., Campbell-Sills, L., Sullivan, G., et al. (2009). Computer-assisted delivery of cognitive behavioral therapy for anxiety disorders in primary-care settings. *Depress Anxiety*, 26(3), 235–242.

Craske, M. G., Stein, M. B., Sullivan, G., Sherbourne, C., Bystritsky, A., Rose, R. D., et al. (2011). Disorder-specific impact of coordinated anxiety learning and management treatment for anxiety disorders in primary care. *Arch Gen Psychiatry*, 68(4), 378–388.

Cuijpers, P., Marks, I. M., van Straten, A., Cavanagh, K., Gega, L., & Andersson, G. (2009). Computer-aided psychotherapy for anxiety disorders: a meta-analytic review. *Cogn Behav Ther*, 38(2), 66–82

Davidson, J. R., Stein, D. J., Shalev, A. Y., & Yehuda, R. (2004). Posttraumatic stress disorder: acquisition, recognition, course, and treatment. *J Neuropsychiatry Clin Neurosci*, 16(2), 135–147.

Engel, C. C., Litz, B., Magruder, K. M., Harper, E., Gore, K., Stein, N., et al. (2015). Delivery of Self Training and Education for Stressful Situations (DESTRESS-PC): a randomized trial of nurse assisted online self-management for PTSD in primary care. *Gen Hosp Psychiatr*, 37(4), 323–328.

Eysenbach, G. (2005). The law of attrition. *J Med Internet Res*, 7(1), e11.

Farvolden, P., Denisoff, E., Selby, P., Bagby, R. M., & Rudy, L. (2005). Usage and longitudinal effectiveness of a Web-based self-help cognitive behavioral therapy program for panic disorder. *J Med Internet Res*, 7(1), e7.

Field, M. (1996). *Telemedicine: a guide to assessing telecommunications in health care*. Washington, DC: National Academies Press.

Fry, J. P., & Neff, R. A. (2009). Periodic prompts and reminders in health promotion and health behavior interventions: systematic review. *J Med Internet Res*, 11(2), e16.

Gellatly, J., Bower, P., Hennessy, S., Richards, D., Gilbody, S., & Lovell, K. (2007). What makes self-help interventions effective in the management of depressive symptoms? Meta-analysis and meta-regression. *Psychol Med*, 37(9), 1217–1228.

Graff, L. A., Kaoukis, G., Vincent, N., Piotrowski, A., & Ediger, J. (2012). New models of care for psychology in Canada's health services. *Can Psychol*, 53(3), 165–177.

Hedman, E., Ljotsson, B., & Lindefors, N. (2012). Cognitive behavior therapy via the Internet: a systematic review of applications, clinical efficacy and cost-effectiveness. *Expert Rev Pharmacoecon Outcomes Res*, 12(6), 745–764.

Hilgart, M., Thorndike, F. P., Pardo, J., & Ritterband, L. M. (2012). Ethical issues of Web-based interventions and online therapy. In A. Ferrero, Y. Korkut, M. M. Leach, G. Lindsay, & M. J. Stevens (Eds.), *The Oxford handbook of international psychological ethics* (pp. 161–175). New York, NY: Oxford University Press.

Hirai, M., & Clum, G. A. (2005). An Internet-based self-change program for traumatic event related fear, distress, and maladaptive coping. *J Trauma Stress*, 18(6), 631–636.

Hirai, M., & Clum, G. A. (2006). A meta-analytic study of self-help interventions for anxiety problems. *Behav Ther*, 37(2), 99–111.

Hobfoll, S. E., Blais, R. K., Stevens, N. R., Walt, L., & Gengler, R. (2016). VETS PREVAIL online intervention reduces PTSD and depression in veterans with mild-to-moderate symptoms. *J Consult Clin Psychol*, 84(1), 31–42.

Hoge, C. W., Castro, C. A., Messer, S. C., McGurk, D., Cotting, D. I., & Koffman, R. L. (2004). Combat duty in Iraq and Afghanistan, mental health problems and barriers to care. *New Engl J Med*, 351(1), 13–22.

International Telecommunication Union. (2013). *2013 ICT facts and figures*. Geneva, Switzerland: International Telecommunication Union.

Ivarsson, D., Blom, M., Hesser, H., Carlbring, P., Enderby, P., Nordberg, R., et al. (2014). Guided Internet-delivered cognitive behavior therapy for post-traumatic stress disorder: a randomized controlled trial. *Internet Interv*, *1*, 33–40.

Jaycox, L. H., Marshall, G. N., & Schell, T. (2004). Use of mental health services by men injured through community violence. *Psychiatr Serv*, *55*(4), 415–420.

Kaltenthaler, E., Sutcliffe, P., Parry, G., Beverley, C., Rees, A., & Ferriter, M. (2008). The acceptability to patients of computerized cognitive behaviour therapy for depression: a systematic review. *Psychol Med*, *38*(11), 1521–1530.

Kim, P. Y., Thomas, J. L., Wilk, J. E., Castro, C. A., & Hoge, C. W. (2010). Stigma, barriers to care, and use of mental health services among active duty and National Guard soldiers after combat. *Psychiatr Serv*, *61*(6), 582–588.

Kimerling, R., & Calhoun, K. S. (1994). Somatic symptoms, social support, and treatment seeking among sexual assault victims. *J Consult Clin Psychol*, *62*(2), 333–340.

Klein, B., Mitchell, J., Abbott, J., Shandley, K., Austin, D., Gilson, K., et al. (2010). A therapist-assisted cognitive behavior therapy Internet intervention for posttraumatic stress disorder: pre-, post- and 3-month follow-up results from an open trial. *J Anxiety Disord*, *24*(6), 635–644.

Klein, B., Mitchell, J., Gilson, K., Shandley, K., Austin, D., Kiropoulos, L., et al. (2009). A therapist-assisted Internet-based CBT intervention for posttraumatic stress disorder: preliminary results. *Cogn Behav Ther*, *38*(2), 121–131.

Knaevelsrud, C., & Maercker, A. (2007). Internet-based treatment for PTSD reduces distress and facilitates the development of a strong therapeutic alliance: a randomized controlled clinical trial. *BMC Psychiatry*, *7*(1), 13.

Knaevelsrud, C., & Maercker, A. (2010). Long-term effects of an Internet-based treatment for post-traumatic stress. *Cogn Behav Ther*, *39*(1), 72–77.

Lange, A., Rietdijk, D., Hudcovicova, M., van de Ven, J. P., Schrieken, B., & Emmelkamp, P. M. (2003). Interapy: a controlled randomized trial of the standardized treatment of posttraumatic stress through the Internet. *J Consult Clin Psychol*, *71*(5), 901–909.

Lange, A., van de Ven, J. P., Schrieken, B., & Emmelkamp, P. M. (2001). Interapy, treatment of post-traumatic stress through the Internet: a controlled trial. *J Behav Ther Exp Psychiatry*, *32*(2), 73–90.

Lewis, C., Pearce, J., & Bisson, J. I. (2012). Efficacy, cost-effectiveness and acceptability of self-help interventions for anxiety disorders: systematic review. *Br J Psychiatry*, *200*(1), 15–21.

Litz, B. T., Bryant, R., Williams, L., Engel, C. C., & Wang, J. (2004). A therapist-assisted Internet self-help program for traumatic stress. *Prof Psychol Res Pr*, *35*(6), 628–634.

Litz, B. T., Engel, C. C., Bryant, R. A., & Papa, A. (2007). A randomized, controlled proof-of-concept trial of an Internet-based, therapist-assisted self-management treatment for posttraumatic stress disorder. *Am J Psychiatry*, *164*(11), 1676–1683.

Luxton, D. D., McCann, R. A., Bush, N. E., Mishkind, M. C., & Reger, G. M. (2011). mHealth for mental health: integrating smartphone technology in behavioral healthcare. *Prof Psychol Res Pr*, *42*(6), 505–512.

Marks, I. M., Cuijpers, P., Cavanagh, K., van Straten, A., Gega, L., & Andersson, G. (2009). Meta-analysis of computer-aided psychotherapy: problems and partial solutions. *Cogn Behav Ther*, *38*(2), 83–90.

Marks, I. M., Mataix-Cols, D., Kenwright, M., Cameron, R., Hirsch, S., & Gega, L. (2003). Pragmatic evaluation of computer-aided self-help for anxiety and depression. *Br J Psychiatry*, *183*, 57–65.

Martin, S. P., & Robinson, J. P. (2007). The income digital divide: trends and predictions for levels of Internet use. *Soc Probl*, *54*(1), 1–22.

Miniwatts Marketing Group. (2015a). *Internet world stats*. From www.Internetworldstats.com.

Miniwatts Marketing Group. (2015b). *Internet world stats: usage and population statistics*. From http://www.Internetworldstats.com/stats.htm.

Ormel, J., Petukhova, M., Chatterji, S., Aguilar-Gaxiola, S., Alonso, J., Angermeyer, M. C., et al. (2008). Disability and treatment of specific mental and physical disorders across the world. *Br J Psychiatry*, *192*(5), 368–375.

Ouimette, P., Vogt, D., Wade, M., Tirone, V., Greenbaum, M. A., Kimerling, R., et al. (2011). Perceived barriers to care among veterans health administration patients with posttraumatic stress disorder. *Psychol Serv, 8*(3), 212–223.

Pew Research Center. (2015). *Internet activities*. From http://www.pewInternet.org/topics/Internet-activities/.

Possemato, K., Ouimette, P., & Knowlton, P. (2011). A brief self-guided telehealth intervention for post-traumatic stress disorder in combat veterans: a pilot study. *J Telemed Telecare, 17*(5), 245–250.

Proudfoot, J., Goldberg, D., Mann, A., Everitt, B., Marks, I., & Gray, J. A. (2003). Computerized, interactive, multimedia cognitive–behavioural program for anxiety and depression in general practice. *Psychol Med, 33*(2), 217–227.

Proudfoot, J., Ryden, C., Everitt, B., Shapiro, D. A., Goldberg, D., Mann, A., et al. (2004). Clinical efficacy of computerised cognitive–behavioural therapy for anxiety and depression in primary care: randomised controlled trial. *Br J Psychiatry, 185*(1), 46–54.

Reger, M. A., & Gahm, G. A. (2009). A meta-analysis of the effects of Internet- and computer-based cognitive–behavioral treatments for anxiety. *J Clin Psychol, 65*(1), 53–75.

Riley, W. T., Rivera, D. E., Atienza, A. A., Nilsen, W., Allison, S. M., & Mermelstein, R. (2011). Health behavior models in the age of mobile interventions: are our theories up to the task? *Transl Behav Med, 1*(1), 53–71.

Robinson, E., Titov, N., Andrews, G., McIntyre, K., Schwencke, G., & Solley, K. (2010). Internet treatment for generalized anxiety disorder: a randomized controlled trial comparing clinician vs. technician assistance. *PLoS One, 5*(6), e10942–e10942.

Roy-Byrne, P., Craske, M. G., Sullivan, G., Rose, R. D., Edlund, M. J., Lang, A. J., et al. (2010). Delivery of evidence-based treatment for multiple anxiety disorders in primary care: a randomized controlled trial. *JAMA, 303*(19), 1921–1928.

Ruggiero, K. J., Resnick, H. S., Acierno, R., Coffey, S. F., Carpenter, M. J., Ruscio, A. M., et al. (2006). Internet-based intervention for mental health and substance use problems in disaster-affected populations: a pilot feasibility study. *Behav Ther, 37*(2), 190–205.

Spek, V., Cuijpers, P., Nyklicek, I., Riper, H., Keyzer, J., & Pop, V. (2007). Internet-based cognitive behaviour therapy for symptoms of depression and anxiety: a meta-analysis. *Psychol Med, 37*(3), 319–328.

Spence, J., Titov, N., Dear, B. F., Johnston, L., Solley, K., Lorian, C., et al. (2011). Randomized controlled trial of Internet-delivered cognitive behavioral therapy for posttraumatic stress disorder. *Depress Anxiety, 28*(7), 541–550.

Spence, J., Titov, N., Johnston, L., Jones, M. P., Dear, B. F., & Solley, K. (2014). Internet-based trauma-focused cognitive behavioural therapy for PTSD with and without exposure components: a randomised controlled trial. *J Affect Disord, 162*, 73–80.

Spoont, M. R., Murdoch, M., Hodges, J., & Nugent, S. (2010). Treatment receipt by veterans after a PTSD diagnosis in PTSD, mental health, or general medical clinics. *Psychiatr Serv, 61*(1), 58–63.

Tate, D. F., Jackvony, E. H., & Wing, R. R. (2006). A randomized trial comparing human e-mail counseling, computer-automated tailored counseling, and no counseling in an Internet weight loss program. *Arch Intern Med, 166*(15), 1620–1625.

Titov, N., Andrews, G., Davies, M., McIntyre, K., Robinson, E., & Solley, K. (2010). Internet treatment for depression: a randomized controlled trial comparing clinician vs. technician assistance. *PLoS One, 5*(6), e10939.

Titov, N., Andrews, G., Kemp, A., & Robinson, E. (2010). Characteristics of adults with anxiety or depression treated at an Internet clinic: comparison with a national survey and an outpatient clinic. *PLoS One, 5*(5), e10885.

Titov, N., Dear, B. F., Johnston, L., Lorian, C., Zou, J., Wootton, B., et al. (2013). Improving adherence and clinical outcomes in self-guided Internet treatment for anxiety and depression: randomised controlled trial. *PLoS One, 8*(7), e62873.

Trusz, S. G., Wagner, A. W., Russo, J., Love, J., & Zatzick, D. F. (2011). Assessing barriers to care and readiness for cognitive behavioral therapy in early acute care PTSD interventions. *Psychiatry 74*(3), 207–223.

U.S. Census Bureau. (2013). *Computer and Internet use in the United States: population characteristics.* Washington, DC: U.S. Census Bureau.

U.S. Department of Veterans Affairs. (2015). *PTSD: National Center for PTSD: mobile applications.* From http://www.ptsd.va.gov/professional/materials/apps/.

Von Korff, M., Gruman, J., Schaefer, J., Curry, S. J., & Wagner, E. H. (1997). Collaborative management of chronic illness. *Ann Intern Med, 127*(12), 1097–1102.

Wang, P. S., Lane, M., Olfson, M., Pincus, H. A., Wells, K. B., & Kessler, R. C. (2005). Twelve-month use of mental health services in the United States: results from the National Comorbidity Survey Replication. *Arch Gen Psychiatry, 62*(6), 629–640.

Zatzick, D. (2003). Posttraumatic stress, functional impairment, and service utilization after injury: a public health approach. *Semin Clin Neuropsychiatr, 8*(3), 149–157.

FIFTEEN

Mobile Apps to Improve Outreach, Engagement, Self-management, and Treatment for Posttraumatic Stress Disorder

JULIA E. HOFFMAN, ERIC KUHN, JASON E. OWEN, AND JOSEF I. RUZEK

WITHIN THE PAST DECADE, THE EMERGENCE AND PERVASIVENESS OF MOBILE technology across all socioeconomic groups in most parts of the world has enabled myriad opportunities to engage trauma survivors in novel approaches to treatment, self-management, and symptom monitoring. While the World Wide Web has continued its explosive growth, reaching more than 40% of the world's population, the availability of mobile phones has kept pace and there are now almost as many mobile phone subscriptions as there are people on the planet (International Telecommunications Union, 2014). These highly sophisticated devices are always on and always accessible, enabling previously unheard-of opportunities for patient engagement, connection with providers and systems, objective measures of functioning and change, and innovative enhancements to evidence-based treatment (EBT) tools. The potential for mobile technology to ease delivery of medical care has led to the release of hundreds of thousands of software and hardware applications ("apps"). The National Center for PTSD has been at the forefront of app development for posttraumatic stress disorder (PTSD), including the PTSD Coach. Various publicly available, free apps from our team are highlighted throughout this chapter because these are the ones with which we are most familiar and thus can attest to their being informed by the evidence base, but many more exist as well, some of which we also mention here.

In this chapter, we describe the advantages of novel mobile technologies—in particular for addressing some of the most pervasive difficulties in the effective and efficient provision of care for trauma survivors with PTSD. We review the relevant challenges to standard posttrauma care and map them to available and evolving mobile resources. Solutions for self-management and supporting engagement with trained practitioners are presented, as well as some considerations for thoughtful integration into existing care practices, including necessary precautions related to privacy and contraindications.

KEY AFFORDANCES OF MOBILE APPS

Mobile devices of various kinds and capabilities are carried in nearly every country on Earth. The most basic of these, the feature phones, enable phone calls, short message exchange, and interactions via text with previously unavailable services for supporting daily living (e.g., banking). These are used even in many remote areas that were previously without any telecommunications infrastructure. The past decade has seen the rise of the smartphone, small computing devices that can accomplish numerous complex tasks, including various forms of communication (e.g., talking, texting, instant messaging, e-mailing, video calling), social interactions (e.g., microblogging, social network engagement), Web browsing to connect with nearly any piece of human knowledge, active and passive self-tracking, and use of software apps for everything from management of daily logistics (e.g., navigation, shopping) to streaming of entertainment to self-management of health conditions. The dominance of the worldwide mobile market has become so important that the Internet, initially conceived as a stationary desktop experience, has been tuned increasingly to the realities of mobile browsing. Currently, smartphones are carried by more than two-thirds of adults in the United States, with no apparent differences in prevalence across racial, ethnic, or socioeconomic groups (Pew Research Center, 2015). Smartphones have given way to other classes of mobile app-compatible devices, such as tablets and e-readers, which have many, if not all, of the same capabilities with slightly different form factors.

Mobile apps have affordances that are uniquely suited to supporting medical and behavioral health uses. First, owners of mobile phones rarely turn them off and are rarely separated from their devices. This always-on, always-available reality allows for users to be reached and to access information, treatment tools, and other resources whenever they are needed, unconstrained by the realities of clinic or provider availability. Interventions in various forms can be delivered *just in time*, better meeting the needs of trauma survivors whose acute reactions and needs for coping tools are significantly more likely to occur outside of clinic appointments. Such tools can enable active self-care, or various sensors and algorithms can drive triggered interventions so that less motivated or less insightful users can be offered coping tools without identifying current or ongoing dysfunctional behaviors or emotional experiences as disorder specific symptoms per se.

The privacy and personalization of mobile apps is a primary driver of their value. Most individuals have their own device, which is largely unshared, and tools can be accessed discreetly. Self-entered or passively collected data from phones or connected wearable and placeable sensors can be stored and transmitted without identification. It is notable that, despite their size, mobile devices have significant computing power; they can support highly customized and very flexible applications. Although a mobile app cannot replace the expertise, self-presentation strategies, sensory capabilities, interpersonal connection, and dexterity of a trained mental health care provider, it can be personalized heavily to meet—or adjust to continuously—the specific needs of an individual trauma survivor.

Game mechanics, which rely on basic behavioral reinforcement principles, and multimedia presentations of content can enhance the experience of basic treatment tasks (e.g., psychoeducation) whereas integration with the numerous built-in reference and logistical management tools (e.g., calendar, contacts lists) can aid in meeting treatment obligations. The initial purpose of these devices—social connection—can be used to enrich clinical care, either through connecting with providers, supportive others, or communities of others with shared experiences.

Finally, it is worth noting that mobile apps are *nonconsumable*. Unlike a tablet of medication or an hour of a trained provider's time, the costs of delivery in time and money do not increase on a per-patient-treated basis. In fact, given the scalability and reach of these interventions, the marginal cost for each additional individual treated decreases until it eventually approaches zero (Muñoz, 2010). This is particularly useful when large populations of users require minimal-cost interventions, such as after a disaster or in rural or other underserved areas (e.g., developing nations) that lack sufficient mental health care resources.

APPS TO MITIGATE BARRIERS TO TRADITIONAL PTSD TREATMENT

Although gold standard treatments based on decades of evidence exist for PTSD (Foa, Keane, Friedman, & Cohen, 2009), there are various barriers to standard care delivery that can potentially be mitigated by mobile apps. First, reluctant consumers of mental health care may fear stigma for either experiencing PTSD symptoms or seeking mental health treatment for it (e.g., Vogt, 2011), resulting in treatment avoidance and/or refusal of referral to mental health care. Although it is clear that high-quality treatment from a trained professional is preferable to app-based alternatives, mobile apps can provide a stigma-free alternative when consumers or their families reject traditional treatment approaches. Ideally, in these cases, apps can provide motivational features aimed at supporting a stepped-care model, in which users are moved gradually into the appropriate level of care based on a combination of their needs and their tolerance.

Successful engagement with PTSD treatment can be hindered by poor problem recognition as well (Sayer et al., 2009). Many survivors are unaware of what constitutes a problematic response after trauma exposure, which can lead to suboptimal treatment-seeking behavior. Mobile apps can aid in identifying pathological responses through integration of diagnostic tools, tracking measures, and psychoeducation, possibly leading to engagement in treatment.

Various circumstances make it likely that large swaths of prospective patients may be unable to access appropriate treatment resources. Individuals who live in rural areas may find it difficult to identify sufficiently local providers (e.g., Morland et al., 2010). Disaster survivors may quickly outnumber local resources, and circumstances related to the disaster itself may limit availability of treatment options. Even for individuals in relatively well-resourced areas, a limited workforce of specialists, operating within the constraints of clinic hours, may be difficult to access, both for the basic requirements of a course of treatment and for potential between-session needs for coaching and/or urgent intervention. Logistical problems (e.g., cost, transportation considerations, timing of clinic availability relative to other obligations) can also disrupt the possibility of engaging in needed care. Mobile apps can provide the basic elements of care to those without access, and can supplement existing care between sessions, when opportunities to reinforce clinical learning and behavioral strategies are most likely to arise (Marks, Kenwright, McDonough, Whittaker, & Mataix-Cols, 2004). They may also enable providers without advanced degrees to deliver high-quality care by guiding users and providers alike through evidence-based protocols for PTSD, thus decreasing costs and increasing treatment availability (Foa, et al., 2009).

Under ideal conditions, EBT options would be available to all trauma survivors in need, and these treatments would represent a good fit with patient characteristics and preferences. In reality, some patients may find the time commitment and rigor of more intensive therapies to be problematic, and may refuse to engage or remain in care. As is the case with many psychotherapeutic interventions, attrition is a significant problem for psychotherapies for PTSD (Hernandez-Tejada, Zoller, Ruggiero, Kazley, & Acierno, 2014). For those who remain engaged, ideal courses of treatment involve providers and patients who adhere to the prescribed activities of care. As is detailed later in this chapter, mobile apps can be used to enhance evidence-based care through increasing motivation to remain in treatment, decreasing the burden of assignment requirements for both patients and providers, and guiding participants to a more adherent course of treatment.

Finally, as noted by the Institute of Medicine (2014) a current limitation of typical PTSD care is the lack of ongoing assessment of clinical outcomes to ensure treatment gains are being made and maintained. Mobile apps can be integrated into care to provide this tracking feature, so that both patients and providers can optimize treatment plans as needed.

MOBILE APPLICATIONS FOR SELF-MANAGEMENT OF PTSD

Because most trauma survivors with PTSD are not receiving evidence-based care (Aakre, Himmelhoch, & Slade, 2014; Hoge et al., 2014; Mott, Hundt, Sansigiry, Mignongna, & Cully, 2014; Spoont, Murdoch, Hodges, & Nugent, 2010), it is essential to understand more completely whether and how mobile apps can be used to support them in self-managing their PTSD symptoms. Mobile apps have shown substantial promise (Donker et al., 2013), both for improving early detection of mental health problems (Reid et al., 2013) and for managing symptoms and quality of life in those who are living with a health or mental condition (Proudfoot et al., 2013). In some studies, mobile apps have been shown to be effective for detecting symptoms rapidly, such as treatment complications and side effects (Weaver et al., 2007), and may be superior to text messaging for monitoring symptoms remotely (Ainsworth et al., 2013). Early evidence from other behavioral health studies suggests that mobile self-management apps can be effective for improving a number of health conditions, including depression (Watts et al., 2014), anxiety and stress (Proudfoot et al., 2013; Villani et al., 2013), fatigue and sleep in airline pilots (van Drongelen et al., 2014), physical activity (Maddison et al., 2015), and weight management (Fukuoka, Gay, Joiner, & Vittinghoff, 2015; Liu et al., 2015).

With respect to mobile self-management apps for PTSD, emerging studies suggest that PTSD Coach (Hoffman et al., 2011a, Hoffman et al., 2011b), a mobile app for self-management of PTSD symptoms, can improve trauma symptoms (Kuhn, Greene, et al., 2014; Miner et al., 2016). PTSD Coach has high user satisfaction ratings (Kuhn,

TABLE 15.1 Mobile Apps Designed for PTSD Self-Management from the mHealth App Repository

	Platform	Average User Rating (# of Ratings)	App Price	Developer	App Description	Supporting Evidence
PTSD Coach	iOS & Android (Health & Fitness)	4.5 (85)	*Free*	US Department of Veteran Affairs/ NCPTSD	App provides evidence-informed psychoeducation about PTSD and treatment, symptom management tools, valid tools for self-monitoring distress and trauma, and support for finding more intensive care.	Kuhn, Greene, et al., 2014; Owen et al., 2015; Miner et al. 2016
PTSD Eraser	iOS (Health & Fitness)	4.5 (30)	$5.99	Pamela Turner	App is designed to deliver a single 12-minute audio. The developers describe the app as "based on EmoTrance (Emotional Transformation) . . . based on the harmonization of the human energy system."	*n/a*
PTSD Help	iOS & Android (Medical)	— (0)	$9.99	TRE LLC	App provides "tension and trauma releasing exercises" and self-monitoring capabilities.	*n/a*
Bust PTSD	iOS & Android (Medical)	— (0)	$9.99	CCEI Psychotherapy	App provides self-monitoring tools and relaxation exercises.	*n/a*
PTSD and Traumatic Stress—Anxiety Recovery Strategies	iOS (Health & Fitness)	— (0)	.99	Involution Weight Management, LLC	App provides a 16-minute video, 2 guided imagery audios, a "soundscape" audio, and 10 additional in-app purchases.	*n/a*
PTSD Free	iOS (Health & Fitness)	— (0)	Free	Stress is Gone, LLC	App provides self-monitoring and meditation exercises.	*n/a*

Source: Xu and Liu (2015).

Greene, et al., 2014) and is among the most widely downloaded self-management apps, reaching more than 50,000 trauma survivors and family members a year (Owen et al., 2015). Importantly, PTSD Coach is free of charge and does not require in-app payments to access the full content of the app. Although much work remains to be done, phase 1 trials of PTSD Coach have been encouraging. Specifically, use of PTSD Coach has been associated with a statistically significant decrease in PTSD symptoms (7 to 8 points on the PTSD Checklist (PCL) after only 1 month of use [Miner et al., 2016]), whereas a wait-list control group showed no significant change in symptoms. Moreover, the app has reached a large number of trauma survivors ($N = 153,834$ downloads) living with moderate to high levels of PTSD symptoms (mean PCL score, 57.2 points), and appears to be effective at reducing momentary distress ratings in those who use at least one app-supplied symptom management tool (Owen et al., 2015).

There are only a handful of PTSD self-management apps widely available to the general public. In early 2015, Xu and Liu (2015) compiled a descriptive database of all existing apps available in the United States related to mobile health ($n = 47,883$ in Apple's App Store and $n = 8,335$ in Google Play Store), making it possible to see which apps are accessible to people seeking a mobile app for self-management of PTSD symptoms. Of the available trauma-specific apps (Table 15.1), very few use evidence-based components of mHealth intervention (Mendiola, Kalnicki, & Lindenauer, 2015; Payne, Lister, West, & Bernhardt, 2015), only one other app has received multiple positive reviews from users, and none (other than PTSD Coach) have been evaluated scientifically. There are many existing apps that target anxiety and other mood disorders more broadly, and also provide features that could be helpful to those with PTSD, including general symptom tracking (e.g., whatsmyM3, Self-help for Anxiety Management), diaphragmatic breathing exercises (e.g., Breathe2Relax), mindfulness exercises (e.g., Mindfulness Coach, Stop Breathe & Think), and general education (e.g., Mental Illness: Facts About Anxiety, About Phobias).

Mendiola et al. (2015) used self-determination theory (Ryan & Deci, 2000) to catalogue a number of mobile self-management features thought to be critical to a positive user experience and better health outcomes over time. These key features include demonstrated usability, self-monitoring trackers, general education, tools for managing symptoms, data export, and personal reminders. Although additional features, such as gamification, social media connectivity, data export, training plans, personal tailoring of education, and community forums, may provide additional benefit, the most commonly available features in reputable mobile apps for self-management are trackers for self-monitoring symptoms (72.6%), general or tailored education (49.5%), specific tools for self-managing symptoms (33.8%), and reminders (31.6%) (Mendiola et al., 2015; Payne et al., 2015), all of which are provided by PTSD Coach.

Self-Monitoring

Providing trauma survivors with the capability to self-monitor their distress and trauma symptoms allows them to track their progress over time, to receive reinforcement and tailored feedback about their symptoms over time, and, potentially, to identify means of developing self-control over symptoms (Bornstein, Hamilton, & Bornstein et al., 1986; Korotitisch & Nelson-Gray, 1999). Although some studies have suggested the potential efficacy of self-monitoring alone for reducing PTSD symptoms (Reynolds & Tarrier, 1996), it is unclear whether self-monitoring provides benefit above and beyond other forms of treatment (Brown et al., 2014). Regardless, self-monitoring is a component of most EBTs for PTSD, and there is substantial evidence that mobile apps for self-monitoring can be validated against standard self-report instruments (Huguet, 2015; Tourous et al., 2015) and trauma checklists in particular (Price, Kuhn, Hoffman, Ruzek, & Acierno, in press). Many of those who access self-monitoring tools may have not yet been diagnosed with PTSD, and use of standardized assessment measures, such as the PCL (Weathers et al., 1993), and personalized feedback could be particularly helpful for improving symptom recognition or symptom exacerbation and encouraging use of professional treatment resources.

Tools for Self-management

Relaxation and mindfulness training are among the most commonly available mobile app self-management tools, and there is evidence for the face-to-face analogues of these techniques for reducing trauma-related symptoms (Gallegos, Lytle, Moynihan, & Talbot, 2015; King et al., 2013; Stapleton, Taylor, & Asmundson, 2006). PTSD Coach implements a number of self-management tools—including progressive muscle relaxation, breath training, positive imagery, cognitive–behavioral exercises, problem-solving tools, and encouragement to seek out social support—and preliminary research suggests use of these tools can reduce in-the-moment distress (Owen et al., 2015). However, very little research has been done to evaluate specific mobile self-management tools or to understand how to maximize their efficacy for trauma survivors with PTSD symptoms.

General Education about PTSD

Providing trauma survivors with information about how PTSD develops, the factors that can maintain PTSD, and the types and availability of effective treatments for PTSD is essential to helping them understand their experience, achieve a sense of normalcy and shared experience with others with PTSD, and increase self-efficacy for managing PTSD (Phoenix, 2007). Psychoeducation plays a prominent role in every EBT for PTSD and is also a core component of many self-management interventions (e.g., Engel et al., 2015) and apps. PTSD Coach provides detailed information about PTSD (e.g., risk factors, symptoms), EBTs for PTSD, and how to access those treatments, along with other questions and concerns reported frequently by trauma survivors. In addition, PTSD Coach provides information about support resources, and encouragement to connect with friends and family to reduce the negative effects of low social support (Brewin, Andrews, & Valentine, 2000) and social isolation.

Next Steps for Mobile Self-management Apps for PTSD

Research on mobile apps for self-management of mental health conditions such as PTSD is clearly in its infancy, with promising early findings but few randomized trials. A wave of published trials is expected soon; many randomized trials are currently underway, having been registered with clinicaltrials.gov or published as a trial protocol (e.g., Atreja et al., 2015; Baskerville et al., 2015; Compare et al., 2012). Future studies should target next-generation mobile apps that incorporate some of the additional features recommended by Mendiola et al. (2015), such as gamification, social networking, and guided training plans, which have the potential to improve effectiveness by promoting deeper and more consistent engagement with mobile interventions. In addition, it will be important to understand ways in which clinical care providers can make the best use of self-management apps, and whether the effectiveness of self-management apps can be improved by adding local or even remote clinician involvement. Mobile apps may have particular promise in primary care settings (Bauer et al., 2014; Shaw, Bonnet, Modarai, George, & Shahsahebi, 2015), where many trauma survivors present for treatment and may have only limited access to specialized mental health services (Institute of Medicine, 2014; Perez Benitez et al., 2012). In fact, findings from a recently conducted pilot randomized control trial suggests that including PTSD Coach in a Veterans Affairs primary care setting may improve PTSD symptoms and promote acceptance to specialty mental health treatment for PTSD (Possemato et al., in press). Finally, research is needed to evaluate the cost-effectiveness of mobile self-management apps for PTSD symptoms. Given relatively low costs and high reach, mobile apps are likely to be highly cost-effective, even if their effect sizes prove to be small in magnitude, but need to be tested with formal cost-effectiveness models (Crombie et al., 2014; de la Torre-Diez, Lopez-Coronado, Vaca, Aguado, & de Castro, 2015).

MOBILE APPLICATIONS TO SUPPORT
EVIDENCE-BASED TREATMENTS FOR PTSD

An especially exciting area where mobile apps may have great benefit is as adjuncts to EBTs for PTSD. Because most of these EBTs are cognitive–behavioral therapies, they are time limited, structured, and follow manualized protocols. Cognitive–behavioral therapies typically require patients to attend weekly sessions and complete between-session homework to reinforce development of skills and engage in therapeutic exercises (e.g., in vivo exposure). Among the most widely used and studied EBTs are prolonged exposure (PE) therapy, eye movement desensitization and reprocessing (EMDR), cognitive processing therapy (CPT), and stress inoculation training (SIT) (Foa et al. 2009). Unfortunately, similar to other forms of psychotherapy for other patient populations, EBTs for PTSD are plagued by issues of patients missing appointments, not following therapy recommendations (e.g., homework) consistently, and dropping out of treatment prematurely (Imel, Laska, Jakupcak, & Simpson, 2013). Ultimately, these adherence issues result in suboptimal clinical outcomes for many patients, and an inefficient use of scarce and costly treatment resources.

Companion mobile apps for EBTs for PTSD may help improve the delivery of therapy and address patient engagement issues. Common features of smartphones such as scheduling reminders can be used within apps to cue patients of appointments, homework assignments, and prescribed coping tool practice, combating forgetfulness or avoidance associated with PTSD. App-based therapy materials can make psychoeducational materials more engaging and may offer enhanced and more frequent opportunities to interact with these materials to facilitate learning. Apps could also improve homework completion through increased convenience and reduced barriers to assignment completion. The fact that mobile devices are carried routinely and are rarely farther than an arms-reach away can virtually eliminate problems of misplaced or lost symptom monitoring and homework forms. Given the ubiquitous public use of smartphones, patients may find on-app homework completion easier to accomplish than paper-based therapy materials without drawing unwanted attention. Having enduring EBT materials on a mobile device may help patients to maintain skills and benefits after treatment has formally ended.

Apps may confer additional but less tangible benefits. For example, having high-quality, professionally designed apps could possibly increase the credibility of psychotherapies and overcome patients' perceptions that therapy will not be effective for them (Elbogen et al., 2013). Having an app readily available with normalizing information, motivational content, and coping skills may increase patients' self-efficacy to accomplish the challenging but necessary therapy activities associated with exposure to painful trauma memories. Apps can provide an easy-to-understand and enduring framework of the therapy to help patients grasp and revisit the rationale for what they are being asked to do and how it is helpful. Having such tools in the hands of patients can support their responsibility, autonomy, and partnership, which makes care more patient centered.

Providers, too, may benefit from using mobile apps as adjuncts to EBTs for PTSD. For example, apps can provide most, if not all, necessary supplemental patient materials, thereby reducing or eliminating the burden of producing workbooks or photocopy handouts. Apps with customized recording functions can remove the requirement of PE to obtain audio-recording equipment and to navigate the logistical challenges of having to manage and share digital files or purchase cassette tapes. Apps can also facilitate providers' use of measurement-based care by administering required assessments while limiting patient data entry errors (e.g., inputting responses outside of the acceptable range), and scoring and graphing results automatically, thus reducing use of valuable session time, easing interpretation, and enabling timely response to the data. Apps can document homework adherence by time-stamping completion and duration of assignments, helping to ensure patients are practicing emerging skills consistently and adequately, thus increasing patient adherence through enhanced accountability. Mobile apps for EBTs may also serve to improve provider fidelity to the EBT protocol, helping to ensure patients are receiving truly evidence-based care.

There are several examples of mobile apps for EBTs for PTSD currently available to the public. Our team has built two of the most widely used of these—PE Coach (Reger, Hoffman, Rothbaum et al., 2013) and CPT Coach (Hoffman et al., 2014)—which are available at no cost in the iOS and Android marketplaces and are described in further detail here.

PE Coach (Reger et al., 2013) was released in spring 2012 and its two versions (iOS and Android) have since been downloaded more than 39,000 times. PE Coach is comprised of psychoeducation about the onset and maintenance of PTSD symptoms, an anxiety-reducing breathing retraining skill, and two forms of exposure therapy—in vivo and imaginal—which allow patients to overcome experiential avoidance and to process trauma memories emotionally. Various between-session requirements of PE Treatment manual include completing in vivo exposure exercises with self-monitoring of distress, listening to audio-recorded sessions and trauma narratives, and monitoring PTSD symptoms. These activities are replicated and facilitated by PE Coach with the intention of increasing the convenience, acceptability, and likelihood of completing these necessary tasks. PE Coach replaces paper-based components of

PE (e.g., readings, worksheets, assessments) with digital versions without adapting the content except when enhancement (e.g., multimedia presentations) may benefit patients (e.g., interactive coaching through the breathing retraining). Activities such as constructing an in vivo fear hierarchy and selecting items subsequently from it for exposure assignments can all be handled securely and conveniently on the app. The required symptom tracking throughout the course of treatment is also app enabled; the PCL (Weathers et al., 1993) is included with relevant reminders. Accomplishing the familiar tasks of treatment is enhanced by the exploitation of preexisting mobile device features, such as triggered reminders for completing homework and attending appointments, and integration with calendars and contact lists to reach providers easily.

CPT Coach (Hoffman et al., 2014) was released in 2014 for iOS and has been downloaded more than 8000 times since then. CPT Coach is comprised of psycho-education about how PTSD develops and is maintained, and a variety of treatment-aligned cognitive restructuring tools for challenging "stuck points" or beliefs that conflict with the acceptance of the trauma, or are extremely negative and prevent recovery from PTSD (Resick et al., 1993; 2008). There is also an optional exposure component that involves writing a detailed account of the traumatic event and reading it daily until the distress it causes is no longer disruptively intense. Similar to PE Coach, CPT Coach replicates the required educational and interactive elements of care (e.g., homework assignments, worksheets, readings, assessments) to ease the burden on patients and providers. Beyond creating a digital versions of therapy tasks, the app provides reminders for assignments and appointments, and automatic scoring of the integrated PCL; allows users to take pictures of the written trauma narrative assignments; and keeps track of all completed work.

Regarding apps for other EBTs for PTSD, a search of the major app market-places turned up a number of apps particularly for EMDR (e.g., EMDR Helper, EMDR Elite), but none specifically for SIT. Because SIT includes a mix of anxiety management skills, some of which can be found in PTSD Coach (e.g., coping self-statements), providers practicing this EBT may need to seek out other apps that can facilitate the delivery of other SIT components (e.g., PE Coach for in vivo exposure).

Mobile apps for EBTs for PTSD have only recently emerged, so have yet to realize their full potential. Ideally, in the near future, apps for EBTs will be sending and receiving data, and interfacing with provider Web-based dashboards, allowing providers insight into patient activities between sessions and easy, virtually real-time monitoring of their entire panel of patients. Such systems have already shown great value in identifying patients who are on track for success versus those who are in need of a modified course of treatment to prevent treatment failure (Lambert, 2011).

MOBILE APPLICATIONS TO EXPAND
THE SCOPE OF PTSD TREATMENT

Individuals with PTSD frequently exhibit co-occurring problems, ranging from additional diagnosable conditions such as depression or substance abuse, to diagnoses that are secondary to the PTSD itself, such as insomnia, or even problems in functioning that may or may not warrant a diagnostic label such as relational distress (Galatzer-Levy, Nickerson, Litz, & Marmar, 2013). Realities of clinical care require that providers focus on one issue at a time, and many choose to engage in a course of EBT that may eliminate the possibility of attending to additional concerns that are not central to maintaining the PTSD itself. In this context, mobile apps can expand the scope of care a patient is receiving so additional problems can be addressed and/ or tracked with the aid of outside-of-session mobile tools. Apps such as CBT-I Coach (Hoffman et al., 2013) aim to support the provision of evidence-based care for insomnia, whereas self-management apps can be used to supplement the themes and activities of ongoing care with a provider.

CONSIDERATIONS FOR INTEGRATION OF MOBILE
APPLICATIONS INTO PTSD CARE

Although adoption of smartphones continues to increase (Pew Research Center, 2015), and they are used at high rates by psychiatric patients (Ben-Zeev, Davis, Kaise, Krzsos, & Drake, 2014), including those with PTSD (Erbes et al., 2014), not all patients have these devices and not all devices may be compatible with the versions of the mobile apps available. Likewise, although many providers may readily adopt apps in care, some may be reluctant to adopt mobile apps in care because of concerns they will be too complicated to use (Kuhn, Greene, et al., 2014). In principle, they can be delivered by a range of kinds of helpers, including mental health clinicians, physicians/nurses, Employee Assistance Program professionals, and peer coaches. Those using the technology must be familiar with its content and process, and trained and competent to deliver and support the material or intervention included in the technology.

Training is needed in such issues as how to select good candidates for use of the technology, explain the technologies, encourage use, and support their delivery. Clearly, if the patient is in crisis or a risk to himself, herself, or others, technology-based intervention should not be offered as the first-line or exclusive type of treatment. Likewise, patients who are severely disordered or have challenging co-occurring problems, including severe personality disturbance and uncontrolled substance use disorders, would most likely require more intensive, traditionally delivered care. That being acknowledged, apps can be used as a powerful adjunct to care and could be reconsidered as patient conditions stabilize.

As noted earlier, an important potential role for mobile apps involves support for delivery of EBTs. Initial findings suggest that clinicians value this support. A survey on perceptions of PE Coach completed by 163 Veterans Affairs mental health clinicians found that perceptions of the relative advantage, compatibility with care, and complexity of using the app were favorable but not very strong (Kuhn, Greene et al., 2014). The study was conducted before the launch of the app, thus ratings were obtained in response to written descriptions of app capabilities rather than experiences with use. Younger clinicians (<40 years old) rated PE Coach significantly more favorably than older clinicians and reported greater levels of intention to use the app.

Successful integration of mobile apps into clinical care requires some general principles and steps, as listed in Figure 15.1. Foremost among these is that providers should familiarize themselves thoroughly with the app they intend to use before recommending it to patients. Providers should inquire about the type of device and familiarity with technology of their patient, because many patients with smartphones and other smart devices are not familiar with how to download and use apps. Providers should be prepared to review the app's core functions and features, and be ready to answer patient questions. A handout would be helpful to facilitate this overview and to serve as a reference if needed between sessions. It is also worthwhile to ask patients to attempt a few common tasks in the app to ensure they have the basic knowledge and skills to use it on their own. If the app timestamps review or completion of exercises, this should be pointed out to patients so they know their provider will know if and when they complete assignments. For patients who are app novices, it may be helpful to schedule a brief check-in call a few days after the session to ensure they are able to use the app meaningfully. After it is established that the patient is proficient using the app as intended, it should be an integral part of each session, without distracting from session activities. The provider should praise and reinforce app use, and should address concerns or issues regarding app use if they arise. Because technology is not 100% effective, it is prudent to prepare for possible problems (e.g., back up paper forms so work is not lost).

Therapists using such apps should consider possible unintended or even countertherapeutic effects. Smartphones are notoriously effective at distracting one from their current surroundings, which may undermine the effectiveness of exposure-based exercises (e.g., in vivo exposure) (Clough & Casey, 2011) and assignments intended to increase real-world social connection and intimacy. Likewise, even just having helpful apps available could serve as a safety signal and reduce anxiety, which

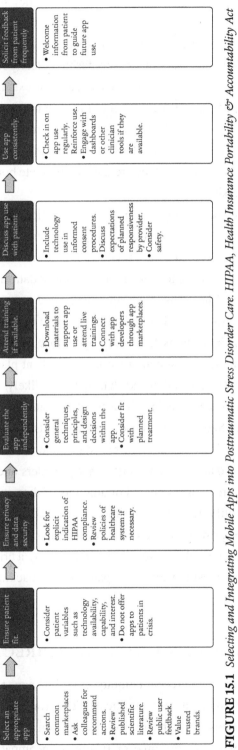

FIGURE 15.1 *Selecting and Integrating Mobile Apps into Posttraumatic Stress Disorder Care. HIPAA, Health Insurance Portability & Accountability Act*

again might impair the benefits of exposure to avoided stimuli. Therefore, patients should be given clear guidance from the outset on when they should and should not use the companion app.

Having the capacity to know when patients are adhering to therapy recommendations and completing homework in a timely fashion clearly has advantages, but it might also have unintended negative consequences. For example, patients may be more likely to skip appointments or drop out of treatment because of feeling shame around clear nonadherence. Obviously, how providers responded to such issues is key to preventing untoward outcomes. This could include letting patients know from the start that regardless of whether they are able to complete homework, they should always attend their sessions.

When technologies begin to gather patient information for purposes of informing care decisions, additional issues are likely to emerge. Patients entering data are likely to expect their providers are reviewing their results and monitoring their well-being. Providers will need to make time to monitor data and incorporate it into the treatment process. Clinicians using apps will need to ensure these technologies are secure and private to feel confident using these modalities to treat patients ethically. Looking for indications from developers that apps are Health Insurance Portability & Accountability Act–compliant is an excellent place to start as current trends make invisible data collection and sharing highly likely.

Providers often indicate concerns about liability issues related to integration of apps into clinical care. Specifically, the new requirements to intervene on novel data or app-identified safety issues is an often-raised consideration. Although there have been no legal cases to date, it is noteworthy that providers and healthcare systems are now in receipt of previously unheard of amounts of data and are correct to consider this carefully. Notifying patients during the informed consent process about the limitations of planned provider responsiveness and the risks of engaging with new technologies is essential. Furthermore, if the app is to play a critical role in a course of treatment, providers must always be prepared with a backup solution in case of system failure.

CONCLUSIONS AND FUTURE DIRECTIONS

Various factors have led to the recent ubiquity of mobile apps to support behavioral health broadly and PTSD treatment specifically. The availability of these tools has enabled previously impossible capacity for reach to consumers reluctant to engage in care, individuals with low-resource or treatment-incompatible conditions, and those patients and systems who could benefit from enhancements to best-case care scenarios. Although apps are not intended to replace high-quality clinical care, they allow for never-before-imagined flexible, scalable, patient-centered care for those whose preferences or capabilities may render them underserved by existing treatment options.

Although the promise of mobile apps for PTSD is great, it is important to underscore the various challenges ahead that need to be addressed to enable the possibilities of mobile technology more fully. First, we must not be lured into a false sense of progress based on superficial and entertaining aspects of mobile technologies. An understanding of PTSD, as well as the mechanisms by which it is maintained or modified, is decades old, and novel technologies should reflect rather than reject the field of existing scientific and clinical knowledge. Second, relatedly, we must not lose track of the value of human interaction and insight in the treatment of psychological disorders. Although cognitive and behavioral tools are powerful, they are much less so outside the context of various other factors such as a healthy therapeutic alliance, a well-structured and personalized rationale for treatment, and a thoughtful provider who can aid those with entrenched and difficult problems. Third, a significant amount of effort is required to integrate mobile apps successfully into existing contexts of care. As described here, clinicians ranging from doctoral-level therapists to primary care providers or even lower degree providers and paraprofessionals must be trained adequately and provided with the correct supplementary materials (e.g., dashboards for app data, manuals) to unleash the power of a hybrid human–technology treatment model. Fourth, this implies the necessity of data transfer, so that engagement and successful use of apps can be tracked and integrated into care. Fifth, considerations related to privacy and security must be held as paramount. Last, mobile apps should continue to evolve rapidly, with accompanying rigorous program evaluation and research to validate innovations, to leverage all the available and forthcoming affordances of this platform to aid those best with PTSD. The aim here should not only be to improve the apps themselves, but also to create bidirectional improvement whereby existing treatments are improved by an increased understanding of mechanisms of change and decreased barriers to success.

Despite these challenges, a growing range of mobile app resources is now available for incorporation into PTSD care. Many of these tools can supplement aspects of face-to-face care effectively and strengthen between-session support. Their just-in-time availability and interactivity render them more valuable and engaging than traditional paper-and-pencil resources, and initial work suggests that both clinicians and patients find value in these tools.

KEY POINTS

- Within the past decade, the worldwide emergence and pervasiveness of mobile technology across all socioeconomic groups has enabled myriad opportunities to engage trauma survivors in novel approaches to treatment, self-management, and symptom monitoring.

- A range of mobile app resources is now available for increased reach, convenience, and effectiveness of PTSD care that are always accessible, enabling previously unheard-of opportunities for patient engagement, connection with providers and systems, objective measures of functioning and change, and innovative enhancements to EBT tools.

- Under certain circumstances, PTSD symptom reduction may be possible from self-management using mobile apps that offer self-assessment, cognitive and behavioral tools that can be used on a just-in-time basis, psychoeducation, and opportunities to receive support.

- Just-in-time interventions can be valuable for patients between sessions, as a support to ongoing behavioral skill practice.

- Apps can enhance existing evidence-based psychotherapies with objective measures of change, opportunities to reinforce behavioral strategies between sessions, reminders to engage in necessary treatment tasks, decreased dependencies on older technologies (e.g., notebooks, tape recorders), and designs aimed at minimizing adherence deviations by both patients and providers.

- Providers should familiarize themselves with apps before bringing them into care. Training may be needed in such issues as how to select good candidates for use of the technology, explain the technologies, encourage use, and support their delivery.

- Providers should consider potential unintended or countertherapeutic effects of apps carefully, such as distraction that undermines exposure-based approaches or increased dropout resulting from interference of objective measures of treatment adherence.

- Privacy and security considerations should be taken seriously, because it is possible for transmission of personal data to be entirely invisible to users and clinicians. Reliance on products from trusted organizations and indications that a product is Health Insurance Portability &Accountability Act compliant are the simplest ways to identify safe apps.

- The nascent evidence for mobile enhancement of PTSD care indicates both patients and providers value these tools as an alternative to standard treatment options, and they can use them successfully to improve various outcomes from insight to symptomatology.

- Apps may be contraindicated in patients in crisis, who are severely disordered, or who have challenging co-occurring problems, including severe personality disturbance or uncontrolled substance use disorders.

REFERENCES

Aakre, J. M., Himelhoch, S., & Slade, E. P. (2014). Mental health service utilization by Iraq and Afghanistan veterans after entry into PTSD specialty treatment. *Psychiatric Services*, *65*, 1066–1069.

Ainsworth, J., Palmier-Claus, J. E., Machin, M., Barrowclough, C., Dunn, G., Rogers, A., et al. (2013). A comparison of two delivery modalities of a mobile phone-based assessment for serious mental illness: Native smartphone application vs text-messaging only implementations. *Journal of Medical Internet Research*, *15*, e60.

Atreja, A., Khan, S., Rogers, J. D., Otobo, E., Patel, N. P., Ullman, T., et al. (2015). Impact of the mobile health PROMISE platform on the quality of care and quality of life in patients with inflammatory bowel disease: Study protocol of a pragmatic randomized controlled trial. *JMIR Research Protocols*, *4*, e23.

Baskerville, N. B., Struik, L. L., Hammond, D., Guindon, G. E., Norman, C. D., Whittaker, R., et al. (2015). Effect of a mobile phone intervention on quitting smoking in a young adult population of smokers: Randomized controlled trial study protocol. *JMIR Research Protocols*, *19*, e10.

Bauer, A. M., Rue, T., Keppel, G. A., Cole, A. M., Baldwin, L. M., & Katon, W. (2014). Use of mobile health (mHealth) tools by primary care patients in the WWAMI region Practice and Research Network (WPRN). *Journal of the American Board of Family Medicine*, *27*, 780–788.

Ben-Zeev, D., Davis, K. E., Kaiser, S., Krzsos, I., & Drake, R. E. (2013). Mobile technologies among people with serious mental illness: Opportunities for future services. *Administration and Policy in Mental Health and Mental Health Services Research*, *40*, 340–343.

Bornstein, P. H., Hamilton, S. B., & Bornstein, M. T. (1986). Self-monitoring procedures. In A. R. Ciminero, K. S. Calhoun, & H. E. Adams (Eds.), *Handbook of behavioral assessment* (2nd ed.). New York: Wiley.

Brewin, C. R., Andrews, B., & Valentine, J. D. (2000). Meta-analysis of risk factors for posttraumatic stress disorder in trauma-exposed adults. *Journal of Consulting and Clinical Psychology*, *68*, 748–766.

Brown, A. J., Bollini, A. M., Craighead, L. W., Astin, M. C., Norrholm, S. D., & Bradley, B. (2014). Self-monitoring of re-experiencing symptoms: A randomized trial. *Journal of Traumatic Stress*, *27*, 519–525.

Clough, B. A., & Casey, L., M. (2011). Technological adjuncts to increase adherence to therapy: A review. *Clinical Psychology Review*, *31*, 697–710.

Compare, A., Kouloulias, V., Apostolos, V., Pena, W. M., Molinari, E., Grossi, E., et al. (2012). WELL.ME: Wellbeing therapy based on real-time personalized mobile architecture, vs. cognitive therapy, to reduce psychological distress and promote healthy lifestyle in cardiovascular disease patients: A study protocol for a randomized controlled trial. *Trials*, *13*, 157.

Crombie, I. K., Irvine, L., Williams, B., Sniehotta, F. F., Petrie, D., Evans, J. M., et al. (2014). A mobile phone intervention to reduce binge drinking among disadvantaged men: Study protocol for a randomised controlled cost-effectiveness trial. *Trials*, *15*, 494.

de la Torre-Diez, I., Lopez-Coronado M., Vaca, C., Aguado, J. S., de Castro, C. (2015). Cost-utility and cost-effectiveness studies of telemedicine, electronic, and mobile health systems in the literature: A systematic review. *Telemedicine and e-Health*, *21*, 81–85.

Donker, T., Petrie, K., Proudfoot, J., Clarke, J., Birch, M. R., & Christensen, H. (2013). Smartphones for smarter delivery of mental health programs: A systematic review. *Journal of Medical and Internet Research*, *15*, e247.

Elbogen, E. B., Wagner, H. R., Johnson, S. C., Kinneer, P., Hang, H., Vasterling, J. J., et al. (2013). Are Iraq and Afghanistan veterans using mental health services? New data from a national random-sample survey. *Psychiatric Services*, *64*, 134–141.

Engel, C. C., Litz, B., Magruder, K. M., Harper, E., Gore, K., Stein, N., et al. (2015). Delivery of Self-training and Education for Stressful Situations (DESTRESS-PC): A randomized trial of nurse assisted online self-management for PTSD in primary care. *General Hospital Psychiatry*, *37*, 323–328.

Erbes, C. R., Stinson, R., Kuhn, E., Polusny, M., Urban, J., Hoffman, J., et al. (2014). Access, utilization, and interest in mHealth applications among veterans receiving outpatient care for PTSD. *Military Medicine*, *179*, 1218–1222.

Foa, E. B., Hembree, E. A., & Rothbaum, B. O. (2007). *Prolonged exposure therapy for PTSD: Emotional processing of traumatic experiences: Therapist guide*. New York, NY: Oxford University Press.

Foa, E. B., Keane, T. M., Friedman, M. J., & Cohen, J. A. (Eds.). (2009). *Effective treatments for PTSD: Practice guidelines from the International Society for Traumatic Stress Studies*. New York, NY: Guilford Press.

Fukuoka, Y., Gay, C. L., Joiner, K. L., & Vittinghoff, E. (2015). A novel diabetes prevention intervention using a mobile app: A randomized controlled trial with overweight adults at risk. *American Journal of Preventive Medicine, 49*(2), 223–237.

Galatzer-Levy, I. R., Nickerson, A., Litz, B. T., & Marmar, C. R. (2013). Patterns of lifetime PTSD comorbidity: A latent class analysis. *Depression and Anxiety*, *30*(5), 489–496.

Gallegos, A. M., Lytle, M. C., Moynihan, J. A., & Talbot, N. L. (2015). Mindfulness-based stress reduction to enhance psychological functioning and improve inflammatory biomarkers in trauma-exposed women: A pilot study. *Psychological Trauma: Theory, Research, Practice, and Policy*, *7*(6), 525.

Hernandez-Tejada, M. A., Zoller, J. S., Ruggiero, K. J., Kazley, A. S., & Acierno, R. (2014). Early treatment withdrawal from evidence-based psychotherapy for PTSD: Telemedicine and in-person parameters. *International Journal of Psychiatry in Medicine*, *48*(1), 33–55.

Hoffman, J. E., Kuhn, E., Chard, K., Resick, P., Greene, C., Weingardt, K., et al. (2014). *CPT Coach (version 1.0)* [mobile application software]. Retrieved from http://itunes.apple.com.

Hoffman, J. E., Taylor, K., Manber, R., Trockel, M., Gehrman, P., Woodward, S., et al. (2013). *CBT-I Coach (version 1.0)* [mobile application software]. Retrieved from http://itunes.apple.com.

Hoffman, J. E., Wald, L. J., Kuhn, E., Greene, C., Ruzek, J.I. & Weingardt, K. (2011a). *PTSD Coach (version 1.0)* [mobile application software]. Retrieved from http://itunes.apple.com.

Hoffman, J. E., Wald, L. J., Kuhn, E., Greene, C., Ruzek, J. I. & Weingardt, K. (2011b). *PTSD Coach (version 1.0)* [mobile application software]. Retrieved from https://play.google.com/store.

Hoge, C. W., Grossman, S. H., Auchterlonie, J. L., Riviere, L. A., Milliken, C. S., & Wilk, J. E. (2014). PTSD treatment for soldiers after combat deployment: Low utilization of mental health care and reasons for dropout. *Psychiatric Services*, *65*, 997–1004.

Huguet, A., McGrath, P. J., Wheaton, M., Mackinnon, S. P., Rozario, S., Tougas, M. E., et al. (2015). Testing the feasibility and psychometric properties of a mobile diary (myWHI) in adolescents and young adults with headaches. *JMIR mHealth uHealth*, *3*, e39.

Imel, Z. E., Laska, K., Jakupcak, M., & Simpson, T. L. (2013). Meta-analysis of dropout in treatments for posttraumatic stress disorder. *Journal of Consulting and Clinical Psychology*, *81*, 394–404.

Institute of Medicine. (2014). *Treatment for posttraumatic stress disorder in military and veteran populations: Final assessment*. Washington, DC: National Academies Press.

International Telecommunications Union. (2014). *Key 2005–2013 ICT indicators for developed and developing countries and the world (totals and penetration rates)* [data file]. Retrieved from http://www.itu.int/en/ITU-D/Statistics/Pages/stat/default.aspx.

King, A. P., Erickson, T. M., Giardino, N. D., Favorite, T., Rauch, S. A., Robinson, E., et al. (2013). A pilot study of group mindfulness-based cognitive therapy (MBCT) for combat veterans with posttraumatic stress disorder (PTSD). *Depression and Anxiety*, *30*, 638–645.

Korotitisch, W. J., & Nelson-Gray, R. O. (1999). An overview of self-monitoring and research in assessment and treatment. *Psychological Assessment, 11*, 415–425.

Kuhn, E., Eftekhari, A., Hoffman, J. E., Crowley, J. J., Ramsey, K. M., Reger, G. M., et al. (2014). Clinician perceptions of using a smartphone app with prolonged exposure therapy. *Administration and Policy in Mental Health and Mental Health Services Research, 41*, 800–807.

Kuhn, E., Greene, C., Hoffman, J., Nguyen, T., Wald, L., Schmidt, J., et al. (2014). Preliminary evaluation of PTSD Coach, a smartphone app for post-traumatic stress symptoms. *Military Medicine, 179*, 12–18.

Lambert, M. J. (2011). What have we learned about treatment failure in empirically supported treatments? Some suggestions for practice. *Cognitive and Behavioral Practice, 18*(3), 413–420.

Liu, F., Kong, X., Cao, J., Chen, S., Li, C., Huang., J., et al. (2015). Mobile phone intervention and weight loss among overweight and obese adults: A meta-analysis of randomized controlled trials. *American Journal of Epidemiology, 181*, 337–348.

Maddison, R., Pfaeffli, L., Whittaker, R., Stewart, R., Kerr, A., Jiang, Y., et al. (2015). A mobile phone intervention increases physical activity in people with cardiovascular disease: Results from the HEART randomized controlled trial. *European Journal of Preventive Cardiology, 22*, 701–709.

Marks, I. M., Kenwright, M., McDonough, M., Whittaker, M., & Mataix-Cols, D. (2004). Saving clinicians' time by delegating routine aspects of therapy to a computer: a randomized controlled trial in phobia/panic disorder. *Psychological Medicine, 34*, 9–18.

Mendiola, M. F., Kalnicki, M., & Lindenauer, S. (2015). Valuable features in mobile health apps for patients and consumers: Content analysis of apps and user ratings. *JMIR mHealth uHealth, 3*, e40.

Miner, A., Kuhn, E., Hoffman, J. E., Owen, J. E., Ruzek, J. I., & Taylor, C. B. (2016). Feasibility, acceptability, and potential efficacy of the PTSD Coach app: A Pilot Randomized Controlled Trial With Community Trauma Survivors. *Psychological Trauma: Theory, Research, Practice, and Policy.*

Morland, L. A., Greene, C. J., Rosen, C. S., Foy, D., Reilly, P., Shore, J., et al. (2010). Telemedicine for anger management therapy in a rural population of combat veterans with posttraumatic stress disorder: A randomized noninferiority trial. *Journal of Clinical Psychiatry, 71*, 855–863.

Mott, J. M., Hundt, N. E., Sansigiry, S., Mignongna, J., & Cully, J. A. (2014). Changes in psychotherapy utilization among veterans with depression, anxiety, and PTSD. *Psychiatric Services, 65*, 106–112.

Muñoz, R. F. (2010). Using evidence-based Internet interventions to reduce health disparities worldwide. *Journal of Medical Internet Research, 12*, 60.

Owen, J. E., Jaworski, B. K., Kuhn, E., Makin-Byrd, K. N., Ramsey, K. M., & Hoffman, J. E. (2015). mHealth in the Wild: Using Novel Data to Examine the Reach, Use, and Impact of PTSD Coach. *JMIR Mental Health, 2*(1), e7.

Payne, H. E., Lister, C., West, J. H., & Bernhardt, J. M. (2015). Behavioral functionality of mobile apps in health interventions: A systematic review of the literature. *JMIR mHealth uHealth, 3*. e20.

Perez Benitez, C. I., Zlotnick, C., Stout, R. I., Lou, F., Dyck, I., & Weisberg, R. (2012). A 5-year longitudinal study of posttraumatic stress disorder in primary care patients. *Psychopathology, 45*, 286–293.

Pew Research Center. (2015). *The smartphone difference.* Retrieved from http://www.pewinternet.org/2015/04/01/chapter-one-a-portrait-of-smartphone-ownership/.

Phoenix, B. J. (2007). Psychoeducation for survivors of trauma. *Perspectives in Psychiatric Care, 43*, 123–131.

Possemato, K., Kuhn, E., Johnson, E. M., Hoffman, J. E., & Brooks, E. (in press). Development and refinement of a clinician intervention to facilitate primary care patient use of the PTSD Coach app. *Translational Behavioral Medicine*, 1–11.

Price, M., Kuhn, E., Hoffman, J. E., Ruzek, J. I., & Acierno, R. (2015). Comparison of the PTSD Checklist (PCL) administered via mobile device relative to a paper form. *Journal of Traumatic Stress, 28*(5), 480–483.

Proudfoot, J., Clarke, J., Birch, M. R., Whitton, A. E., Parker, G., Manicavasagar, V., et al. (2013). Impact of a mobile phone and Web program on symptom and functional outcomes for people with mild-to-moderate depression, anxiety, and stress: A randomised controlled trial. *BMC Psychiatry*, *13*, 312.

Reger, G. M., Hoffman, J., Riggs, D., Rothbaum, B. O., Ruzek, J., Holloway, K. M., & Kuhn, E. (2013). The "PE coach" smartphone application: An innovative approach to improving implementation, fidelity, and homework adherence during prolonged exposure. *Psychological Services*, *10*(3), 342.

Reger, G. M., Skopp, N. A., Edwards-Stewart, A., & Lemus, E. L. (2015). Comparison of prolonged exposure (PE) coach to treatment as usual: A case series with two active duty soldiers. *Military Psychology*, *27*(5), 287.

Reid, S. C., Kauer, S. D., Hearps, S. J. C., Crooke, A. H. D., Khor, A. S., Sanci, L. A., et al. (2013). A mobile phone application for the assessment and management of youth mental health problems in primary care: Health service outcomes from a randomised controlled trial of mobiletype. *BMC Family Practice*, *14*, 84.

Resick, P. A., & Schnicke, M. K. (1993). *Cognitive processing therapy for rape victims: A treatment manual*. Newbury Park, CA: Sage Publications.

Reynolds, M., & Tarrier, N. (1996). Monitoring of intrusions in post-traumatic stress disorder: A report of single case studies. *British Journal of Medical Psychology*, *69*, 371–379.

Ryan, R. M., & Deci, E. L. (2000). Self-determination theory and the facilitation of intrinsic motivation, social development, and well-being. *American Psychologist*, *55*, 68–78.

Sayer, N. A., Friedemann-Sanchez, G., Spoont, M., Murdoch, M., Parker, L. E., Chiros, C., et al. (2009). A qualitative study of determinants of PTSD treatment initiation in veterans. *Psychiatry*, *72*(3), 238–255.

Shaw, R. J., Bonnet, J. P., Modarai, F., George, A., & Shahsahebi, M. (2015). Mobile health technology for personalized primary care. *American Journal of Medicine*, *128*, 555–557.

Spoont, M. R., Murdoch, M., Hodges, J., & Nugent, S. (2010). Treatment receipt by veterans after a PTSD diagnosis in PTSD, mental health, or general medical clinics. *Psychiatric Services*, *61*, 58–63.

Stapleton, J. A., Taylor, S., & Asmundson, J. G. (2006). Effects of three PTSD treatments on anger and guilt: Exposure therapy, eye movement desensitization and reprocessing, and relaxation training. *Journal of Traumatic Stress*, *19*, 19–28.

Torous, J., Staples, P., Shanahan, M., Lin, C., Peck, P., Keshavan, M., et al. (2015). Utilizing a personal smartphone custom app to assess the Patient Health Questionnaire-9 (PHQ-9) depressive symptoms in patients with major depressive disorder. *JMIR Mental Health*, *2*, e8.

van Drongelen, A., Boot, C. R. L., Hynek, H., Twisk, J. W. R., Smid, T., & van der Beek, A. J. (2014). Evaluation of an mHealth intervention aiming to improve health-related behavior and sleep and reduce fatigue among airline pilots. *Scandinavian Journal of Work and Environmental Health*, *40*, 557–568.

Villani, D., Grassi, A., Cognetta, C., Toniolo, D., Cipresso, P., & Riva, G. (2013). Self-help stress management training through mobile phones: An experience with oncology nurses. *Psychological Services*, *10*, 315–322.

Vogt, D. (2011). Mental health-related beliefs as a barrier to service use for military personnel and veterans: A review. *Psychiatric Services*, *62*, 135–142.

Watts, S., Mackenzie, A., Thomas, C., Griskaitis, A., Mewton, L., Williams, A., et al. (2014). CBT for depression: A pilot RCT comparing mobile phone vs. computer. *BMC Psychiatry*, *13*, 49.

Weathers, F. W., Litz, B. T., Herman, D. S., Huska, J. A., & Keane, T. M. (1993, October). The PTSD Checklist (PCL): Reliability, validity, and diagnostic utility. In *annual convention of the international society for traumatic stress studies*. San Antonio: International Society for Traumatic Stress Studies.

Weaver, A., Young, A. M., Rowntree, J., Townsend, N., Pearson, S., Smith, J., et al. (2007). Application of mobile phone technology for managing chemotherapy-associated side effects. *Annals of Oncology, 18,* 1887–1892.

Xu, W., & Liu, Y. (2015). mHealth apps: A repository and database of mobile health apps. *JMIR mHealth uHealth, 3,* e28.

PART
5

CONCLUSION

SIXTEEN

Toward a More Comprehensive Approach to the Management of PTSD

DAVID M. BENEDEK AND GARY H. WYNN

IN THIS VOLUME, AFTER A BRIEF DISCUSSION OF PHENOMENOLOGY OF POSTTRAUMATIC stress disorder (PTSD), the current guidelines and clinical consensus surrounding treatment, and the limitations of available treatment supported by sufficient evidence necessary to receive endorsement in practice guidelines, we describe emerging treatments that demonstrate varying degrees of promise for relieving the suffering associated with PTSD. Both clinical experience and the most current practice guidelines support the notion that successful treatment requires a partnership between patient and provider, and a concerted effort by the clinician to "meet the patient where he or she is at" in terms of treatment approaches. Therefore, we hope the modalities described in the preceding chapters encourage creative treatment approaches tailored to individual patient needs and desires based on a mutual understanding of the potential benefits and limitations of available alternatives.

The fact that there are hundreds of thousands of potential combinations of symptoms that may define any given case of PTSD makes it clear that PTSD is, in fact, a highly individualized disorder. It follows logically that no single treatment may be effective for all combinations that comprise the illness. A careful and thorough history is thus the first step toward creating a thoughtful and targeted treatment approach. However, even after a patient's history of current illness, associated symptoms, pertinent "positives" and "negatives"; past psychiatric, medical/surgical, and developmental history; current social, occupational, educational, and interpersonal functioning; and individual preferences are carefully assessed, the current practice guidelines and gold standard scientific evidence limit patient and provider choices at two classes of medications, two or three varieties of psychotherapy, and eye movement desensitization and reprocessing. But where does a provider (or a treatment team) turn after those are exhausted or if patient preference dictates something else? Further research may provide a more specific and clear-cut road map for successful next steps. However, we hope this compendium provides some guidance with regard to possible choices for those requiring alternatives to current practices. For those considering alternative paths to successful treatment of PTSD, we ask that you remember the following:

- Acceptance and commitment therapy (ACT) is a behavioral intervention that focuses on the pursuit of valued goals and the process, rather than the content of thoughts. ACT has proved effective for some physical health conditions and depression—which is often comorbid—but additional research is needed to determine the extent to which ACT may reduce specific symptoms of PTSD effectively.
- Meditation in its various forms appears to be a safe, easy-to-learn, portable, and cost-effective self-management approach to PTSD. Mantram repetition and mindfulness-based forms have been demonstrated to reduce PTSD symptoms on the Clinician-Administered PTSD Scale and PTSD Checklist. These forms and others have demonstrated efficacy in comorbidities, including chronic pain, depression, and substance use disorders. Randomized controlled trials of sufficient number or power preclude recommendation as first-line therapy for PTSD at this time.
- Transcranial magnetic stimulation (TMS) is a U.S. Food and Drug Administration–approved noninvasive brain stimulation technique for modulating neural activity in targeted brain regions depending on the placement of magnetic coils as well as frequency, duration, strength, and total number of magnetic pulses delivered. TMS has demonstrated efficacy for depression refractory to medication and pain conditions associated with types of trauma that may precipitate PTSD. Specific brain regions to target for PTSD have been identified; however, the results of research currently underway will help clarify the role of TMS in PTSD treatment.
- Acupuncture is the complementary and alternative medication modality with the best evidentiary support for efficacy in PTSD. Indeed, several well-designed randomized controlled trials provide support for its use. Moreover, populations

of patients at high risk for PTSD, including military service members and law enforcement personnel, have engaged in treatment for PTSD actively, as well as multiple other psychiatric and physical health conditions. The extent to which needle placement versus other aspects of the holistic approach to the patient afforded by acupuncture contributes to efficacy remains debatable. Nonetheless, various forms of acupuncture appear to be viable complements or even alternative PTSD treatments endorsed by current practice guidelines.

• Although medications approved by the U.S. Food and Drug Administration for the treatment of PTSD are extremely limited, off-label use of medications approved for other indications is commonplace. Whether atypical neuroleptics are effective as augmentation therapy is not firmly established. Alpha-1 antagonists (approved for hypertension), other antihypertensive medications, nonbenzodiazepine sedative–hypnotic agents, and drug classes acting on *N*-methyl-D-aspartate receptors and γ-aminobutyric acid modulators may have a role in symptom relief. Thus far, trials of agents that might enhance or expedite exposure-based therapies through facilitation of extinction learning have proved disappointing, but initial success with other anxiety disorders has spurred ongoing trials.

• Animal-assisted therapies (such as equine therapy or canine-assisted therapy) have gained widespread popularity—particularly within the military community. Although methodological flaws preclude any conclusions regarding efficacy for specific PTSD symptoms, models suggesting the mechanisms by which animal–patient bonding may enhance treatment have been identified, and the anecdotal evidence supporting growth of this augmentation strategy is impressive.

• Like other chronic and debilitating illnesses, the presence of PTSD in a family member has ripple effects for significant others, including spouses and children living in the same household. PTSD can affect parenting style negatively, caregiver burden has been well documented, and rates of psychological distress, depression, and other indices of impaired social function are elevated in children with a parent with PTSD. Family-focused strategies may help to build shared understanding, develop and master interpersonal skills such as conflict resolution and problem solving, reduce caregiver burden, and enhance safety in households that include a person suffering from PTSD.

• Recreational or adventure therapy for persons with PTSD (including hiking, skiing, climbing, and fishing) have gained popularity, particularly in veteran groups, perhaps because they appeal to the traditional interests and values of veterans. Although small sample size and methodological flaws limit the evidence supporting any such program, the fact that these programs are often offered to veterans for free and there have been no demonstrated negative effects suggest that clinicians should consider encouraging their patients to participate if and when their patients voice interest. Further research may help identify the mechanisms by which such participation reduces specific symptoms or enhances functioning.

- Like acupuncture, there is clear evidence that specific yoga interventions can alleviate symptoms of PTSD including anxiety, depression, and avoidance, and that these modalities may lead to enhanced quality of life. Because yoga incorporates elements of meditation, mindfulness, positivity, social cohesion, and cognitive appraisal, the potential mechanisms contributing to symptom relief are varied. Because there have been no significant side effects, and efficacy across multiple domains has been apparent in small and otherwise limited studies, yoga appears to be a safe and well-accepted augmentation strategy in patients who are only partially responsive to other treatments.

- Just as ACT focuses on the process rather than the content of thoughts, *resilience* may be conceptualized as a process whereby specific behaviors or attitudes may lead to a more positive outcome in the face of adversities such as traumatic stressors. Specific topics including optimism, relationship building, cognitive skills, energy management, and emotional regulation are often the targets of resilience training programs. Training modules focusing on these components may be customized to specific individuals or groups. Although there is face validity to the notion that a focus on these processes might affect PTSD positively, the timing of such training modules and the degree to which specific symptoms of PTSD may be reduced by such models are areas for future research.

- Virtual reality exposure therapy (VRET) provides an alternative to imaginal exposure therapy (e.g., prolonged exposure) for PTSD, which may be particularly appealing to younger, more technologically savvy patients. To date, there is more experience with VRET in combat-related PTSD than with civilian trauma. A number of studies have demonstrated the effective use of virtual reality in the treatment of PTSD and anxiety disorders. Because VRET represents a vehicle for the delivery of evidence-based exposure therapy, it is best considered as a mechanism for augmenting this traditional approach. Whether VRET can be facilitated by pharmacological strategies, its applicability to less tech-savvy patients, and the specific mechanisms by which it may offer improvement over imaginal exposure are yet to be clarified. However, where it is available, it should be considered an option.

- Online therapies may be another option for patients who are even moderately technologically inclined. Adaptations of traditional cognitive or exposure-based treatments as well as stress management techniques are widely available at limited or no cost. The portability, cost, self-paced, and self-timed nature of these programs offer great appeal, but the extent to which treatment occurs outside the boundaries of the traditional clinic/office or doctor–patient relationship raises questions related to the monitoring of patient safety and of clinician liability. In addition, smartphone applications have been developed for real-time measurement and self-management of symptoms of PTSD, including panic, anxiety, and anger management. Although the boundary and liability questions regarding their use are, in many ways, similar to those surrounding Internet-based therapies, an active partnership between patient and therapist, and an agreement between the two with regard to how and when these real-time applications may provide insight into symptom triggers and management techniques can lead to immediate relief if not remission.

The complementary and alternative modalities just reviewed here, and described in more detail in the preceding chapters, represent those emerging interventions for which there is the most emerging evidence or for which mounting clinical experience suggests efficacy. Other new treatments are being explored or identified as these first approaches are gaining an evidence base. The editors and authors of *Complementary and Alternative Medicine for PTSD* encourage students, residents, clinicians of all levels of experience—and their patients—to remain alert to the possibility of these and other opportunities to reduce the suffering and improve the quality of life for those persons whose intimate relationships, educational and occupational function, and capacity for building meaningful relationships are impacted by the burden of PTSD.

We thank you for your open mind, and your continued application of critical thinking and clinical judgment. We wish you success in your efforts to meet the needs of your patients.

DMB and GHW

Index